Global Corruption Report 2006

D1501390

Global Corruption Report 2006

Transparency International

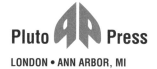

Pluto Press

LONDON • ANN ARBOR, MI

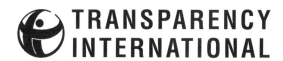

TRANSPARENCY INTERNATIONAL

First published 2006 by Pluto Press
345 Archway Road, London N6 5AA
and 839 Greene Street, Ann Arbor, MI 48106, USA

www.plutobooks.com

in association with
Transparency International
Alt Moabit 96, 10559 Berlin, Germany

www.globalcorruptionreport.org

British Library Cataloguing in Publication Data
A catalogue record for this book is available from the British Library

ISBN   hardback 0 7453 2509 2
ISBN   paperback 0 7453 2508 4

ISSN 1749–3161

Library of Congress Cataloging in Publication Data applied for.

Edited by Jana Kotalik and Diana Rodriguez
Contributing editors: Taslima Ahmed, Michael Griffin, Robin Hodess, Caroline Tingay and Marie Wolkers

Every effort has been made to verify the accuracy of the information contained in this report, including allegations. All information was believed to be correct as of July 2005. Nevertheless, Transparency International cannot guarantee the accuracy and the completeness of the contents. Nor can Transparency International accept responsibility for the consequences of its use for other purposes or in other contexts. Contributions to the *Global Corruption Report 2006* by authors external to Transparency International do not necessarily reflect the views of Transparency International or its national chapters.

10 9 8 7 6 5 4 3 2 1

Designed and produced for Pluto Press by
Chase Publishing Services, Fortescue, Sidmouth, EX10 9QG, England
Typeset from disk by Stanford DTP Services, Northampton, England
Printed and bound in the European Union by Gutenberg Press, Malta

Contents

Part three: Research on corruption

Acknowledgements

The editors of the *Global Corruption Report 2006* would like to thank all the individuals who made the production of this report possible, above all our authors.

We are particularly grateful to our Editorial Advisory Panel for their ongoing commitment to the *Global Corruption Report* and in particular for their large contribution to the thematic section of this year's report: Sir George Alleyne, Harvey Bale, Zainab Bangura, John Bray, Sarah Burd-Sharps, Laurence Cockcroft, Dennis de Jong, Jean de Kerguiziau de Kervasdoué, John Makumbe, Anke Martiny, Phil Mason, Devendra Raj Panday, William D. Savedoff, Frank Vogl and Alexandra Wyke.

Many thanks are due to the countless colleagues across the Transparency International movement, from the Secretariat in Berlin to national chapters around the world, who made our challenging task easier with their ideas and advice. TI national chapters deserve special mention for making a tremendous contribution to the expanded country reports section.

Outside the TI network, thanks are also due to the many people who generously devoted their time and energy to the report: David Abouem, Jens Andvig, Frank Anechiarico, Ben Aris, Salahuddin Aminuzzaman, Guitelle Baghdadi, Manuhuia Barcham, Predrag Bejakovic, Peter Birle, Gerry Bloom, Martin Brusis, Richard Calland, Rowan Callick, Marianne Lala Camerer, Neil Collins, Aurel Croissant, Nicolás Dassen, Luis de Sousa, Phyllis Dininio, Gideon Doron, Tim Ensor, Aleksandar Fatic, Judith February, Mark Findlay, Ursula Giedion, Åse Grødeland, Djilali Hadjadj, Clement Henry, Paul Heywood, Sorin Ionita, Fernando Jiménez, Claude Kabemba, Nancy Kane, John-Mary Kauzya, Stuti Khemani, Grazyna Kopinska, Joe Kutzin, Johann Graf Lambsdorff, Peter Larmour, Azzedine Layachi, Nelson Ledsky, Robert Leonardi, Henrik Lindroth, Joan Lofgren, Roy Love, Xiaobo Lu, Stephen Ma, Muiris MacCarthaigh, Charles Manga Fombad, Susan Foster, Martin McKee, Timo Moilanen, Philippe Montigny, James Mormon, Ed Mountfield, Gregory Mthembu-Salter, Olga Nazario, Naison Ngoma, Jeremiah Norris, Abissama Onana, Katarina Ott, Heiko Pleines, Pierina Pollarolo, Gail Price, Miroslav Prokopijevic, Véronique Pujas, Gabriella Tuason Quimson, Mouin Rabbani, Vivek Ramkumar, Bernd Rechel, Peter Roberts, Nicholas Rosen, Alan Rousso, Greg Salter, Olaf Schmitz-Elvenich, Peter Schönhöfer, Amy Schultz, Hubert Sickinger, Leo Sisti, Bruno Wilhelm Speck, Gopakumar K. Thampi, Rajib Upadhya, Nubia Uruena, Shyama Venkateswar, Marcin Walecki, Steve Weiss, Laurence Whitehead and Tom Zanol.

A special thank you to Gerard Waite for his work during the early stages of commissioning the report, and to TI interns Conny Abel, Sarah Hees, Tom Lavers, Hazel Mowbray, Georg Neumann, Mathilde Piard, Amber Poroznuk and Aaron Rajania.

Finally, we thank our publisher, Pluto Press, for their ongoing enthusiasm for our publication, and our external editor, Michael Griffin, for his flair, diligence and unfailing talent.

The *Global Corruption Report* receives financial support from the government of Germany.

Preface

David Nussbaum, Chief Executive, Transparency International

'When my wife went to the hospital they examined her and prescribed some pills. They said that none were available there, but if we paid 20 or 30 dirhams, someone could provide the "free medication". The problem is we can't afford the drugs.'

These are the words of a man in Casablanca interviewed by Transparency International Morocco, but they could have been uttered by any number of people in any number of countries. This simple example illustrates the serious consequences of corruption in the health sector. Corruption might mean the difference between life and death for those in need of urgent care. It is invariably the poor in society who are affected most by corruption because they often cannot afford bribes or private health care. But corruption in the richest parts of the world also has its costs. Hundreds of millions of dollars are lost each year to insurance fraud and corruption in rich countries, including the United States and the United Kingdom.

Fighting corruption in the health sector is a complex challenge. At one end of the scale are doctors and nurses who charge small informal payments to patients to supplement inadequate incomes. At the other end, and far more pernicious, are the corrupt suppliers who offer bribes, and the health ministers and hospital administrators who accept bribes, or siphon millions of dollars from health budgets, skewing health policy and depleting funds that should be spent building hospitals, buying medicines or employing staff.

Three of the UN's eight Millennium Development Goals – intended to halve poverty by 2015 – relate directly to health: reducing child mortality, improving maternal health and combating HIV/AIDS, malaria and other diseases. Transparency International's *Global Corruption Report 2006* demonstrates that fulfilment of these goals by the target date is severely hampered by the pervasiveness of corruption in the health care system.

Transparency International's work around the world includes analysing and reducing corruption in the health sector, principally by redressing the information imbalance between governments and service providers on the one hand, and patients on the other. TI's national chapters in Argentina, Germany, Niger and Senegal, to name a few, have done pioneering work in this field. As highlighted in this volume, dedicated journalists and representatives of watchdog bodies are other inspirational figures: they dared to confront powerful government and industry figures, often at great personal risk.

In addition to exploring the health sector, the *Global Corruption Report* in its annual country overviews, takes stock of corruption-related developments. One especially encouraging recent development is the entry into force of the UN Convention against Corruption, which provides a common framework for all countries in tackling corruption. Particularly noteworthy are its provisions on cross-border cooperation, reflecting the increasingly international nature of corruption and the movement of its illicit gains.

A pervasive challenge is to ensure that lessons on how to fight corruption are adopted with rigour and commitment by the people entrusted with power around the world. Too often anti-corruption rhetoric is not followed up with action. The *Global Corruption Report 2006* charts the corruption-driven collapse of a number of regimes that rose to power promising moral integrity and fiscal probity. It also shows how institutions, laws and mechanisms, ostensibly aimed at fighting corruption, can be rendered toothless if they are not granted the resources and independence necessary to perform.

Another challenge is to build stronger ties between the anti-corruption movement and movements concerned with other aspects of good governance. This report shows that, although money lost directly to corruption is the most obvious and immediate cost, the negative effects of corruption in terms of quality of government and the well-being of a population are much longer term. The potential gains from fighting corruption – such as more and better health care, stronger judiciaries and legitimate politics – are immense.

The challenges facing the anti-corruption movement have changed markedly over the last decade. When Transparency International was formed in 1993, national and international leaders wilfully ignored calls to tackle corruption; it was a challenge even to be heard. Now the body of evidence is too large, and the pervasive impact of corruption recognised as too great, to ignore. In countries rich and poor around the world, corruption ruins lives.

Corruption is a powerful force, but it is not inevitable or unavoidable. Diminishing its impact restores diverted resources to their intended purpose, bringing better health, nutrition and education to victims of corruption around the world, and with them, opportunity and hope.

Foreword

Mary Robinson[1]

The human rights community needs to pay even more attention to corruption.

The highest attainable standard of health is one of the fundamental rights of every human being, incorporated in article 12 of the International Covenant on Economic, Social and Cultural Rights. Corruption – alongside poverty, inequity, civil conflict, discrimination and violence – is a major issue that has not been adequately addressed within the framework of these basic rights. It leads to the skewing of health spending priorities and the leaching of health budgets, resulting in the neglect of diseases and those communities affected by them; it also means that poor people often decide against life-saving treatment, because they cannot afford the fees charged for health services that should be free.

Corruption in the health sector affects people all over the world, as the essays featured in the *Global Corruption Report 2006* reflect. Money that should be spent on alleviating poverty and illness ends up instead in private pockets. In this way, corruption literally violates human rights, as people are denied the care that their governments are obliged to provide.

But while the concern is global, there are populations for whom the consequences of ill health are particularly bleak. If corruption and a lack of transparency are not addressed as integral to health care strategies, HIV/AIDS and other infectious diseases threaten to reverse hard-won development gains, especially in Africa. In many of these countries, it is women who suffer most through discrimination in service provision, and because they lack the capacity to access adequate health care or to act upon prevention information.

Central to a human rights approach to health is ensuring that essential medicines are available, accessible and of good quality. Availability means that these drugs must be on offer in sufficient quantity within countries where there is a need for them. Accessibility means that they should be easily obtainable on a non-discriminatory basis to those who require them. Good quality signifies that the drugs have to be scientifically and medically approved.

Corruption hampers compliance with each of these obligations. The unpredictability of disease, coupled with opaque spending decisions and aggressive marketing practices by medicines producers and suppliers, generate ample opportunities for corruption. This affects the quality of medicines, for example, when regulators are bribed to exercise less than rigorous checks or hospital administrators purchase cheaper, less effective drugs and embezzle the proceeds. The consequences may be further reaching than failure to treat today's patients: the use of poor-quality medicines stimulates drug-resistant strains of killers such as malaria.

The *Global Corruption Report 2006* unpacks the issues related to corruption and health, that as members of governments, international institutions, the private sector and civil society, we need to take into account if we are serious about safeguarding the right to health. The challenge is immense, and can only be tackled if we work together, making use of the moral and legal arguments provided by the international human rights framework, as well as the practical tools and strategies, many of which are highlighted in this book, that are needed to address the problems associated with ill health around the world effectively.

There is a particular urgency about the issues in this 2006 report. For the years up to 2015 we will see a steep increase in the aid budgets of donor countries, and much of this aid will go to support health areas in developing countries. Unless we improve donor coherence, transparency and the willingness of developing countries to have rigorous systems of accountability, we could see corruption becoming more of a problem, and miss out on an important opportunity to strengthen primary health care systems.

This book should be on the table of every policy-maker who cares about development.

Note

1. Mary Robinson is former UN High Commissioner for Human Rights and former president of Ireland. She is the founder and president of Realizing Rights: The Ethical Globalization Initiative.

Executive summary

Transparency International

Every year, the world spends more than US $3 trillion on health services, most of which is financed by taxpayers. These large flows of funds are an attractive target for abuse. The stakes are high and the resources precious: money lost to corruption could be used to buy medicines, equip hospitals or hire badly needed medical staff.

The diversity of health systems worldwide, the multiplicity of parties involved, the paucity of good record keeping in many countries, and the complexity in distinguishing among corruption, inefficiency and honest mistakes make it difficult to determine the overall costs of corruption in this sector around the globe. But the scale of corruption is vast in both rich and poor countries. In the United States, which spends more on health care – 15.3 per cent of its GDP – than any other industrialised nation, the two largest US public health care programmes, Medicare and Medicaid, estimate that 5–10 per cent of their budget is lost to 'overpayment'. In Cambodia, health practitioners interviewed for the *Global Corruption Report 2006* estimate that more than 5 per cent of the health budget is lost to corruption before it even leaves the central government.

Corruption deprives people of access to health care and can lead to the wrong treatments being administered. Corruption in the pharmaceutical chain can prove deadly: in the words of Dora Akunyili, head of Nigeria's Food and Drug Authority and a winner of the TI Integrity Award in 2003, 'drug counterfeiting, facilitated by corruption, kills en masse and anybody can be a victim'. The authority she heads has found cases of water being substituted for life-saving adrenaline and of active ingredients being diluted by counterfeiters, triggering drug-resistant strains of malaria, tuberculosis and HIV, the world's biggest killers.

The poor are disproportionately affected by corruption in the health sector, as they are less able to afford small bribes for health services that are supposed to be free, or to pay for private alternatives where corruption has depleted public health services. A study of health care delivery in the Philippines finds that poor and middle-income municipalities report longer waiting times at public clinics than rich ones, and a higher frequency of being denied vaccines when corruption is rampant.

Corruption affects health policy and spending priorities. Examples in this year's *Global Corruption Report* from Mexico and Kenya illustrate how public officials have abused their power to divert funds to 'pet' projects, regardless of whether they are in line with agreed health policy. There are also incentives for a distortion in payments at the service delivery level. When caregivers are paid on a fee-for-service basis, they have incentives to provide unnecessary treatment to maximise their revenue. If instead they are paid 'per patient', they can profit by failing to provide needed services.

Reducing corruption can inject revenues back into the health sector. In the United Kingdom, the National Health Service's anti-fraud unit reports it has stopped corruption totalling more than £170 million (US $300 million) since 1999, and the total financial benefits to the NHS (which also includes recovery of losses due to fraud and reduction in measured losses due to intervention by the counter-fraud service) have been four times that. That is enough to build 10 new hospitals.

Transparency International defines corruption as 'the abuse of entrusted power for private gain'. In the health sphere corruption encompasses bribery of regulators and medical professionals, manipulation of information on drug trials, the diversion of medicines and supplies, corruption in procurement, and overbilling of insurance companies. It is not limited to abuse by public officials, because society frequently entrusts private actors in health care with important public roles. When hospital administrators, insurers, physicians or pharmaceutical company executives dishonestly enrich themselves, they are not formally abusing a public office, but they are abusing entrusted power and stealing precious resources needed to improve health.

Why is the health sector so prone to corruption?

Certain characteristics make all health systems – whether public or privately funded, in rich and poor countries – vulnerable to corruption:

- An *imbalance of information* prevails in health systems: health professionals have more information about illness than patients, and pharmaceutical and medical device companies know more about their products than public officials entrusted with spending decisions. Making information available can reduce losses to corruption. A study from Argentina showed that the variation across hospitals in prices paid for medical supplies dropped by 50 per cent after the ministry began to disseminate information about how much hospitals were paying for their supplies.

- The *uncertainty in health markets* – not knowing who will fall ill, when illness will occur, what kinds of illnesses people get and how effective treatments are – is another challenge for policy-makers, as it makes it difficult to manage resources, including the selection, monitoring, measuring and delivery of health care services and the design of health insurance plans. The risk of corruption is even higher in humanitarian emergency situations when medical care is needed urgently and oversight mechanisms are often bypassed.

- The *complexity of health systems*, particularly the large number of parties involved, exacerbates the difficulties of generating and analysing information, promoting transparency, and detecting and preventing corruption. The relationships between medical suppliers, health care providers and policy-makers are often opaque and can lead to distortions of policy that are bad for public health.

The types of corruption in health

Regulators, payers, health care providers, suppliers and consumers face a complex mix of incentives that can lead to corruption. Forms of corruption in the health sector include:

- *Embezzlement and theft* from the health budget or user-fee revenue. This can occur at central or local government level or at the point of allocation to a particular health authority or health centre. Medicines and medical supplies or equipment may be stolen for personal use, use in private practice or resale.

- *Corruption in procurement.* Engaging in collusion, bribes and kickbacks in procurement results in overpayment for goods and contracted services, or in failure to enforce contractual standards for quality. In addition, hospital spending may include large investments in building construction and purchase of expensive technologies, areas of procurement that are particularly vulnerable to corruption.

- *Corruption in payment systems.* Corrupt practices include waiving fees or falsifying insurance documents for particular patients or using hospital budgets to benefit particular favoured individuals; illegally billing insurance companies, government or patients for services that are not covered or services not actually provided, in order to maximise revenue; falsification of invoice records, receipt books or utilisation records, or creation of 'ghost' patients. Other forms of corruption that relate to payment structures are: buying business from physicians by creating financial incentives or offering kickbacks for referrals; physicians improperly referring public hospital patients to their private practice; and performing unnecessary medical interventions in order to maximise fee revenue.

- *Corruption in the pharmaceutical supply chain.* Products can be diverted or stolen at various points in the distribution system; officials may demand 'fees' for approving products or facilities for clearing customs procedures or for setting prices; violations of industry marketing code practices may distort medical professionals' prescribing practices; demands for favours may be placed on suppliers as a condition for prescribing medicines; and counterfeit or other forms of sub-standard medicines may be allowed to circulate.

- *Corruption at the point of health service delivery* can take many forms: extorting or accepting under-the-table payments for services that are supposed to be provided free of charge; soliciting payments in exchange for special privileges or treatment; and extorting or accepting bribes to influence hiring decisions and decisions on licensing, accreditation or certification of facilities.

Recommendations for the health sector

Anti-corruption measures must be tailored to fit the particular context of a country's health system. As with any sector, health system corruption is less likely in societies where there is broad adherence to the rule of law, transparency and trust, where the public sector is ruled by effective civil service codes and strong accountability mechanisms, and where there is an independent media and strong civil society. Preventative measures – including procurement guidelines; codes of conduct for operators in the health sector, both institutional and individual; and transparency and monitoring procedures – are all pressure points for honest behaviour which are not part of the law but which can be effective mechanisms to combat corruption.

Transparency

- It is essential that governments and health authorities publish regularly updated information on the Internet on health budgets and performance at the national, local and health delivery centre levels. Government departments, hospitals, health insurance entities and other agencies handling health service funds must be subject to independent audits.

- Governments and health authorities have responsibility to ensure that information about tender processes, including offers to tender, terms and conditions, the evaluation process and final decisions, is publicly available on the Internet.

- Effective nationwide systems for reporting adverse drug effects must be implemented wholeheartedly by governments, in order to provide a mandate and an incentive for physicians to report such information.

- A public database listing the protocols and results of all clinical drug trials needs to be developed. Reporting by the drug industry on clinical drug trials should be mandatory, as well as the disclosure of all financial contributions made to medical research units from pharmaceutical companies.

- Donors must be open and explicit about what they are giving, when and to whom, and should evaluate their programmes in terms of health outcomes and not level or speed of disbursement. Donors also have the duty to coordinate their support to the health sector, using the same accounting and auditing mechanisms to reduce transaction costs, improve efficiency and reduce risks of corruption.

Codes of conduct

- The introduction and promotion of codes of conduct, through continued training across the health system, is a must for regulators, medical practitioners, pharmacists and health administrators. These codes ought to make explicit reference to preventing corruption and conflicts of interest that can lead to corruption, detail sanctions for breaches and be enforced by an independent body.

- It is imperative for pharmaceutical, biotech and medical device companies to adopt the Business Principles for Countering Bribery, through which a company commits to refraining from bribery in its operations and implementing a comprehensive anti-corruption programme.[1]

Civil society participation and oversight

- Health authorities must introduce avenues for public oversight, which improve accountability and transparency. These should oversee procurement and drugs selection at facility level and health delivery at community and local health board level.

- It is essential for public policies, practices and expenditures to be open to public and legislative scrutiny, while all stages of budget formulation, execution and reporting should be fully accessible to civil society.

Whistleblower protection

- Governments need to introduce whistleblower protection for individuals working in procurement bodies, health authorities, health service providers and suppliers of medicines and equipment.

- Pharmaceutical companies must also introduce whistleblower mechanisms and protection.

Reducing incentives for corruption

- In order to ensure that treatment is dictated by patient need and not by opportunities for profit, governments must continuously monitor payment mechanisms (whether fee-for-service, salary, capitation, global budgeting or other).

- Doctors, nurses and other health professionals have to be paid a decent wage, commensurate with their education, skills and training.

Conflict of interest rules

- Regulators have the responsibility to adopt conflict of interest rules that disqualify individuals or groups with an interest in the manufacturer from participating in clinical drug trials.

- Governments must push for transparency in drug regulation processes, reduction in the excessive promotion of medicines, tougher restrictions on doctors overprescribing drugs, and closer monitoring of relationships between health departments and the drugs industry.

- Medical licensing authorities need to define the specific rules for physician behaviour regarding conflicts of interest (in particular in relationships with the pharmaceutical and medical device industries) and obtain the necessary resources to enforce these rules.

Integrity pacts and debarment

- An Integrity Pact – a binding agreement by both bidders and contracting agencies not to offer or accept bribes in public contracting – needs to be applied to major procurement in the health sector.[2]

- Companies found to have engaged in corrupt practices must be debarred by governments from participating in tender processes for a specified period of time.

Rigorous prosecution

- It is essential for prosecuting authorities to strengthen the message that corruption has consequences by rigorously pursuing corrupt acts that are clearly proscribed by law. Producers of counterfeit drugs and the public officials who collude with them must be prosecuted and duly sanctioned.

- Special anti-corruption and fraud agencies to detect corruption and promote preventative measures in the health sector must be equipped with the necessary expertise, resources and independence to carry out their functions, and be backed by functioning independent courts.

Health is a major global industry, a key responsibility and budget expense for governments and businesses; but more than that, it is a global human right. Corruption deprives people of access to health care and leads to poor health outcomes. There are no simple remedies for tackling corruption in the health sector, but the recommendations outlined above and the initiatives highlighted in the *Global Corruption Report* could prevent, reduce and control corruption. These are addressed as a call to action to researchers, governments, the private sector, the media and citizens the world over.

Notes

1. For more on the Business Principles for Countering Bribery and its supporting guidance document and suite for implementation and monitoring tools, see www.transparency.org/building_coalitions/private_sector/business_principles.html
2. For more on the TI Integrity Pact, see www.transparency.org/integrity_pact/index.html

Part one

Corruption and health

1   The causes of corruption in the health sector: a focus on health care systems

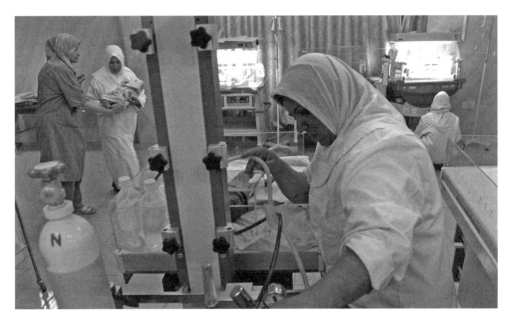

An Iraqi trainee nurse works with newborns in the special care baby unit of Yarmouk Hospital on 10 May 2005 in Baghdad, Iraq. Despite spending hundreds of millions of dollars on the health ministry, endemic corruption has led to a lack of drugs and helped keep infant mortality and malnourishment rates as high as during the Saddam Hussein era. (Scott Peterson/ Getty Images)

Corruption exists in all types of health care systems. William Savedoff and Karen Hussmann look at the reasons why the health sector is especially vulnerable to corruption, and ask whether the vulnerabilities are different in kind and in magnitude, depending on the type of system chosen. An analysis of Colombia and Venezuela shows that very different manifestations of corruption emerged as the two countries' health care models diverged.

If there is corruption, no matter which system is opted for, and how well it is funded, health spending may not lead to commensurate health outcomes. In the United States, Americans spend more on health care than many other industrialised countries, yet health outcomes are arguably no better. At the opposite end of the scale is Cambodia, which is reliant on hundreds of millions of dollars per year in overseas development assistance to prop up its health care system, and where known cases of tuberculosis are increasing.

Why are health systems prone to corruption?
William D. Savedoff and Karen Hussmann[1]

Corruption in the health sector is not exclusive to any particular kind of health system. It occurs in systems whether they are predominantly public or private, well funded or poorly funded, and technically simple or sophisticated. The extent of corruption is, in part, a reflection of the society in which it operates. Health system corruption is less likely in societies where there is broad adherence to the rule of law, transparency and trust, and where the public sector is ruled by effective civil service codes and strong accountability mechanisms.

These general factors affect the extent of corruption in any sector, but the health sector has a number of dimensions that make it particularly vulnerable to abuse. No other sector has the specific mix of uncertainty, asymmetric information and large numbers of dispersed actors that characterise the health sector. As a result, susceptibility to corruption is a systemic feature of health systems, and controlling it requires policies that address the sector as a whole.

Two other factors that contribute to corruption in health care are worth mentioning. First, the scope of corruption in the health sector may be wider than in other sectors because society frequently entrusts private actors in health with important public roles. When private pharmaceutical companies, hospitals or insurers act dishonestly to enrich themselves, they are not formally abusing 'public office for private gain'. Nevertheless, they are abusing the public's trust in the sense that people and organisations engaged in health service delivery are held to a higher standard in the interests of protecting people's health. The medical profession, in particular, is given great latitude in most countries to police itself in return for assuming professional responsibility to act in the best interests of patients (see 'Fighting corruption: the role of the medical profession', Chapter 5, page 94).

Second, the health sector is an attractive target for corruption because so much *public* money is involved. The world spends more than US $3.1 trillion on health services each year, most of it financed by governments. European members of the OECD collectively spend more than US $1 trillion per year and the United States alone spends US $1.6 trillion.[2] In Latin America, around 7 per cent of GDP, or about US $136 billion, is consumed by health care annually, of which half is publicly financed. In lower-income countries, private health spending is often greater than public health spending, although the latter is still a significant amount. The share of total government revenues spent on health care ranges from under 5 per cent in Ethiopia, Egypt, Indonesia and Pakistan to more than 15 per cent in Ireland, Germany, the United States and Costa Rica. These large flows of funds represent an attractive target for abuse.

Why are health systems prone to corruption?

No other sector of society has the specific mix of uncertainty, asymmetric information and large numbers of dispersed actors that characterise the health sector. These features combine in ways that systematically create opportunities for corrupt behaviour, while making it difficult to ensure the transparency and accountability that would inhibit this.

Uncertainty is a central feature of the health sector and has far-reaching implications, as was first argued by Kenneth Arrow in 1963.[3] Arrow showed that uncertainty regarding who will fall ill, when illness will occur, what kinds of illnesses people get and how efficacious treatments are make the market for health care services very different from other markets in terms of the scope for *market failure*. Due to uncertainty, medical care service markets and health insurance markets are both likely to be inefficient.

Uncertainty pervades the health care sector. People may not even know that they are ill or that they could benefit from health care services – as frequently happens to people with high blood pressure, anaemia or the early stages of diabetes. When people fall ill and seek medical care, they cannot judge whether the prescribed treatment is appropriate. If they get better, they may not know whether the treatment was necessary for their recovery. For example, people with viral infections are often prescribed antibiotics that are useless against viruses.

This uncertainty makes it difficult for those demanding medical care – patients or their families – to discipline suppliers of medical care, as occurs in other markets. Patients cannot shop around for the best price and quality when they are ignorant of the costs, alternatives and precise nature of their needs. In such situations, consumer choices do not reflect price and quality in the normal fashion, and other mechanisms – such as the licensing of professionals and facilities or even direct public provision – are introduced to allocate resources and determine what kinds of care are provided. As an additional consequence, the poor functioning of markets creates opportunities for corruption, and the uncertainty inherent in selecting, monitoring, measuring and delivering health care services makes it difficult to detect and assign responsibility for abuses.

The uncertainty surrounding health care leads people to insure themselves against illness. But the functioning of voluntary insurance markets leaves too many people without insurance and encourages the provision of too much health care for those who have it.[4] A common social response has been to establish mandatory health insurance coverage, which may resolve the market failures in health insurance but also introduces problems associated with ineffective public sector functioning.[5] The resulting engagement of public policy in the provision or regulation of health insurance is another significant avenue for corruption.

But the degree of uncertainty is not identical for everyone in the health sector, leading to a second systemic feature, namely *asymmetric information*. Information is not shared equally among health sector actors and this has significant implications for a health system's efficiency and its vulnerability to corruption. Health care providers are better informed of the technical features of diagnosis and treatment than patients; pharmaceutical companies know more about their products than the doctors who prescribe them; individuals have certain kinds of information about their health that are not available to medical care providers or insurers; and providers and insurers may have better information about the health risks faced by certain categories of individuals than the individuals themselves.

When combined with differing interests among health sector actors, asymmetric information leads to a series of problems that are usefully analysed within the framework of *'principal–agent' relationships*.[6] In such a framework, the 'principal' hires an 'agent' to perform some function. When the agent has interests that differ from those of the principal *and* when the principal cannot get complete information about the agent's output, it is difficult to find contracts that are optimal. These two characteristics – diverging interests and incomplete information – are inherent and widespread in the health sector. For example, doctors have an interest in improving the health of their patients, but their choices of treatments and medications also may affect their income, professional status and working conditions. Whether doctors are hired by patients in the private sector or by public health services, they are entrusted with making decisions in the best interest of the patient, but may be tempted to provide substandard services or prescribe expensive treatments. Doctors are not the only agents in the health system. Those who manage health facilities, pharmaceutical companies, equipment suppliers or insurance agencies face complex incentives that may encourage them to reduce the quality of care, or promote the use of unnecessary diagnostics or treatments. When political interests are involved, any of these agents may be pressured to take actions that undermine health care or increase its costs.

While principal–agent problems in the health sector have mainly been analysed in terms of their impact on health system efficiency, these same problems increase opportunities for corruption. Furthermore, the difficulty of fully monitoring the actions of doctors, hospitals, pharmaceutical companies and regulators makes it hard to hold them accountable for the results of their actions. For example, patients usually lack information to monitor decisions made on their behalf, or judge whether they have been appropriately billed; insurance auditors have a hard time assessing whether billing is accurate and whether services rendered were necessary; regulatory agencies are hard-pressed to assure the quality of drugs and medical equipment, and the accuracy of labels and expiration dates. All of this establishes a system that is prone to corruption, and in which identifying and punishing corrupt practices is inherently difficult.

Finally, health systems are prone to corruption because of the *large number of actors* involved and the complexity of their multiple forms of interaction. These actors can be classified into five main categories (see Figure 1.1): government regulators (health ministries, parliaments, specialised commissions); payers (social security institutions, government office, private insurers); providers (hospitals, doctors, pharmacists); consumers (patients); and suppliers (medical equipment and pharmaceutical companies). The presence of so many actors exacerbates the difficulties of generating and analysing information, promoting transparency and even identifying corruption when it occurs. It increases the number of opportunities for corruption; for example, funds can be diverted or misallocated at a ministry, state hospital board or local clinic by individuals working as managers, procurement officers, health professionals, dispensers, clerks or patients. And the involvement of so many actors multiplies the number and kinds of interests that might encourage corrupt behaviour. Actors may be tempted to abuse their positions for direct financial gain, to increase their prestige, political influence and power, or to expand their market share. When corruption is detected, it may be difficult to attribute it to a particular individual, or to distinguish corruption from a misjudgement or error.

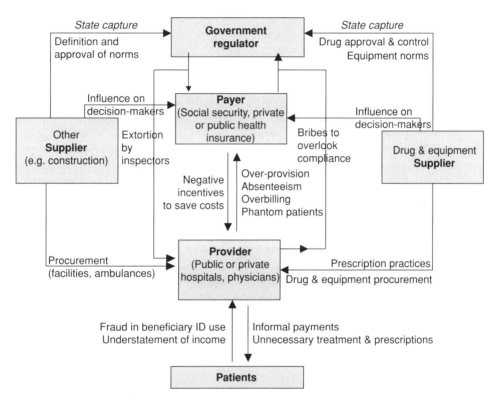

Figure 1.1: Five key actors in the health system

These three features – uncertainty, asymmetric information and large numbers of actors – systematically increase the likelihood that corruption will occur and that it will be difficult to detect, punish and deter in three distinct ways. First, they impair the normal functioning of a competitive market that might otherwise be harnessed to constrain illicit behaviour.[7] Second, they encourage the involvement of the public sector as a direct provider of health services, as insurer and/or as regulator, opening additional opportunities for corruption. Finally, these three features constrain efforts to generate reliable information, establish transparency and enforce accountability.

How are corruption and fraud manifested in the health sector?

Roles and responsibilities within health systems are split between regulators, payers, health care providers, suppliers and consumers in ways that make good decision-making difficult, even when everyone is thoroughly honest. When individuals who are willing to take advantage of this system are factored in, things become even more entangled. To see how this works, it is useful to consider, in turn, how each actor can use its position to defraud others.

Regulators (ministries of health, parliaments, supervisory commissions)

The basic uncertainty in health care services creates a potential role for government to protect consumers through supervision and improved information. It is common for governments to assume the role of verifying that medications are safe and effective, that health care practitioners have completed approved courses or have proven skills, and that facilities are adequately staffed and equipped. However, the existence of regulations opens avenues for corrupt activities. Pharmaceutical companies can skew research studies, influence review boards or simply bribe regulators to approve or speed up the processing of their applications. Health care providers and facilities may be tempted to pay a regulator to overlook lapses in licensing requirements. As in any sector, government inspectors can be tempted to abuse their position to extract bribes even when providers are in compliance.

Payers (social security organisations, health insurers)

Payers can be defrauded by other actors, but they can also engage in corrupt practices themselves. The public sector can act as a payer either through direct provision of care or as a public insurance agency. In the private sector, payers include commercial insurance firms and non-profit insurance organisations. Individuals can also be considered 'payers' when they pay fees directly to providers (see 'Patients' below).

When the public sector provides services directly, it generally allocates resources through the normal public budgetary process. This creates opportunities for political interests to contravene decisions that are in the best interest of patients. For example, decisions may be made to favour regions governed by political allies, rather than following criteria of equity and efficiency.

When the public sector manages an insurance fund, as is common in countries with mandatory social insurance, corruption can occur when officials embezzle funds. The public insurer can also allocate resources for political gain and at the expense of patients or taxpayers.

Private insurers, whether for-profit or non-profit, can engage in corrupt activities when they collaborate in public programmes, or are subjects of regulation. They may defraud public sector programmes that subsidise health care through fraudulent billing. They may reject insurance claims that they are committed to reimburse by law. And they may bribe insurance regulators to ignore illegal practices.

Health care providers (hospitals, doctors, nurses, pharmacists)

Health care providers have a wide range of opportunities to engage in corruption because they have such a strong influence over medical decisions, including prescribing medications, determining the length of a hospital stay, ordering tests and referring patients for additional consultations or services. In making these decisions, health care providers may act in ways that are not in their patients' best interests, whether motivated by direct financial gain, increased prestige, greater power or improved working conditions. These risks are one of the reasons that health care professionals are generally bound by professional standards and ethical codes that are expressly aimed at deterring corruption.

Patients generally defer to health care professionals in determining what course of action should be taken to treat an illness. Consequently, health care providers are in the unique position of telling the 'consumer' what service 'to buy'. When providers are paid 'fee-for-service' (that is, a fee for each service that they provide), it is in their financial interest to provide more services, and more costly services, than might otherwise be indicated by the individual's health condition. When providers are paid on a 'capitated' basis (that is, a single fee to cover any services required by a patient enrolled in their care, regardless of how many are actually provided) then it is in their financial interest to provide fewer services than would otherwise be indicated by the individual's health condition alone. When providers are paid a fixed salary, independent of the volume of services provided, there are no financial incentives to oversupply or undersupply services, but there is a tendency to be less productive and provide less care.[8]

In the case of publicly employed health providers, a wide range of abuses can occur. They can abuse their public sector job by referring patients to their parallel private practice (or use public facilities and supplies to serve their private patients). They may defraud the public sector by accepting a full salary while absenting themselves to provide private consultations elsewhere. They may steal drugs and medical supplies for resale or use in other places, and solicit bribes from patients for services that are supposed to be free. Although these practices are generally illegal, they may be excused in many countries by people who see them as acceptable strategies for coping with low pay and poor working conditions.[9]

Health care providers are also in a position to defraud payers in several ways. Most payment systems have to rely on the honesty of providers to state the kind and intensity of services that have been provided. Health providers may create 'phantom' patients to claim additional payments. They can order tests to be conducted at private laboratories in which they have a financial stake, or prescribe expensive drugs in exchange for kickbacks or bribes from pharmaceutical companies.

In addition to health care providers, health facility officials may accept kickbacks to influence the procurement of drugs and supplies, infrastructure investments and medical equipment. In so doing, they may pay higher prices or overlook shoddy work.

Patients

Consumers or patients can also participate in corrupt behaviour. In many systems, patients try to get free or subsidised care by underreporting their personal or family income. In other systems, patients misrepresent their enrolment in an insurance plan by using the insurance cards of friends or family members. This has been documented in Canada where the province of Ontario detected numerous people using forged cards to gain access to free public care.[10] A patient may bribe a doctor to obtain benefits for non-health issues, such as a health certificate to obtain a driver's licence, to avoid military service or to obtain disability payments.

Paying bribes to get privileged access to public care is also a common form of corruption. In some countries, such bribes are socially acceptable and excused as a way to compensate poorly paid, public sector health professionals, or as an understandable response by people who may be in dire need of care. When such bribes become 'institutionalised', however, it creates a situation in which wealthier people are likely to get better attention than those who are poorer and unable to pay bribes (see Chapter 3, 'Corruption in hospitals').

Suppliers (producers of medical equipment, pharmaceutical companies)

Medical equipment suppliers and pharmaceutical companies have privileged information about their own products and deliveries that assist them to corrupt the health care system. Suppliers can skimp on the quality of equipment or repackage expired medications. They can short-change deliveries and bribe procurement officers to authorise higher prices. They can induce providers to use their products at inflated prices, even when cheaper, equally effective alternatives are available. In the mid-1990s, Germany investigated 450 hospitals and more than 2,700 doctors on suspicion of taking bribes from manufacturers of heart valves, life support equipment, cardiac pacemakers and hip joints.[11] Suppliers can bribe public health authorities in any of their normal procurement processes, including kickbacks from companies that want to win lucrative hospital construction tenders (see *Global Corruption Report 2005*).

Finally, suppliers can bribe regulatory agencies to develop policies in their favour. For example, pharmaceutical companies may influence governments to impede competition from generic drug manufacturers, or equipment producers may try to change regulations so that licensed facilities will be required to purchase their products.

Proving intent is difficult

Though all five actors are generally present in each system, their relative power and incentives will vary dramatically. For example, doctors paid on a salaried basis have no way to overcharge insurers, and systems that prohibit insurers from establishing exclusive provider networks have less leeway to control costs and billing practices.

In all cases, however, detecting corruption in the health system is difficult. As strange as it sounds, distinguishing an act of self-enrichment from systemic inefficiency, human error or just poor judgement is hard. The line between abuse and honest mistakes is frequently blurred. For example, when providers bill the government for treatments that are not medically indicated (or not even provided), it may still be difficult to determine whether the decision represented an intentional effort to defraud the government, poor training or a simple mistake.

These difficulties in proving intent encourage a situation in which impunity is commonplace. Efforts to convict individuals or firms for corruption can be further stymied when professional medical associations or industrial lobby groups use political pressures to shield their members from what may be viewed or characterised as prosecutorial zealotry.[12] One response can be to sidestep prosecution and instead use public leverage to induce more transparent and honest behaviour. For example, the US Department of Health and Human Services sought to reduce fraudulent billing of Medicare (the United States' public health insurance for the elderly) by documenting discrepancies and developing 'compliance programmes'. Thus, whether the practices of 'upcoding', 'miscoding' or 'unbundling' that led to overpayments were due to errors, misinterpretations or intentional malfeasance was simply sidestepped in favour of assuring that future billing would be in compliance with the law. The compliance programmes required a hospital to develop written standards of conduct, train staff in the appropriate use of codes, establish hotlines for complaints and monitor its own compliance, among a wide range of measures.[13]

Does corruption vary across health systems?

Though health care providers, payers, consumers, regulators and suppliers are active in all health systems, the actual relationships, responsibilities and payment mechanisms will vary. Some countries have relatively well financed public health services that are directly provided by national or local governments (Sweden, Spain). In other high-income countries, the public sector pays for health services that are provided by private and public health care providers (Canada, Germany). In most low- and middle-income countries, the health system is fragmented. It may include a public insurance scheme for formal sector workers; direct public provision of health care for the indigent; private insurers and providers contracted by wealthier households; and a large share of private practitioners who are paid directly by their patients, both rich and poor (Mexico, South Africa).[14]

Abuses in the health system aimed at personal gain are not exclusive to any particular country or health system. But the forms of abuse may differ depending on how funds are mobilised, managed and paid. For this reason, it is useful to classify health systems into two broad categories based on their institutional structure: systems in which the public sector finances and directly provides health care services, and systems that separate public financing from provision.

In the case of direct public provision of health care services, the most common forms of abuse involve kickbacks and graft in procurement, theft, illegally charging patients, diverting patients to private practice, reducing or compromising the quality of care, and absenteeism. In systems that separate public financing from provision, the most common forms of abuse involve excessive or low-quality medical treatment, depending on the payment mechanism used, and fraud in billing government or insurance agencies.

Systems with direct public provision

In many countries, public health systems have been established to provide health care to the population at little or no cost at time of service. The most common structure for such systems involves a health ministry, or its equivalent, which hires the necessary administrative, medical and support staff, builds facilities, and organises the purchase and distribution of medications, equipment and supplies. Many European countries follow this model. Integrated public health systems display a wide range of structural differences, whether through decentralisation (as in Spain) or experimenting with autonomous health facilities (Sweden), but they share common approaches to allocating budgets and delivering services.

In developing countries, successes involving direct public provision of health care services are rare. In the most effective ones, health services do reach the bulk of the population (Chile, Cuba, Malaysia). In most cases, however, the public systems have been unable to reach large segments of the population, or to provide adequate services (Venezuela, Indonesia). In the absence of complete coverage, countries sometimes finance, or at least subsidise, non-profit health care institutions, such as mission hospitals in Africa or NGO health clinics in the Americas.

The evidence available on corruption in health systems with direct public provision is largely focused on informal, or illegal, payments for services in developing or transitional economies. This form of corruption has a particularly negative impact on access to care for the poor when they cannot afford these payments. In China and many former communist countries of Eastern Europe and Central Asia, the apparent existence of such illegal payments has led observers to conclude that the health care system has been 'privatised', that it functions like a private health care market and is only nominally public.[15]

The next most common focus for studies of corruption in health systems with direct public provision is theft by employees, self-referral of patients, absenteeism and the illicit use of public facilities for private practice. Kickbacks and graft in the purchase of medical supplies, drugs or equipment have also been studied in health systems with direct public provision, but these forms of corruption are more difficult to detect and document. Some studies have been able to estimate the magnitude of overcharges to the public sector for medical supplies and drugs by comparing prices paid by different hospitals.[16]

Systems that separate public financing from provision

In many health systems, the entity that finances health services is separate from the entity providing those services. This is common in countries with social insurance systems such as France and Germany, in large federated countries such as Brazil and Canada, and in systems with public safety nets such as Medicaid and Medicare in the United States. This separation of public financing and provision is rare in low-income countries, but is common in high-income countries and in the middle-income countries of Latin America and Asia.

When public financing is separated from provision, the character of abuses is likely to change, focusing on ways to divert the flow of payments and reimbursements. One central aspect influencing the type of abuse is the payment mechanism chosen by the financers to pay providers for their services. For example, medical professionals who are reimbursed on a fee-for-service basis have no incentive to be absent from work, but dishonest ones may be tempted to overcharge for services, bill for services that were not provided, or order tests and procedures that are not medically indicated. Provider payments on a capitation basis may introduce the right incentives for providers to focus more on preventive than on curative care, but it may also motivate the dishonest ones to neglect the provision of necessary care or to reduce quality below acceptable standards.

The public financing agent itself may be a focus for corruption, with officials diverting funds to improper uses or for personal financial gain. Furthermore, public reimbursement of private providers, in systems where this is permitted, raises a wide range of regulatory issues. The government frequently establishes regulations to assure that private providers meet minimum quality standards. Such regulations create opportunities for corruption in licensing procedures and inspections.

Whether countries directly provide health services or separate public financing from provision, their systems are not immune to corruption. Only the forms and scale of corruption are likely to vary (see Box 1.1).

Common forms of corruption in all health systems

Cutting across both types of systems are forms of abuse in the processes of allocating public funds and transferring public funds between national and sub-national entities. Sometimes there is large-scale diversion of funds at the ministerial or senior management levels of a health system; in other cases, funds are diverted from their intended purposes when they are transferred to lower-level political administrators. Though these forms of embezzlement can potentially cost the system more than other forms of corruption that occur at the facility level, they are studied less often and are poorly documented.

Both types of health systems share the vulnerability to abuses related to counterfeit drugs, selling faulty equipment, misrepresenting the quality or necessity of medical supplies and conflicts of interest between purchasers, providers, suppliers and researchers.

Conclusion

Health systems are prone to corruption because uncertainty, asymmetric information and large numbers of actors create systematic opportunities for corruption. These three factors combine to divide information among different actors – regulators, payers, providers, patients and suppliers – in ways that make the system vulnerable to corruption and that hinder transparency and accountability.

When regulations are put in place to remedy these problems, efforts to influence regulators become a new potential source of corruption. Powerful interest groups, including suppliers, payers and health providers, may 'capture' regulators in order to evade their responsibilities, or further their interests at public expense. Consumers generally lack the organisation and power to discipline other actors by voicing criticism or choosing different health care providers. In addition, abuses can be hidden behind simple administrative inefficiencies or, if challenged, be justified by claiming that the

Box 1.1 A tale of two health systems

A closer look at two countries demonstrates how corruption manifests itself differently across health systems. Colombia and Venezuela are neighbouring Latin American countries with comparable incomes that share many similarities in history, culture and language. Until 1990, the two countries also had similarly fragmented health systems, comprised of a large social security institution serving the formal sector, national or state-level governments that directly provided health care services to the rest of the population, and an active private sector which relied predominantly on direct payment for services by patients and their families.

In the early 1990s, Colombia engaged in a series of dramatic health reforms that decentralised public services to the municipal level and, in parallel, created a mandatory universal insurance system with the participation of non-governmental insurers (for-profit and non-profit). Under the new insurance system, individuals were given the option of choosing their insurer. The content and price of the benefit package was defined at the national level with the hope that insurers would compete on quality of care and service.

To make the system more equitable, the reform created a national fund that taxed away a portion of the relatively high contributions made by upper-income individuals so as to subsidise the relatively low contributions made by lower-income individuals. As a result of this system, insurers are now guaranteed a fixed premium for each member, adjusted by age and sex, which should be invariant to the individual's actual income. In this way, Colombia shifted from a segmented system dominated by large public institutions with integrated provision, to an increasingly universal system dominated by a separation of payers and providers.

Unfortunately, both countries have experienced a great deal of corruption across sectors, and the health system is no exception. A comparison between the two countries in the late 1990s suggested that corruption was widespread, but had taken somewhat different forms as their health systems diverged. For example, a large share of staff in public hospitals in both countries reported a range of irregularities, including theft, graft, absenteeism and bribe taking.[1] However, 59 per cent of staff surveyed in Bogotá's public hospitals reported that such irregularities had declined since implementation of the health reform. Staff in Venezuelan hospitals reported that doctors were absent from work about 37 per cent of the time while absenteeism in Colombia's public hospitals apparently accounted for less than 6 per cent of doctors' time. Although the available evidence is sparse, and certainly not conclusive, the differences suggest that public hospitals under the new system in Colombia may have been characterised by fewer irregularities.

On the other hand, Colombia's health reform opened an entirely new avenue for corrupt activities. The large flows of funds involving contributors, non-governmental insurers and government subsidies for low-income subscribers became targets for abuse. In the mid-1990s, Bogotá's Secretariat of Health – responsible for administering subsidies for low-income subscribers – began to audit the lists of members submitted by insurers for reimbursement. They found that benefits were being received by 114,000 new affiliates, far beyond the increase that could be expected through the extension of universal coverage. Instead, the Secretariat found that insurers kept individuals on their books, so they could continue to receive government subsidies, even after the same individuals had signed on to a new insurer.

▶

The practice was facilitated by the fact that individuals were often unfamiliar with the insurance system and did not understand the implications of signing a new application. Some insurers failed to issue their members with the required documentation, undermining their ability to access the services to which they were entitled. Finally, some insurance agents simply submitted false applications. As a result, Bogotá was defrauded of millions of dollars until it established a unified database, and began to scrutinise and investigate claims more intensely. Similar practices, however, were likely to have continued in the rest of the country where claims were less actively scrutinised.

William D. Savedoff

Note
1. Rafael Di Tella and William D. Savedoff, *Diagnosis Corruption: Fraud in Latin America's Public Hospitals* (Washington, DC: Inter-American Development Bank, 2001).

medical professional or procurement officer should not be 'second-guessed' by someone who is less informed of the circumstances of a case. As a result, opportunities to divert funds, sell favours, solicit bribes or otherwise corrupt the application of resources may be widespread.

These problems emerge in all kinds of health systems around the world. The particular institutional structures of the health system may make particular forms of corruption more or less attractive, but no system is immune to abuses and fraud. Understanding how a country's health system functions, reviewing the underlying incentives for provision of care and analysing its particular vulnerabilities are the first steps toward designing holistic strategies to tackle corruption from a systemic point of view, and implementing measures that will be effective in reducing the extent of abuse and fraud.

Notes

1. William D. Savedoff is a senior partner at Social Insight and formerly senior economist at the World Health Organization (WHO) and the Inter-American Development Bank. Karen Hussmann is a public policy consultant specialising in health economics and governance, and formerly programme officer at Transparency International.
2. These figures are the authors' estimates for 2001 from a variety of sources, including WHO, the Pan American Health Organization (PAHO), the World Bank and the US Department of Health and Human Services.
3. Kenneth J. Arrow, 'Uncertainty and the Welfare Economics of Medical Care', *American Economic Review* 53 (1963). For a discussion of Arrow's article and its impact on health economics, see William D. Savedoff, '40th Anniversary: Kenneth Arrow and the Birth of Health Economics', *Bulletin of the World Health Organization* 82(2), February 2004.
4. The detailed economic explanations for these problems involve adverse selection and moral hazard and are explained in most health economics textbooks. See, for example, T. Getzen, *Health Economics: Fundamentals and Flow of Funds* (New York: Wiley, 1997).
5. Public choice models and government failure literature includes Dennis C. Mueller (ed.), *Perspectives on Public Choice* (Cambridge: Cambridge University Press, 1997), and Torsten Persson and Guido Tabellini, *Political Economy: Explaining Economic Policy* (Cambridge, MA: MIT Press, 2002).

6. For principal–agent model literature, see D. E. Sappington, 'Incentives in Principal–Agent Relationships', *Journal of Economic Perspectives* 5(2), 1991, and William D. Savedoff, 'Social Services Viewed Through New Lenses', in William D. Savedoff (ed.), *Organization Matters: Agency Problems in Health and Education in Latin America* (Washington, DC: Inter-American Development Bank, 1998).
7. Alberto Ades and Rafael Di Tella, 'Rents, Competition and Corruption', *American Economic Review* 89(4), 1999.
8. For a discussion of different payment mechanisms and their impact on provider behaviour, see H. Barnum, J. Kutzin and H. Saxenian, 'Incentives and Provider Payment Methods', *International Journal of Health Planning and Management* 10, 1995, and J. C. Robinson, 'Theory and Practice in the Design of Physician Payment Incentives', *Milbank Quarterly*, November 2001.
9. See Chapter 3, 'Corruption in hospitals', page 54.
10. N. Inkster, 'A Case Study in Health Care Fraud in Ontario, Canada', *Corruption in Health Services*. Papers presented at the 10th International Anti-Corruption Conference Workshop 'Corruption and Health', Prague, Czech Republic, October 2001 (Washington, DC: Inter-American Development Bank, 2002).
11. *British Medical Journal* 312, 13 January 1996.
12. William D. Savedoff's interview with Leslie Aronovitz, US Department of Health and Human Services, 17 December 2000.
13. L. Aronovitz, 'Allegations of Inaccurate Billing in the Medicare System in the United States', *Corruption in Health Services*. Papers presented at the 10th International Anti-Corruption Conference Workshop 'Corruption and Health', Prague, Czech Republic, October 2001 (Washington, DC: Inter-American Development Bank, 2002).
14. *World Development Report 2004: Making Services Work for Poor People* (Washington, DC: World Bank, 2004), and *The World Health Report 2000. Health Systems: Improving Performance* (Geneva: WHO, 2000).
15. Gerald Bloom, 'Primary Health Care meets the Market: Lessons from China and Vietnam', IDS Working Paper 53 (Brighton, UK: Institute of Development Studies, 1997), and Tim Ensor, 'What Role for State Health Care in Asian Transition Economies?' *Health Economics* 6 (5), 1997.
16. Rafael Di Tella and William D. Savedoff, *Diagnosis Corruption: Fraud in Latin America's Public Hospitals* (Washington, DC: Inter-American Development Bank, 2001).

Corruption in health care systems: the US experience

Malcolm K. Sparrow[1]

The United States spends more on health care than any other industrialised country, with national health expenditures in 2003 exceeding US $1.6 trillion.[2] This represents 15.3 per cent of the country's GDP, up from 5.7 per cent in 1965, and 8.8 per cent in 1980.[3] Despite the extraordinary level of spending, health care economists have traditionally paid very little attention to corruption, fraud, waste and abuse in the US health care delivery system. They do not factor it into their cost models, they say, because 'there is no data on that'. There is certainly a paucity of reliable data on the extent of corruption in the system, and few reliable estimates of how much of each health care dollar is actually lost to criminal enterprise.

As a risk to be controlled, fraud and corruption in the health care system exhibits all the standard challenges of white-collar crime: well orchestrated criminal schemes are invisible by design and often go undetected. Investments in control are based on the visible (that is, detected) sliver of the problem, rather than on its underlying scale or any valid statistical or scientific estimates of its magnitude.

Despite the essentially invisible nature of the problem, health care fraud in the United States was deemed sufficiently serious by the Clinton administration (based on cases revealed) that in 1993, Attorney General Janet Reno declared it America's 'number two crime problem', second only to violent crime. This signalled a level of concern over health industry integrity without precedent in the United States, and perhaps around the world.

Characteristics of the US system

Despite high levels of public sector spending on health care,[4] the health system involves comparatively few public sector officials or employees in frontline service delivery roles. Therefore, if one adopts a definition of corruption restricted to 'abuse of *public* authority', most health care fraud issues do not quite fit. But the broader definition, 'abuse of *entrusted* authority', does cover dishonest actions of physicians, hospitals and other health care professionals, who are generally afforded high social and professional status and are expected to exercise professional medical judgement unbiased by private financial interests. The majority of fraud within the system, perpetrated by medical providers, can therefore be understood as corruption under this definition. For example, when physicians accept payment to hand out unnecessary prescriptions as part of pharmaceutical recycling scams, 'con' patients into treatments they don't need, or submit bills to public programmes for services that were never provided, they would surely be seen by most members of the public as having abused the trust placed in them as medical professionals.

The US health system has a number of distinct features that make it vulnerable to corruption:

- **Health care delivery is largely contracted out.** Health care is mostly delivered by the private sector, or independent, not-for-profit entities. But the services are *paid for* by government programmes such as Medicare (federal programme for the elderly) or Medicaid (state-run programmes for the poor), or by commercial insurers who offer health insurance to individuals, to groups or to employers (who buy coverage for their employees as an employment benefit). This means that payers have no reliable information about which services were performed, or were necessary, other than the word of the providers.
- **Fee-for-service structure and payment on trust.** The majority of services are reimbursed on a *fee-for-service* basis, despite the recent development of alternative structures such as capitation (where the entity contracts to deliver necessary care in exchange for a fixed revenue stream per patient per month), and other 'managed care' systems. Under the fee-for-service structure, health care providers (doctors, hospitals, specialists, and so on) are trusted to determine the appropriate levels of care, and then trusted to bill the insurer for the services they perform.

- **Medical suppliers and providers constitute main loci of corruption.** The principal opportunity for theft lies with providers rather than patients. Patients can only cheat on their own accounts, and to a limited extent if they are to avoid tripping various flags or alarms. So the prevalence of patient-orchestrated fraud is constrained to some degree by the proportion of dishonest patients. By contrast, providers and their billing agents are in a position to submit false or inflated bills in high volumes, spreading the activity across hundreds or thousands of patient accounts. Providers thus have a *business opportunity* in dishonest conduct, and relatively few dishonest actors can do disproportionate amounts of economic damage to the system. Most significant cases of corruption have involved medical professionals, providers and corporations in the health care delivery supply chain.
- **Highly automated payment systems.** Fee-for-service payment systems are now consolidated into massive, highly automated payment systems. Electronic submissions transmitted into the system (in the form of claims for services rendered) result in computerised dispatch of electronic payments. The bulk of such claims are paid through *auto-adjudication*, which means the claim was received, subjected to a rules-based examination, approved and paid, all electronically, with no human scrutiny. Such payment systems make very attractive targets for fraud. An extraordinary range of actors have been found lining up to defraud these systems, ranging from blue-collar individuals (who can sign on as suppliers of medical equipment for a small fee, without any training, and proceed to submit bills without ever seeing a patient); to major corporations, such as hospital chains and pharmaceutical companies; to drug traffickers (reported by the FBI as switching to health care fraud because it was safer and more lucrative than trafficking, and with lower chances of detection); to organised crime groups and gangs.[5]
- **Absence of verification and focus on processing accuracy.** The bulk of claims are therefore paid electronically, and on trust. The whole system is designed with honest physicians in mind, incorporating the values of speed, efficiency, accuracy, predictability and transparency. The edits and audits (automated sets of rules) built into computerised claims-processing systems serve the purpose of checking pricing, policy coverage and medical orthodoxy (based on the diagnosis reported in the claim). But the control systems generally assume the claim itself to be true, and do little or nothing to verify that the patient actually received the services claimed, or even that the diagnosis was real. To exploit these systems, those intent on stealing need only to ensure that they *bill correctly*. If they do that, they can fabricate or alter diagnoses, or invent entire medical episodes. If, by some mischance their claims are selected for audit, they need only create and submit medical records that support the fictitious billing, and – provided perpetrators are capable of lying twice, and consistently – they will survive such audit scrutiny without much fear of detection. The controls in place within the industry therefore deal better with billing errors and with honestly reported medical unorthodoxy than they do with outright criminal deception in the form of falsified claims. They deal better with poorly documented services than with well documented

lies. Investigators in the industry are starting to use a broader range of controls to address this problem (see below).

- **Multiple methods of cheating, and centrality of the false claims problem.** The incentives produced by the fee-for-service payment structure lead to submission of false or inflated bills. Other more sophisticated scams involve illegal kickbacks for referral of patients, physicians' acceptance of bribes for prescribing particular pharmaceuticals, inflating cost reports in systems where reimbursement rates for services depend on the reported costs and self-referral (referring business to other entities in which the referrer has an ownership or other financial interest), among others. Nevertheless, submission of *false claims* (claims that contain some material deception) represents perhaps the central and most persistent form of cheating in the US system.

- **Poor measurement of overpayment rates.** The Medicare programme and several Medicaid programmes have conducted measurement studies recently,[6] producing loss rates varying from 3 per cent to 15 per cent of overall costs, and with most results in the 5–10 per cent range. The studies draw random samples of claims paid, but then tend to apply somewhat weaker audit protocols than those necessary to produce true estimates of overpayment rates. The audit protocols used often replicate document-based or 'desk' audits, which check that the claims were processed correctly, and that they are supported by medical records requested and received by mail. But these audit methods generally include minimal or no attempts to track down the patients and verify that the services were both necessary and actually delivered. Hence the overpayment rates obtained by these measurement programmes generally miss many of the more sophisticated types of fraud, and often miss the ordinary phenomenon of *billing for services not provided* in cases where perpetrators take the precaution of submitting a false medical record to match the claim. These estimates therefore significantly understate the overall loss rates. This deficiency has been recognised by the Government Accountability Office, which acknowledges that use of more rigorous audit protocols designed to detect fraud would have made the derived estimates for overpayment rates 'greater – how much greater nobody knows'.[7]

- **Investments in control do not match the scale of the problem.** Despite loss rates that could easily exceed 10 per cent of programme costs, investments in controls for fraud and corruption remain pitifully low – as is typical of white-collar crime control. In the health industry, levels of investments in programme integrity and fraud control average roughly 0.1 per cent of programme costs. This ratio holds true remarkably consistently across the industry, irrespective of whether the insurer is public, commercial or not-for-profit. Investments in control are therefore woefully lacking, when viewed against potential losses.

Lessons learned from the US experience

The US health system remains vulnerable to attack, and programme integrity and fraud control systems are not yet sufficiently equipped to deal with the problem. Scandalous revelations of medical professionals or companies stealing millions of dollars from the system make almost daily appearances in the media. As a result, important lessons have been learned about controlling fraud and corruption, some of which include:

- **Attractiveness of automated systems as targets for fraud.** Large, highly automated payment systems make dream targets for fraud perpetrators. Their payment behaviour can be studied and their utter predictability exploited. Quality control and process improvement techniques can only guarantee the correct operation of the payment system, but do nothing to validate the information fed into it. In this environment, *fraud works best when processing systems work perfectly*. This vulnerability extends beyond health care programmes to many other major public assistance or payment programmes that share similar characteristics.
- **Importance of measurement.** Failure to measure losses in a scientifically valid and rigorous fashion creates uncertainty about the scale of the problem. This leaves policy-makers unable to justify greater investments in control or enforcement and keeps resources for control at minimal levels.
- **Importance of whistleblower statutes.** Most of the big cases brought against major corporations for defrauding government health care programmes in the past decade arose from, or relied heavily upon, *qui tam* suits (allowing private citizens to file lawsuits charging fraud in government programmes) brought under the federal False Claims Act.[8] Most often the whistleblower was an employee or ex-employee of the offending corporation. Although the False Claims Act was originally designed to reduce corruption in defence contracting, health care fraud cases now routinely account for more than half of the annual volume of *qui tam* cases taken up by the Department of Justice. Whistleblowers receive a share of any eventual settlement. Providing financial incentives and compensation to whistleblowers has turned out to be one of the most powerful weapons available to the US government in tackling health care fraud and corruption. One prominent example involves the Columbia/HCA hospital chain, America's single largest health care provider. A series of whistleblower lawsuits launched against Columbia in the 1990s resulted in aggregate settlements with the Department of Justice exceeding US $1 billion dollars.[9] The practices whistleblowers reported included paying physicians for patient referrals to the hospitals, funnelling of patients to affiliated home-health services even when the patients preferred another provider, setting performance targets in terms of 'complication rates' (which justify higher levels of reimbursement from Medicare), hiding paperwork and accounts from government auditors, and false billing.
- **Dynamic nature of the game**. Investigators and auditors have learned how quickly fraud perpetrators can adapt to changes in the control system. Control strategies that rely on any static set of controls (such as reliance on a particular set of rule-based edits and audits in the processing system) fail utterly. Fraud control is a game of intelligence and counter-intelligence played against conscious, and highly adaptive, opponents.

- **Limitations of transaction-based analysis and detection methods.** Investigators are discovering the importance of moving beyond transaction-level control systems, which are easily circumnavigated by perpetrators who design their scams so that each claim, viewed in isolation, looks perfect. The more successful detection units within the industry are beginning to use a broader range of structural analysis and pattern-recognition methodologies that can search for patterns of coincidence or clustering (across thousands of claims) reflective of computerised billing scams and organised conspiracies – very few of which would ever be detected by examination of individual claims or individual patient histories.
- **The dangers of rushing to structural solutions.** Normally one would applaud policy-makers for seeking long-term structural solutions to integrity problems. Anti-corruption literature emphasises structural changes in incentives as a method of eliminating known forms of corruption and embezzlement. Many officials, concerned about fraud in the fee-for-service health structure, mistakenly assumed the advent of capitated managed care systems would eliminate the fraud problem by removing the financial incentives for overutilisation and overbilling. What they realise now is that changing the structure without removing the bad actors leads to criminal adaptation, and a whole new class of scams.

  With capitated systems, the incentives for overutilisation have been replaced by incentives for underutilisation. Dishonest providers take the monthly capitation payments and find a multitude of creative mechanisms to divert resources into their own pockets and away from frontline service delivery. The new forms of fraud that emerge turn out to be harder to detect, harder to control, more difficult to prosecute (because there is no false claim per se around which to build a case), and more dangerous to human health. Examples of abuses include: embezzlement of capitation funds paid by the state; the use of fraudulent subcontracts as a method of diverting funds to friends or family; improper enrolment or disenrolment practices (such as seriously ill patients being driven out or refused admission to a health care plan, or bribes being paid to secure younger and healthier patients); denial of treatment without proper evaluation; failure to inform patients of their rights and entitlements; failure to provide sufficient medical professionals to meet the needs of the enrolled population; and requiring patients to fight their way through extensive appeals processes in order to obtain necessary treatment. Under the fee-for-service structure, crimes were largely financial, with patients often oblivious to what was being billed in their names. With managed care, diversion of capitation payments results in inaccessible or inadequate patient care.

Looking ahead

The battle against health care fraud and corruption in the United States is not over. The Clinton administration paid more attention to the problem than any previous administration, and made some important financial and legislative investments to enhance control. Despite those investments, levels of resources available for monitoring, validation and enforcement remain completely inadequate when compared with the scope of the problem. The introduction of a new prescription drug benefit for seniors under the Medicare programme,[10] almost guarantees that the federal government will have to pay renewed attention to this issue in years to come, since drug-related fraud remains one of the most prominent fraud threats within other programmes. The recent deceleration of the transition to capitated managed care (and in some regions and segments of the industry, the *reversal* of this transition), means that US health insurers will still have to develop more effective controls within a fee-for-service environment, as there is no prospect of structural change within the industry being able to solve the problem in the near future.

Notes

1. Malcolm K. Sparrow is professor of the practice of public management at Harvard's John F. Kennedy School of Government, and author of *License to Steal: How Fraud Bleeds America's Health Care System* (Denver: Westview Press, 2000), which contains a detailed analysis of the vulnerabilities of the US health system to fraud, waste and abuse.
2. 'Historical National Health Expenditures Aggregate, per Capita, Percent Distribution, and Average Annual Percent Change by Source of Funds: Calendar Years 1960–2003', www.cms.hhs.gov/statistics/nhe
3. Ibid.
4. Public sector spending runs at roughly 45 per cent of national costs. The two largest public programmes are Medicare (federal programme for the elderly) and Medicaid (programme for the poor, administered by the states and jointly funded by federal and state governments). See also national health expenditures in note 2 above.
5. The introduction to *License to Steal* (see note 1) catalogues the extraordinary range of apparent perpetrators and fraud methods seen in the industry over the last decade.
6. Measurement of Medicare overpayment rates was required by the Government Management Reform Act of 1994, instituted by the Office of Inspector General (DHHS) in 1996, and repeated every year until 2002. Derived overpayment rate estimates ranged from a high of 14.1 per cent to a low of 6.3 per cent. For a synopsis of recent measurement studies within Medicaid, see 'Payment Accuracy Measurement Project: Year 2 Final Report', Center for Medicaid and State Operations, Center for Medicare and Medicaid Services, DHHS, April 2004.
7. 'Efforts to Measure Medicare Fraud', Letter to Rep. John R. Kasich (Chair, House Budget Committee), GAO/AIMD-00-69R, 4 February 2000.
8. The 1986 Federal False Claims Act updated Civil War-era laws originally designed to prevent procurement fraud against the Union Army. It became available for use against health care fraud upon its revision in 1986. Penalties for false claims against government programmes were further stiffened by the Health Insurance Portability and Accountability Act of 1996.
9. www.cbsnews.com/stories/2002/12/18/national/main533453.shtml
10. The prescription drug benefit, known as Medicare Part D, comes into full effect in January 2006 under the Medicare Prescription Drug Improvement and Modernization Act of 2003.

Box 1.2 Corruption in Cambodia's health sector[1]

Cambodia's health record is amongst the worst in Asia. The maternal mortality rate is the highest in the region, with 437 deaths per 100,000 live births. Skilled personnel attend less than a third of all births.[2] Almost one in every ten babies does not live to his/her first birthday and more than 60,000 babies die every year of malnutrition or diseases that

▶

can be prevented or cured.[3] Malaria remains a serious problem, and known cases of tuberculosis have increased from approximately 61,000 in 1999 to 108,000 in 2004.[4]

Such a poor state of health exists despite money pouring into Cambodia's health sector over the past decade to reconstruct a health system that was systematically decimated under the Khmer Rouge regime (1975–78) and underfunded in subsequent years. Overseas development aid (ODA) funded a lot of the reconstruction and continues to be an important source of finance for the government. In 2002 the US $490 million ODA Cambodia received accounted for just over 12 per cent of the GDP, some 20 per cent of which was spent on health.

However, government and ODA spending on health are dwarfed by the sums spent privately. Of the 177 countries assessed in the *Human Development Report*, Cambodia has the highest private health expenditure as a percentage of the GDP. Out-of-pocket spending on health care in Cambodia's private clinics or as informal payments for public health services accounts for 10 per cent of the country's GDP.[5]

Corruption is one reason why public investment in health, coupled with high rates of private spending, has not translated into good health outcomes. Anecdotal evidence suggests that corruption takes place at every level of the health system in Cambodia, but there has typically been a reluctance to speak about it. Researchers, health workers and administrators interviewed in July 2005 said it was widely assumed that between 5 and 10 per cent of the health budget disappears before it is paid out by the Ministry of Finance to the Ministry of Health.[6] More money is then siphoned off as funds are channelled down from the national government to the provincial governors and to the directors of operational districts, and then to directors or managers of local hospitals and clinics.

Reports commissioned by the World Bank and USAID indicate that corruption is common in public procurement and contracting processes, public fund management activities at central and district government levels and in health service delivery schemes. It is common for companies to pay bribes for public contracts.[7] Several experts interviewed alleged that health ministry officials and hospital administrators inflate the cost of medical equipment in collusion with private suppliers and share the non-reported difference, which can be as much as five times the true cost.

Another source of concern is that public health services are underutilised due to their poor quality and inaccessibility. With the increase in land prices in Phnom Penh and Siem Reap, this problem threatens to escalate under the government's reported plans to remove hospitals from city centres to outskirts where land is cheaper, but where the hospitals will be less accessible. In Siem Reap, for example, a hospital is in danger of being destroyed to free up prime real estate close to a popular tourist attraction. The government claims that the land is valued at US $4 million. Health programme managers from the private and public health system claim the land is worth many times more than the cost of rebuilding the hospital.

The potential for profit-making through schemes such as this can be the very motivation for entering the health sector. In Cambodia it is considered common practice to pay large sums of money to secure positions as public officials in government: the higher the position, the higher the price.[8] Health workers interviewed reported a going rate of up to US $100,000 for a post as director at the provincial or national offices of the health ministry. A job as a low-level public servant in the health sector may go for US $3,000. These sums represent a large investment considering that government employee salaries are generally very low: on average US $40 per month.

▶

Corruption also takes place at the point of health service delivery, where underpaid health workers request informal payments above the normal cost service, or siphon off public funds from available cash budgets. Informal payments to doctors or nurses in order to receive better and more expedient treatment are common, and the low salary paid to health workers is an important area to reform. In 2001, Médecins Sans Frontières worked with the Ministry of Health and UNICEF on a project in Sotnikum district, Siem Reap province, that topped up salaries for health workers based on performance and commitment to ethical practice. It also tried to initiate an Equity Fund to assist the poor in paying for medical costs and services. These two strategies have been successful and continue in many donor-funded health care projects in Cambodia, though coverage is patchy.

Other important reforms include increasing transparency in procurement, improving links between health policies and budgets, and conducting research to help understand the mechanisms of corruption in the sector. A planned public expenditure tracking survey, initiated by the World Bank for the health sector to identify bottlenecks and leaks in public finances at national and local levels, is an important step towards plugging the information gap surrounding Cambodia's health sector.

Urgent attention also needs to be paid to law enforcement. An extremely weak judiciary, coupled with inadequate laws that are very slowly being reformed, mean that impunity is the norm for cases of corruption. There are 100 prosecutors, 250 private attorneys and 100 judges operating in the country – most of the latter self-selected, having bought their positions.[9] Some progress has been made in training judges and a number of NGOs are developing basic legal services for the weak and poor, but to all intents and purposes there is no redress for those who have suffered from the effects of corruption at the hand of health authorities or staff.

Lisa Prevenslik-Takeda[10]

Notes
1. The article is based on fieldwork and author interviews conducted from May to July 2005.
2. Royal Government of Cambodia, *Cambodia Millennium Development Goals Report 2003*.
3. UNDP, *Human Development Report 2003* (Geneva: UNDP, 2003); UNICEF, *Childhood Under Threat: The State of the World's Children 2005* (New York: UNICEF, 2005).
4. WHO Report, *Global Tuberculosis Control* (Geneva: WHO, 2005). The actual figures are probably much higher since normal tuberculosis testing in medical centres throughout the country is done by sputum tests which detect only 75 per cent of pulmonary tuberculosis infections.
5. Although the constitution enshrines the right to free medical care to all Cambodian citizens, a recent government policy requires all Cambodians to pay 2,000–3,000 riel (US $0.75) to access health care in public health facilities. This entitles the patient to be examined by a doctor, though additional costs for medicine and other medical supplies must be borne by the patient.
6. Author interviews, Phnom Penh, Cambodia, July 2005.
7. Michael Calavan, Sergio Diaz Briqvets and Jerald O'Brien, 'Cambodian Corruption Assessment', report prepared for the World Bank, USA/Cambodia, August 2004; Jean-François Bayart, 'Thermidor au Cambodge', *Alternatives Economiques*, March 2005; Peter Leuprecht, Special Representative of the UN Secretary-General for Human Rights in Cambodia, *Rethinking Poverty Reduction to Protect and Promote the Rights of Indigenous Minorities in Cambodia*, NGO Forum on Cambodia, April 2005.
8. See, for example, Calavan et al., 'Cambodian Corruption Assessment'.
9. Ibid.
10. Lisa Prevenslik-Takeda is a project coordinator in Transparency International's Asia-Pacific department.

2 The scale of the problem

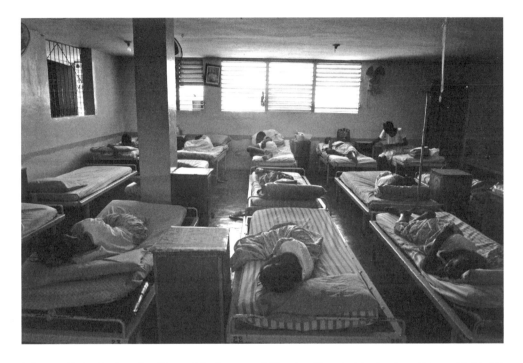

Women lie in bed at the Sisters Missionary of Charity Hospital in Port-au-Prince, Haiti, 22 March 2005. (Shaul Schwarz/Getty Images)

While it is impossible to determine the overall costs of corruption in the health sector worldwide, it is evident that it amounts to tens of billions of dollars. Indeed one US estimate of annual earnings from the sale of counterfeit drugs alone puts the annual cost at more than US $30 billion, which is just the tip of the iceberg of health care corruption.

In this chapter, the World Bank's efforts to track expenditure in health give an indication of costs by tracking how much money dispersed by higher levels of government fails to reach its intended recipients. New data from Central and Eastern Europe finds a strong correlation between perceptions of corruption and an individual's health. A study in the Philippines highlights how local-level corruption undermines health service delivery. The case study on Costa Rica looks higher up in the chain of responsibility for health budgets, and follows the money trail in one of the country's biggest ever corruption scandals. An example from Mexico shows that corruption can affect not only the volume of resources for health care, but also health policy. The UK's National Health Service claims high returns on its investment in anti-corruption and counter-fraud mechanisms.

The real costs, however, cannot be measured in dollar terms alone. The impact of corruption must also be measured in terms of those people who suffer because they cannot afford brown envelope payments to health care workers (see Chapter 4) and those who are forced to pay far more than they should for hospital services and pharmaceuticals due to rampant corruption (see Chapters 3 and 5). Corruption has a direct negative impact on access and quality of patient care and is one reason why, so often, increased spending on health does not correlate with improved health outcomes.

Case study: Grand corruption in Costa Rica
Emilia González (TI Costa Rica)

Costa Rica has one of the best funded health systems in Latin America. Established in 1941, the Caja Costarricense de Seguro Social (CCSS) has been responsible for providing universal health care coverage since 1961. The health care network comprises five health regions, each with hospitals, clinics, health centres and mobile health units. Costa Rica's health indicators are comparable to those of developed countries and better than any Latin American country with the exception of Cuba. Workers pay 5.5 per cent of their salary in health insurance and employers contribute a further 9.25 per cent.

Given the high cost and the high regard in which the CCSS is held, its fall from grace was therefore steep when reports of maladministration and corruption started to seep into the public domain in 2001. Two congressional party commissions were tasked with looking into the matter. Allegations involved corruption at many different levels, most commonly in the purchase of medical services, often at inflated prices; the procurement of medicines and equipment; the provision of private training courses and medical research; the construction of hospitals; and the management of the CCSS pensions system.

The climax of the scandals came in October 2004 when the public prosecutor accused CCSS head Eliseo Vargas, members of the board of directors, several CCSS managers and former president Rafael Angel Calderón of corruption in the running of the agency. They had allegedly skimmed millions off a US $39 million Finnish government loan (see Finland country report, page 156).

The loan to modernise hospitals was conditional on Costa Rica using at least half of it to buy Finnish products. The contract was won by Finnish consortium Instrumentarium Corporation Medko Medical and a commission of US $8.8 million (20 per cent of the value of the loan) was paid to Corporación Fischel, the consortium's Costa Rican representative. It was this commission that found its way into the bank accounts of CCSS directors and senior government officials. The CCSS spent the loan – plus an extra US $7.5 million of its own funds – on equipment that was not needed.

The money trail was uncovered in October 2003 by journalists who found that the head of CCSS, Eliseo Vargas, was living in a house worth US $750,000, which had been paid for by Corporación Fischel (see *Global Corruption Report 2005*).[1] Suspecting that the house was payment for a favour, the reporters looked for a possible motive. They found that two years earlier, as head of the ruling party faction in congress, Vargas had pushed through approval of the tied loan from Finland. Vargas now argues that he was assisted – and encouraged – to do so by then president Calderón. The journalists later uncovered a series of bank accounts in Panama, Costa Rica, the United States and the Bahamas through which 'commissions' had been paid to politicians and CCSS officials. Vargas and the financial director of Fischel resigned when the news hit the headlines in April 2004.

The Finnish loan was not the first to be called into question. In 1997, a US $40 million loan by the Spanish government and Banco Bilbao Vizcaya, also to modernise hospitals, was spent on equipment, much of which has never been used. A group of notable experts named by the government to look into the functioning of CCSS requested that the authorities responsible for executing the loan be investigated for paying above-market rates for the equipment and for failing to prepare the hospitals for the equipment to be installed.

Incidents of opaque procurement processes at CCSS are unfortunately not restricted to the use of the two loans. Complaints of systematic corruption have been made in a series of reports and statements by a special legislative commission, the ombudsman, a group of notable experts and users of the health system. CCSS internal audit reports also point to irregularities.

A majority party congressional investigation report published in April 2001 provided evidence of disorganised purchasing – the results of a decentralisation strategy that was supposed to make procurement processes more efficient.[2] The result was a chaotic network of channels through which millions of colones flowed, swelling the accounts of private pharmaceutical companies at the cost of the CCSS, and ultimately the taxpayer. In addition to the monetary costs involved, there were also the associated health costs resulting from delays in getting medicine to the sick and the use of poorer-quality medicines

The various reports into the CCSS note that a common practice at some hospitals was to purchase excessive quantities of medicines not included on the official list of medicines (defined by the WHO as those necessary to counter the principal causes of morbidity). These were purchased under a budget line reserved for medicines needed for uncommon illnesses or exceptional cases, which are not subject to the usual CCSS controls. Another concern is the readiness with which some CCSS doctors accepted trips paid for by pharmaceutical companies. This was the subject of a Supreme Court ruling in January 2004 stating that acceptance of gifts from providers could lead to a loss of confidence in the doctor and therefore could be cited as grounds for lawful dismissal.[3]

Many examples of overpayment for medical services contracted out to private service providers emerged from the investigations. It is difficult, however, to distinguish between poor management and corruption, where doctors – often with one foot in the public system and the other in private practice – might have unnecessarily contracted out expensive treatments. For example, the CCSS paid a private foundation close to US $1 million in 2000 for 9,600 minor surgical procedures, 37,000 eye and nose consultations and 322 vitrectomies at a cost per intervention of between 40 per cent and 140 per cent above the cost of CCSS providing the treatment at one of its own clinics. A special congressional commission published a report in May 2001 into the procurement of private medical services and the misuse of CCSS resources through offering excessively cheap teaching facilities to private university students.[4]

The CCSS response to these multiple accusations of maladministration and corruption has been to hire consultants and researchers to come up with new strategic plans and new mission and values statements. Complaints mechanisms have been introduced, and the client has been placed at the forefront of the institution's plans.

But the correctives do not go to the root of the problem. With the exception of the investigation into misuse of the Finnish loan, senior CCSS staff have not been asked to take responsibility for wrongdoing. Few are named in the numerous reports and documents written on the cases, and no administrative, criminal or civil action has been taken to sanction those responsible.

Close ties between the board and directors of the CCSS – many party members hold board-level positions at the CCSS – may have stood in the way of judicial and audit bodies, contributing to a situation where the CCSS functions with virtual impunity, unaccountable to users. There are indications that the close relationship between political parties and the CCSS may have led to conflicts of interest that influenced decision-making. The 1999 budget shows, for example, that more than US $160 million of CCSS funds was invested in state bonds at a time of dire need for investment to improve health care facilities.

Scandals have erupted before without responsibility being assigned to the officials involved, while civil society watched on impassively. This time, public pressure and media attention is not abating. There is hope that high- and middle-ranking CCSS staff will be held to account and deep reforms will be made to the management, organisation and structure of CCSS, including the introduction of greater accountability and transparency mechanisms to reduce future opportunities for corruption.

Notes

1. The team of investigative journalists from *La Nación* (Costa Rica) were awarded Transparency International's Journalism for Transparency prize in 2005.
2. Costa Rican Legislative Assembly, 'Informe de Mayoría: Comisión Especial que proceda a analizar la calidad de los servicios, compra de servicios privados, utilización de los recursos de la CCSS para la enseñanza universitaria privada, medicamentos y pensiones' (Majority Report: Special Commission to proceed to analyse the services, purchase of private services, use of CCSS resources for private university teaching, medicines and pensions), File number 13-980, San José, Costa Rica, 26 April 2001.
3. Ruling by the second tribunal of the Supreme Court, Exp: 95-000493-02-LA Res: 2004-00212.
4. A second congressional report co-sponsored by current president Abel Pacheco, a congressman at the time, presented a contrasting view of the CCSS, concluding that: 'There is no legal,

technical, scientific nor strategic reason whatsoever for us to have reservations about the contracting modalities used by CCSS since the end of the 1990s.' See Costa Rican Legislative Assembly, 'Informe de Mayoría: Comisión Especial que proceda a analizar la calidad de los servicios, compra de servicios privados, utilización de los recursos de la CCSS para la enseñanza universitaria privada, medicamentos y pensiones'.

Measuring corruption in the health sector: what we can learn from public expenditure tracking and service delivery surveys in developing countries

Magnus Lindelow, Inna Kushnarova and Kai Kaiser[1]

Most government officials and development practitioners acknowledge that high levels of health spending do not necessarily translate into improved health status. This observation is also borne out by empirical evidence – studies have found that once other factors are controlled for, increased government spending on health is not associated with a reduction in child mortality in cross-country data, at least not in contexts with weak governance.[2] In part, the challenge in transforming resources into improved health outcomes is technical in nature; it concerns the allocation of resources across interventions and programmes, as well as the technical skills of providers responsible for delivering the interventions. The focus of this chapter, however, is on how corruption – defined here as 'the abuse of public office for private gain' – can drive a wedge between what is put into the health system, on the one hand, and what it delivers, on the other.

Some of the evidence on the nature and consequences of corruption in the sector comes from perception-based surveys.[3] While these surveys have generated useful insights, the data suffer from many of the same weaknesses that plague perception-based measures of corruption in general. An alternative approach is to try to develop more direct measures of fiscal leakages, including corruption. This has been the aim of a number of recent Public Expenditure Tracking Surveys (PETS), which aim to answer the question: 'Does public money spent on health and education actually reach frontline health facilities and schools?' They seek to achieve this by tracking the flow of public resources through various layers of the administrative hierarchy to individual service providers, and by developing quantitative estimates of fiscal leakage – that is, the failure of resources intended for frontline service provider (clinics and hospitals) facilities to reach their intended destination.

The World Bank and other organisations have conducted PETS, almost exclusively in the social sectors, in over two dozen countries, beginning with Uganda's education sector in 1995 where it was found that 77 per cent of non-wage funds failed to reach schools. This chapter reviews what has been learnt from tracking surveys in the health sector so far. It shows that while many PETS have generated valuable insights, practical and methodological challenges have often made it difficult to develop firm and comprehensive estimates of leakage.

Moreover, once an estimate of leakage has been arrived at, there are challenges interpreting the data, specifically in how to establish the relationship between leakage and corruption. There are two main reasons for this difficulty. First, it is possible that resources were legitimately diverted from their intended purpose towards other ends. All budget systems allow for some flexibility in the resource allocation process: budgets can be changed, allocation rules can be modified or ignored, and so on. This provides government with the flexibility to adjust plans in response to unexpected events and needs, and means that discrepancies between expenditure outcomes and original allocations (leakage) may be both legitimate and desirable.

Second, facilities or lower levels of government may receive less than intended due to problems in the budget execution or resource distribution process. For example, capacity weaknesses and red tape can result in low levels of budget execution, and a broken down vehicle can disrupt the distribution of drugs. A discrepancy between expenditure allocation and outturn may hence be the consequence of delays in the disbursement or distribution of funds rather than evidence of corrupt acts.

With these caveats in mind, what have tracking surveys revealed about leakage in the health sector? As can be seen from the summary in Table 2.1, the focus of the surveys has varied across countries. Some surveys such as those in Ghana, Tanzania and Rwanda – have generated leakage estimates for overall expenditures. For example, the Ghana PETS found that 80 per cent of non-salary funds did not reach health facilities, with most of the leakage arising between central government and the district. Considering that approximately 65 per cent of total health spending (total spending estimated to be about US $2.24 per capita in 1998) is non-salary recurrent, and assuming that the total of the 35 per cent salary expenditures reached the health facilities, approximately half of the overall amount allocated to clinics and hospitals did not actually reach them. Similar problems were found in Tanzania and Rwanda.

Tracking overall expenditures is often difficult, however. Health facilities typically do not receive a single monthly budget allocation that they proceed to spend and account for. Rather, they receive resources through multiple channels and sources.[4] The upshot of these institutional arrangements is a myriad of complex resource flows, each governed by separate administrative and recording procedures. In each case, there are risks of leakage. Expenditures on drugs and other supplies can leak through the procurement process, or through supplies being stolen, lost or disposed of (such as expired drugs or vaccines) as part of the distribution process. Administrative and logistical procedures tend to be different for other non-salary expenditures, but similar issues arise. Salary budgets can be siphoned off at different levels of government either by simply withholding salary payments, by creating fictitious health workers ('ghosts') and collecting the salaries on their behalf, or by paid staff simply not showing up for work.

Given this complexity, tracking surveys have often been forced to be selective about what resources to track. For example, the survey in Honduras collected individual-level data on 14,454 health professionals, and found that 9.3 per cent did not actually work in the location where they were officially assigned. About a quarter of these individuals

Table 2.1: Overview of findings from Public Expenditure Tracking Surveys in the health sector

Country	Year	Sample	Leakage	Other findings
Ghana[a]	2000	200 facilities; 40 districts	Leakage of non-salary recurrent expenditures is estimated at 80%.	Found greater leakage between centre and district than between district and facility. Service users bear much higher cost than intended primarily due to the non-salary expenditure leakage.
Honduras[b]	2000	805 staff; 35 facilities	2.4% of all workers on the payroll at health facilities considered 'ghosts'.	Absenteeism estimated at 27%. In addition, study found that 5.2% of workers were not actually in the assigned post but had moved to other locations.
Mozambique[c]	2002	90 facilities; 167 staff; 679 users	Some evidence of leakage of drugs in transfer from provinces to districts, within the primary health care system, but no firm estimate.	Documented delays and bottlenecks in budget execution and supply management; inequalities in allocation of resources across districts and facilities; incomplete registering of user-fee revenues by facilities (reported revenue as per cent of expected revenue was 67.6% for consultations and 79.6% for medicines); absenteeism estimated at 19%.
Nigeria[d]	2002	252 facilities; 30 loc. gov.; 700 staff	No firm estimate of leakage (focus was on governance issues in health sector, in particular on flow of resources, provider behaviour and incentives, and the role of local governments and community participation).	42% of staff experience salary delays despite sufficient budget; detailed description of governance and service delivery arrangements, including facility characteristics; evidence of delays in salary payments.
Papua New Guinea[e]	2002	117 facilities	No firm estimate of leakage (main focus on the education sector, but some data on health facilities were collected).	Evidence of poor access to care and limited availability of drugs; absenteeism estimated at 19%.

Country	Year	Sample	Leakage	Other findings
Peru[f]	2001	120 munici-palities	Leakage in 'Glass of Milk' food supplementation programme estimated at 71% (includes 'leakage' of benefits at household level).	Quantified leakage at different levels of government (greater at the higher levels); evidence that poorer municipalities affected the most; diversion of funds to cover operational costs.
Rwanda[g]	2000	351 facilities; 40 districts	Some evidence of leakage between regions and districts, but no firm estimate.	Evidence of delays in budget execution and low execution rates (80% of non-wage funds released at year end); user-fee revenues and drug sales shown to be principal sources of funding.
Senegal[h]	2002	100 facilities; 10 districts; 37 loc. gov.	Some evidence of leakage at regional and communal level in allocation of non-salary resources from the central level to service providers through the decentralisation fund but no firm estimate.	Delays in the decentralisation fund transfers; evidence on extent of discretion by local governments in allocation of resources.
Tanzania[i]	1999	36 facilities; 3 districts	Leakage of non-salary funds estimated at 41% (budget and accounting mechanisms were studied for health and education at district and facility level).	Donor contributions shown to favour better-off districts; leakage attributed to poor record-keeping and lack of audits.
Tanzania[i]	2001	20 facilities; 5 districts	No firm estimate of leakage in primary education and health facilities studied.	Substantial delays at all levels, especially non-wage expenditures; lack of supplies in facilities; some evidence of underreporting of facility revenues.
Uganda[k]	1996	100 facilities; 19 districts	No firm evidence of leakage in flow of resources to primary health care providers but heavy reliance on in-kind flows and poor record-keeping hampered data collection. Qualitative evidence suggests that leakage is limited.	Qualitative evidence suggested that main leakage takes place at facility level, rather than in transfer of resources to facilities.

Uganda[l]	2000 155 facilities	Leakage of specific drugs and supplies estimated at 70% in government, private non-profit facilities studies.	Detailed descriptive data on facility characteristics and performance; overview of accountability arrangements; comparison of government and non-government providers.

Notes

a   Xiao Ye and Sudharshan Canagarajah, 'Efficiency of Public Expenditure Distribution and Beyond: A Report on Ghana's 2000 PETS in the Sectors of Primary Health and Education', World Bank Africa Region Working Paper Series No. 31, 2002.
b   World Bank, 'Honduras: Public Expenditure Management for Poverty Reduction and Fiscal Sustainability', Report No. 22070, World Bank Poverty Reduction and Economic Sector Management Unit, Latin America and the Caribbean Region, 2001.
c   Magnus Lindelow, Patrick Ward et al., 'Primary Health Care in Mozambique: Service Delivery in a Complex Hierarchy', World Bank Africa Region Human Development Working Paper Series No. 69, 2003.
d   Monica Das Gupta, Varun Gauri et al., 'Decentralized Delivery of Primary Health Services in Nigeria: Survey Evidence from the States of Lagos and Kogi', World Bank Africa Region Human Development Working Paper 70, 2004.
e   World Bank, 'Papua New Guinea: Public Expenditure and Service Delivery', unpublished manuscript, 2004.
f   World Bank and Inter-American Development Bank, 'Peru: Restoring Fiscal Discipline for Poverty Reduction: Public Expenditure Review', Report No. 24286-PE, 2002.
g   Hippolyte Fofack, Robert Ngong et al., 'Public Expenditure Performance in Rwanda: Evidence from a Public Expenditure Tracking Study in the Health and Education Sectors', Africa Region Working Paper Series No. 45, 2003.
h   World Bank, 'Expenditure Tracking Survey in Senegal: The Health Sector', unpublished manuscript, 2003.
i   PricewaterhouseCoopers, 'Tanzania Public Expenditure Review: Health and Educational Financial Tracking Study', Final Report, vols I–II (Dar es Salaam, 1999).
j   Research on Poverty Alleviation and Economic and Social Research Foundation, 'Pro-poor Expenditure Tracking', unpublished manuscript, 2001.
k   Emmanuel Ablo and Ritva Reinikka, 'Do Budgets Really Matter? Evidence from Public Spending on Education and Health in Uganda', Policy Research Working Paper 1926, World Bank, 1998.
l   Magnus Lindelow, Ritva Reinikka et al., 'Health Care on the Frontline: Survey Evidence on Public and Private Providers in Uganda', World Bank Africa Region Human Development Working Paper 38, 2003.

were 'ghost' employees, while the remainder were retired or had been transferred without records being updated. The survey also found evidence of dual job-holdings, absenteeism and other human resource management problems.

While most health PETS have managed to generate leakage estimates for overall or specific resource flows to health care providers, the reliability of findings has often been undermined by the quality of administrative records (budgets, expenditure accounts, receipts, drug records, payrolls, and so on). These records are often poorly kept, reflecting a lack of capacity, weak procedures and possibly efforts by staff to 'play' the system. As a result, survey enumerators have to contend with records that are both incomplete and riddled with errors. In Mozambique, provincial health departments could provide complete district-level data for only 40 per cent of their districts. Similarly, complete records were found in less than half of the district health offices surveyed in Ghana, and although the data collected in Rwanda were consistent with high levels of leakage – there were substantial discrepancies between funds recorded as dispersed by higher levels of government and the funds recorded as received by lower levels – these discrepancies may in part be due to poor book-keeping, and no firm leakage estimate could be developed.

Beyond leakage: insights into public expenditure management

Where, due to the paucity of administrative records or the absence of clear allocation rules, it has not been possible to reach firm conclusions concerning leakage, valuable insights may still be gleaned from PETS. An important contribution has been to provide hard evidence on the extent and source of delays and bottlenecks in budget execution and supply management systems. For example, the Nigeria study found that although funds had been released to local government, 42 per cent of the facility workers had not received their salaries for more than six months in the year prior to the survey. Similarly, in the Mozambique survey, 30 per cent of staff said that salaries are always or almost always late, and 15 per cent of staff reported that salaries are sometimes not paid in full. Whatever the source of the problem, delays in payments are likely to have adverse consequences for staff morale, and may contribute to problems of absenteeism, informal charging and other problems.

Problems of the same nature have been documented in the case of non-salary budgets, and in the distribution of drugs and other essential supplies. The Senegal PETS found that it takes an average of 10 months for the resources from the Decentralisation Fund – the main source of government financing for health facilities – to actually reach the providers. In Mozambique, nearly 30 per cent of district health offices received their first budget transfer of the year more than three and a half months late. Delays in budget transfers often conspire with other factors to result in low levels of budget execution. For example, in Mozambique, districts executed an average of only 80 per cent of their budgets, and in some districts execution rates were as low as 35 per cent.

More generally, tracking surveys have contributed to a better understanding of the public expenditure management process, allocation rules, financial management and accounting practices, and accountability arrangements; in particular, at lower levels of government where routine monitoring and reporting systems tend to be weak. For example, the Ghana, Mozambique and Rwanda PETS found evidence that existing user fee rules and regulations are not followed: patients are charged more than they should be, exemptions are not granted, revenues are not used as intended, and so on. In part, these problems probably reflect the problems in the budget and supply systems, that is, user fees become a lifeline for facilities that do not receive adequate funds and resources from government – but opportunistic overcharging by health workers may also be a factor.

The consequences of leakage and other public expenditure management problems

Do problems of leakage, delays and reallocation of resources matter? Many surveys have focused on primary health care services, which often account for a relatively small share of health spending. However, even though dollar values may be small, leakage of resources or delays in budget transfers or drug supplies may seriously undermine the capacity of facilities to deliver services. The costs in terms of poor health, suffering and loss of life may be considerable.

In Ghana, most clinics received fewer resources than intended – some received no cash at all – and had to rely on internally generated funds for their operations. As a result, users were forced to bear higher costs than intended, in part through high charges for drugs. The Nigeria survey found that most facilities were missing essential equipment, medications, vaccines and supplies: 95 per cent did not have microscopes, 59 per cent did not have sterile gloves, 98 per cent did not have a malaria smear, and 95 per cent did not have urine test strips. In Mozambique, over 60 per cent of facilities had been out of stock of one or more essential medicines during the six months preceding the survey, with an average stock-out time of six weeks. The Uganda survey (2000) also found evidence of stock-outs of vaccines and drugs, combined with overuse of antibiotics and other drugs. These problems may have multiple causes, but are clearly a cause for concern.

Tracking surveys thus can help diagnose leakages, delays and other budget execution problems that can seriously undermine service delivery and contribute to an improved understanding of how resources are allocated and used at lower levels of government – issues that often fall outside the purview of routine reporting systems. But PETS also have important limitations. For one thing, most tracking surveys have mainly been implemented in integrated health systems, where public resources are channelled to public providers, and have proven most effective in contexts with clearly identifiable service providers and explicit resource allocation rules. Tracking surveys may be less useful in other contexts, such as where third-party payers (insurers) play an important role, or where private provision and contracting is more widespread. Even within public integrated systems, different tools are needed to diagnose some forms of corruption. This raises questions about how PETS relate to other integrity and accountability tools.[5] It is clear that effective efforts to diagnose and combat corruption will depend on a wide range of internal mechanisms (such as clear rules and procedures, effective accounting and record keeping, internal and external audits) and external ones (transparency, mechanisms for client voice, and so on). PETS may have an important role to play, but this role needs to be determined with an eye on their cost, and with a view to complement rather than replace other parts of the public financial management system.

Ultimately, however, successfully channelling resources to providers is only half the battle. Once there, resources must be used efficiently and as intended in order to have an impact. Tracking surveys have increasingly sought to provide evidence on facility performance, but detailed studies – including facility surveys, case studies and qualitative work – of absenteeism, informal charging and pilfering of drugs and other supplies also have an important role to play.

For example, a recent multi-country study based on multiple, unannounced facility visits reports absenteeism rates ranging from 23 per cent to 40 per cent in the health sector, and finds absenteeism to be related to both the location and the characteristic of the health facility.[6] Evidence from provider and household surveys have shown that informal or unofficial charges add an unintended financial burden on patients in many countries.[7] Finally, there have been attempts to collect facility-level data on theft of drugs and other supplies by health workers through small-scale surveys or case studies.[8] Such studies have revealed serious service delivery problems in many countries, and highlighted the importance not only of getting resources to facilities, but also of ensuring that health workers are provided with incentives and opportunities to perform. But the studies have also helped counter the image of health workers and government administrators as inherently corrupt agents – an unfortunate by-product of single-minded efforts to diagnose corruption in service delivery. Detailed case studies and qualitative work has shown that the majority of health workers are dedicated professionals trying to cope in difficult and frustrating environments with low pay, poor management and support systems, and weak accountability mechanisms.[9] This is an important perspective to keep in mind in any efforts to strengthen the tools for diagnosing corruption in the health sector.

Notes

1. Magnus Lindelow is an economist at the World Bank in East Asia Pacific Human Development, Inna Kushnarova is a consultant with the World Bank, and Kai Kaiser is an economist with the World Bank's Public Sector Group in Poverty Reduction and Economic Management.
2. Deon Filmer and Lant Pritchett, 'Child Mortality and Public Spending on Health: How Much Does Money Matter?', Policy Research Working Papers, World Bank, 1997; Vinaya Swaroop and Andrew Sunil Rajkumar Swaroop, 'Public Spending and Outcomes: Does Governance Matter?', World Bank, Policy Research Working Paper Series, 2002. For a general discussion of the 'weak links' in the chain between public expenditure and outcomes in health and other public services, see World Development Report 2004: Making Service Work for Poor People (Oxford: Oxford University Press and World Bank, 2003).
3. See, for example, Anne Cockcroft, Lorenzo Monasta et al., 'Bangladesh Baseline Service Delivery Survey: Final Report', CIET International, 1999, and 'Filipino Report Card on Pro-Poor Services', World Bank Environment and Social Development Sector Unit East Asia and Pacific Region, May 2001. Evidence of corruption from perception-based service delivery surveys has been linked to child and infant mortality by Sanjeev Gupta, Hamid R. Davoodi and Erwin R. Tiongson, 'Corruption and the Provision of Health Care and Education Services' in George T. Abed and Sanjeev Gupta, Governance, Corruption, and Economic Performance (Washington, DC: IMF, 2002).
4. For example, facilities in Ghana, Rwanda and Mozambique receive practically no cash through the budget process. Salaries are paid directly to staff and other resources are procured at higher level and distributed in kind.
5. Increasingly, both bilateral and multilateral development agencies are channelling aid as general budget or sector support. Shifts in aid modalities, combined with debt reduction initiatives, have led to a growing concern with the transparency and integrity of public financial management in developing countries. In this context, PETS have emerged as an important diagnostic tool. Recently, PETS have also been proposed as a tool for promoting

accountability in public spending. For a discussion of PETS as a tool for tracking poverty-reducing public spending under the Enhanced HIPC Initiative, see *Tracking of Poverty-Reducing Public Spending in Heavily Indebted Poor Countries* (Washington, DC: IMF, 2001). A general discussion is provided in the World Bank's *Public Financial Management: Performance Measurement Framework* (Washington, DC: World Bank, 2005). The jury is still out on whether PETS are a useful and cost-effective tool for preventing corruption.

6. Nazmul Chaudhury, Jeffrey Hammer et al., 'Provider Absence in Schools and Health Centers', *Journal of Economic Perspectives*, (forthcoming).

7. James Killingsworth, Najmul Hossain et al., 'Unofficial Fees in Bangladesh: Price, Equity and Institutional Issues', *Health Policy Plan* 14(2): 152–63, 1999; Maureen Lewis, *Who is Paying for Health Care in Eastern Europe and Central Asia?* (Washington, DC: World Bank, 2000); Tim Ensor and Sophie Witter, 'Health Economics in Low Income Countries: Adapting to the Reality of the Unofficial Economy', *Health Policy* 57(1): 1–13, 2001; Paolo Belli, George Gotsadze, and Helen Shahriari, 'Out-of-Pocket and Informal Payments in Health Sector: Evidence from Georgia', *Health Policy* 70(1): 109–23, 2004; Tim Ensor, 'Informal Payments for Health Care in Transition Economies', *Social Science and Medicine* 58(2): 237–46, 2004.

8. Barbara McPake, Delius Asiimwe et al., 'Informal Economic Activities of Public Health Workers in Uganda: Implications for Quality and Accessibility of Care', *Social Science and Medicine* 49(4): 849–65, 1999; Rafael Di Tella and William D. Savedoff, *Diagnosis Corruption: Fraud in Latin America's Public Hospitals* (Washington, DC: Inter-American Development Bank, 2001).

9. Paulo Ferrinho, Wim Van Lerberghe and Aurélio da Cruz Gomes Ferrinho, 'Public and Private Practice: A Balancing Act for Health Staff', *Bulletin of the World Health Organization* 77(3): 209, 1999; Wim Van Lerberghe, Claudia Conceição, Wim Van Damme and Paulo Ferrinho, 'When Staff is Underpaid: Dealing with the Individual Coping Strategies of Health Personnel', *Bulletin of the World Health Organization* 80(7): 581–4, 2002.

Local-level corruption hits health service delivery in the Philippines

Omar Azfar and Tugrul Gurgur[1]

In the past two decades there has been a widespread devolution of authority to local governments around the world. As local governments increase their share of authority and responsibility vis-à-vis central government, their effectiveness in terms of quality, quantity and the accessibility of public services has become critical. Consequently, the effect of local-level corruption on service delivery has critical relevance for development economists and policy-makers.

The Philippines is an ideal place to study the impact of corruption on service delivery. Five years after the democratic revolution in the Philippines, the Local Governments Act of 1991 devolved both political authority and administrative control of many health and education services to the provincial and municipal level. According to some public survey results and anecdotal evidence, much of the corruption in the Philippines does appear to be at the local level. The large number of municipalities, the significant devolution of authority, and the high and varying levels of corruption make the Philippines an ideal place to study the impact of corruption on service delivery.

Data collected in 2000 from 80 municipalities in the Philippines was used to assess the impact of corruption in local governments on health and education outcomes. The results showed clearly that corruption undermines the delivery of health services. We found a significant partial correlation between 13 dependent variables that measure various aspects of health and education services and corruption perceptions, after controlling for capacity (based on measures of human and physical capital), adult education levels, urban residence, living standards (as proxied by assets), inequality, existence of private sector competition, voting and media exposure, accountability measures and local autonomy.

Corruption levels were measured using corruption perceptions of households and public officials (administrators, health and education services, school principals and health workers). The respondents were asked questions about specific acts of corruption (such as bribery, the sale of jobs and theft of supplies) as well as their general perceptions about the corruption level at each municipal government, public school and public health clinic. Most kinds of corruption were found to be more prevalent in the municipal administrator's office than in other offices, perhaps due to the administrator's office exerting more authority and thus having more opportunity to extract rents. A total of 19 per cent of municipal administrators said there were cases of bribery in their offices in the year preceding the survey (1999), while 32 per cent said there were instances of theft of funds. By contrast, the figures for municipal health officers were 2.5 per cent and 16.5 per cent, respectively.

To measure the quality, quantity, and accessibility of health services, we used seven variables: six of them from a household survey (immunisation of children, delay in vaccination of children, patient waiting times, accessibility of health clinics for treatment, choosing public health clinics for immunisation, and satisfaction with public health clinics) and one from the Ministry of Health (municipal average of immunisation rate of children).

The results showed clearly that corruption undermines the delivery of health services in the Philippines. In each case regression results indicated a significant and negative effect of corruption on the quality of health services. For example, a standard deviation (about 10 per cent) increase in corruption reduces the immunisation rate by around 10–20 per cent, increases waiting time in public health clinics as much as 30 per cent, decreases user satisfaction by 30 per cent, and reduces the odds of completing vaccination by four times and choosing public health facilities by a factor of three.

The results also suggest that corruption does not affect the rural areas the same way it affects the urban areas. In the urban areas demand for public health care is more 'corruption-elastic' (that is, households' use of public health facilities declines more rapidly in response to higher corruption incidence). Households in rural areas, on the other hand, suffer with more waiting at public health clinics, late immunisation of infants, and less satisfaction with public health services as compared to households in urban areas facing the same level of corruption. The presence of alternative health facilities in urban areas, either in the form of private health care providers or other public health facilities, may be the reason for such differences.

We also ran regressions to understand the effect of corruption in rich, middle-income and poor municipalities. Even after controlling for other factors we found that when corruption is endemic, poor and middle-income municipalities report more waiting at public clinics and a higher frequency of being denied vaccines than rich municipalities.

Corruption in public clinics is also more likely to deter households living in poor municipalities and forces them to opt for self-medication.

Robustness checks that control for outliers, sample selection problems and reverse causality concerns (for instance, that some common variable is affecting both corruption and service delivery, or that poor service delivery is causing corruption) confirmed our findings.

Taken together our results suggest that corruption undermines the delivery of services in the Philippines. This complements cross-country findings on the subject, and adds to the expanding list of ways corruption undermines welfare.

Note

1. Omar Azfar (omar@iris.econ.umd.edu) is a research associate at the IRIS Center of the University of Maryland College Park, and Tugrul Gurgur (tgurgur@umd.edu) is a graduate student at the Economics department of the University of Maryland College Park. The article summarises research conducted by the IRIS Center of the University of Maryland on behalf of the World Bank and the Netherlands Trust Fund. The full report was published as: Omar Azfar and Tugrul Gurgur, 'Does Corruption Affect Health and Education Outcomes in the Philippines?', Working Paper (College Park: IRIS Center, University of Maryland College Park, 2004), available at www.iris.umd.edu. The authors thank Satu Kahkonen, Anthony Lanyi, Patrick Meagher and Diana Rutherford for their contributions to this report.

Corruption is bad for your health: findings from Central and Eastern Europe
Richard Rose[1]

Modern medicine offers many treatments that can alleviate pain or restore people to good health. Moreover, in prosperous OECD countries there is the assurance that, if you do get ill, you will be treated by a state-funded health service or through a private health insurance programme. But health care costs money, and in many developing countries the most the state can finance are the rudiments of public health facilities, such as clean water and sewers. In the developing world, individuals needing health care must sometimes turn to traditional remedies or borrow money to pay for private health care. Where corruption is rife, people have the worst of both worlds: paying twice for treatment, once through taxes and once in a brown envelope.

Communist governments in Central and Eastern Europe once promised health care to everyone in need. However, the result was favouritism and corruption in the allocation of medical and hospital treatment. Those who were in the party *nomenklatura* had access to good treatment; those who could pull strings through informal networks (*blat*) also benefited; and people who could offer payments on the side were more likely to get good treatment than those who could not. The corruption that was an integral part of the 'shadow' economies of communist countries has left a legacy of corruption throughout the region, particularly in the health sector.

As part of this legacy, the imposition of a 'corruption tax' for treatment that ought to be free is likely to have negative consequences for the health of citizens. At worst, it may lead to the denial of treatment or even people not seeking treatment because they do not have the money to make payments under the table. Corruption in health inevitably punishes the elderly, who are most likely to need health care, and the poor.

The seventh New Europe Barometer (NEB) of the Centre for the Study of Public Policy has tested the extent to which corruption is bad for a society's health.[2] Between 1 October 2004 and 23 January 2005, it organised nationwide random sample surveys of the adult populations in eight new EU member states (the Czech Republic, Estonia, Hungary, Latvia, Lithuania, Poland, Slovakia and Slovenia); two applicant countries (Bulgaria and Romania); plus Belarus and Russia. National research institutes interviewed 13,499 people face to face, asking questions about their perception of corruption, health care and such influences on health as age, education and social class.

When people assess their physical health, the largest group of 39 per cent, not surprisingly, says it is average; 34 per cent say their health is good; and 10 per cent describe it as excellent. By contrast, only 14 per cent say their health is bad and 3 per cent report it is very bad.[3] In Romania, Slovenia and Slovakia, more than half say their health is good or excellent. Even in Belarus, where one-quarter says their health is bad, the largest group has average health.

However, almost three-quarters of those surveyed have a negative view of their country's health services (Table 2.2). Altogether, 24 per cent describe the system as very bad, and almost half characterise it as not so good, as against 27 per cent who consider it fairly good, or very good. The evaluation of health care varies greatly within the region. In the Czech Republic, an absolute majority gives the health system a positive endorsement and the same is true in Belarus. By contrast, in Russia and Bulgaria fewer than one in twelve is positive. Bulgarians and Russians differ only as to whether their health service is not so good or very bad.

At the same time, there is a widespread perception that the body politic is infected with corruption. When asked how many officials are corrupt, 29 per cent say that practically all officials are corrupt and an additional 44 per cent see a majority of officials as corrupt (Table 2.3). Again, there are big differences between countries. In Romania, a majority perceive practically all officials as corrupt, and in Russia 43 per cent do. By contrast, nearly half of all Estonians and Slovenes polled think corruption affects less than half of public officials.

Where corruption appears widespread, people also see major deficiencies in health care (Figure 2.1). Five out of six people who see nearly all officials as corrupt think their health system is either very bad or not so good; and almost four-fifths who think a majority of officials are corrupt see the health service in negative terms. Among those who think that less than half the public officials are corrupt, three in five still have a negative view of the health service. Even among the small percentage of citizens in the region who see very few officials as corrupt, just under half have a positive view of their health system.

Table 2.2: Health service seen as not very good

Q. How would you evaluate the current system for health care in this country?

	Very good	Fairly good	Not so good	Very bad
Czech Republic	3	51	39	7
Slovenia	4	42	42	11
Belarus	2	49	38	11
Romania	2	14	66	18
Hungary	1	38	46	15
All NEB countries	1	26	49	24
Estonia	1	24	49	26
Lithuania	1	22	56	21
Slovakia	1	21	52	26
Latvia	1	20	47	32
Poland	1	16	48	35
Bulgaria	1	7	55	38
Russia	1	7	53	40

Source: Centre for the Study of Public Policy, *New Europe Barometer VII*. Total number of respondents: 13,499. Fieldwork conducted between 1 October 2004 and 23 January 2005.

Table 2.3: Corruption perceived as widespread

Q. How widespread do you think that bribe-taking and corruption are in this country?
Very few public officials are corrupt; less than half are corrupt; most public officials are engaged in corruption; almost all public officials are engaged in corruption.

	Almost all	Majority	Less than half	Very few
		(% replying)		
Romania	51	34	14	1
Bulgaria	43	45	10	2
Russia	43	46	8	3
All NEB countries	29	44	22	5
Lithuania	32	50	15	3
Slovakia	30	50	18	2
Hungary	27	36	35	1
Belarus	26	44	21	8
Latvia	24	49	22	6
Poland	22	52	24	2
Czech Republic	21	49	26	5
Slovenia	17	36	33	14
Estonia	12	39	36	13

Source: Centre for the Study of Public Policy, *New Europe Barometer VII*. Total number of respondents: 13,499. Fieldwork conducted between 1 October 2004 and 23 January 2005.

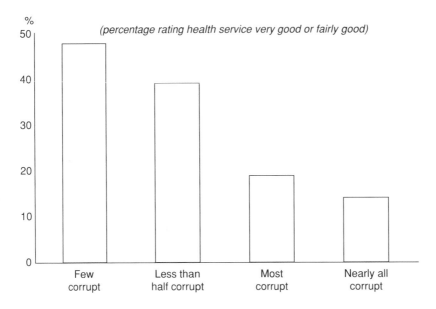

% 50

(percentage rating health service very good or fairly good)

| | Few corrupt | Less than half corrupt | Most corrupt | Nearly all corrupt |

Figure 2.1: As corruption rises, health service gets worse

Source: Answers to questions in Tables 2.2 and 2.3 gamma correlation: –0.36. Centre for the Study of Public Policy, *New Europe Barometer VII*. Total number of respondents: 13,499. Fieldwork conducted between 1 October 2004 and 23 January 2005.

People with below-average health are most likely to be dissatisfied with their country's health system; 78 per cent describe it as not so good or very bad. But being in bad health is not the chief reason why a health service is viewed negatively. More than three-quarters of those who rate their health as average also think that health care is not very good or very bad; and even among those in good or excellent health, two-thirds view the health care available in negative terms.

An individual's health not only reflects the state of the country but also the characteristics specific to that person, such as age and education. The extent to which bad government has a negative effect on individual health, in addition to individual characteristics, can be determined by multiple regression analysis. It identifies conditions that have a statistically significant influence on health, net of the effects of other influences.

Both individual characteristics (age, social status and education) and perceptions of public services significantly – and independently – influence the health of individuals in Central and Eastern Europe and the former Soviet Union. Together, they can account for 26.8 per cent of the variance in self-assessed health. As expected, age is by far the single most important influence: being 60 or over has an even more negative effect on health than the positive effect of being under 30.

Three other socio-economic characteristics give a significant boost to individual health. The higher a person's social status and education, the better his or her health, however old they are. The more durable consumer goods there are in the house – a proxy for income in countries where subsidies and shadow earnings complicate the evaluation of conventional wages – the better a person's health. The statistic that shows men are more likely to be healthy than women is a by-product of the higher rate of male mortality at younger ages, which results in men who do survive into old age on average being healthier.

The perception of corruption has both a direct and an indirect influence on health. After controlling for social characteristics, people who perceive government as more corrupt are more likely to be in worse health. Corruption also has an indirect effect because it correlates with a negative assessment of the health service, and a bad health service is bad for individual health. For individual health, at least, the individual perception of corruption is more significant than the overall national rating.[4]

Notwithstanding the widespread perception of inadequate and even corrupt public services, the welfare values of Central and East Europeans continue to support paying taxes for better services. However, the more corrupt a system actually is, the less benefit that individuals will gain from paying higher taxes. In order to improve health in the region, national governments not only have to spend more money on health care, but also have to spend that money honestly.

Notes

1. Richard Rose is professor at the Centre for the Study of Public Policy, University of Aberdeen, Scotland.
2. The New Europe Barometer survey is financed by a grant from the British Economic & Social Research Council for the analysis of diverging paths of post-communist countries. The health data was collected with the support of a MacArthur Foundation grant to Professor Sir Michael Marmot, Department of Epidemiology and Public Health, University College, London.
3. All percentages are based on pooling the 12 NEB national surveys and weighting each equally, so that each contributes one-twelfth of the total answers reported.
4. The TI Corruption Perceptions Index (CPI) does not register statistical significance due to the fact that the CPI rates the country as a whole; thus the regression analysis assigns the same CPI score to each individual respondent in a country. However, there is never 100 per cent agreement within a country as to the degree to which officials are corrupt. The NEB collects data from individuals and thus can take into account differences in individual perception within a country.

'Citizens' audit' in Mexico reveals paper trail of corruption
Helena Hofbauer[1]

At the end of 2002, as it was discussing the 2003 budget, Mexico's Congress announced it would provide 600 million pesos (US$ 56.5 million) of additional funding for programmes that promoted women's health. The president of the Budget Committee sent instructions to that effect to the Ministry of Health. Included was a statement that 30 million pesos (US$ 2.8 million) were to be reallocated to a private organisation, Provida, as part of the women's health initiative. Originally, the amount had been allocated to HIV/AIDS public health campaigns.

Six Mexican civil society organisations (CSOs) – Consorcio para el Diálogo Parlamentario y la Equidad; Equidad de Género, Ciudadanía, Trabajo y Familia; Fundar, Centro de Análisis e Investigación; Grupo de Información en Reproducción Elegida; Letra S, Sida, Cultura y Vida Cotidiana; and Salud Integral para la Mujer – launched an investigation into why the budget had been altered. The six embarked on a time-consuming piece of detective work lasting 18 months during which they documented evident irregularities. Much of the CSOs' efforts were possible because Mexico implemented a new Transparency and Access to Public Information Law in June 2002.

The organisations uncovered a funding request that Provida presented to the Ministry of Health on 3 December 2002 for 30 million pesos, as well as confirmation from both the ministries of finance and of health that 30 million pesos were given to Provida's national committee. They also uncovered the signed agreement between the grants administrator and Provida, a financial and social impact report presented by Provida on the expenditure of the resources and a 6,525-page financial file containing invoices detailing how the 30 million pesos were spent.

With this knowledge, the CSOs began their own audit trail of how Provida spent 30 million pesos of taxpayers' money in 2003. They found evidence of misuse and corruption. More than 80 per cent of the funds were used to hire the services of a public relations firm for work such as a campaign against provision of emergency contraception for women. Money was also spent on an agency importing overpriced medical equipment, as well as to pay for the rent of a ballroom. The two companies and the owner of the ballroom shared Provida's address, telephone numbers and its administrative director. The CSOs also found that Provida had purchased luxury pens, clothing and groceries with some of the funds. Documents showed serious fiscal inconsistencies. Receipts dated October 2003 related to products acquired in July 2003.

In addition the CSOs made a number of observations about procedural violations that had taken place. First, the president of the Budget Committee is not allowed to speak for the plenary, or to issue instructions to a minister; second, Congress cannot allocate money to private organisations, particularly if it is taken away from public programmes; third, the Ministry of Health can only disburse resources to NGOs through an open, public process, after soliciting proposals; and fourth, Provida's radical stance contradicts significant parts of Mexico's public health policy in that it actively opposes the prevention of HIV/AIDS via the use of condoms, and systematically rejects the right to abortion that was granted to raped women.

Armed with this damning evidence, the CSOs unveiled their 'citizens' audit' at a press conference in June 2004 at which they launched a campaign demanding transparency and accountability, supported by 700 NGOs across Mexico. The campaign demanded that the Ministry of Health publicly explain its reasons for financing a private organisation that advocated health policies contradicting those of the government; that the government carry out an official audit of the 30 million pesos and clarify the responsibilities of the government officials involved and Provida's legal representative; that the 30 million pesos be returned to the state budget; and that legislation be drafted and implemented to prevent similar transgressions with government money.

The campaign became the focus of national attention, occupying the headlines of Mexico's news media for a month. As a result of the mounting public pressure, Congress unanimously voted in July 2004 to call on the Minister of Health to explain the use of the 30 million pesos and speed up an ongoing official audit. Shortly after, the ministry demanded the return of the 30 million pesos and cancelled its contract with Provida, suspending the distribution of additional funds to the organisation for 2004.

In September 2004, the Internal Comptroller, who is responsible for initiating audits within the executive branch of government, issued the results of the official audit, which corroborated the irregularities the CSOs had identified. At the end of March 2005, the earliest permissible date, the Auditor General (of the legislative branch) also issued its results on the case. But the Auditor General's report went further, noting that 90 per cent of the money Provida received from the government had been inappropriately used. As a result, the Senate asked for a judicial process to be started against Provida and its legal representatives.[2]

In April 2005 the Internal Comptroller removed the three officials at the head of the health ministry unit who had handed out the resources without a public process; and banned Provida's legal representative, Jorge Serrano Limón, from occupying public office and fined him 13 million pesos. The 30 million pesos have not been returned, the fine has not been paid and the judicial process is still under way.

Nonetheless, the CSOs have effectively promoted the cause for greater transparency in important ways.

They demonstrated the important role CSOs can play in making government more accountable by using a country's legal framework. In particular, they showed the value of the Transparency and Access to Information Law to enable processes that would not have been possible three years ago.

This was the first time CSOs followed a misallocation of resources and its corrupt expenditure throughout the entire budget process. It was possible to identify what had happened, to audit the exercise of resources and to reach into the oversight stage of the process in order to seek redress. The misuse of resources and the corruption highlighted by CSOs was confirmed by official institutions, and action followed.

A legal precedent was established, since the Law of Responsibilities of Public Officials (in operation since 1982, with several reforms) was applied for the first time to an individual (Serrano Limón), who had made unlawful use of public resources.

Inconsistencies between public health policies and Provida's activities were highlighted, and the care centres that should have been built and run with the 30 million pesos have since been carefully supervised in order to ensure lawful practices.

The administrative unit in the Ministry of Health responsible for distributing resources among CSOs reviewed its policies and for the first time published its procedures in the public domain.

Notes

1. Helena Hofbauer is Executive Director of Fundar, Mexico City.
2. www.senado.gob.mx/sgsp/gaceta/?sesion=2005/04/26/1&documento=60

Fighting fraud and corruption in Britain's National Health Service
Jim Gee[1]

Fraud and corruption represent a pincer movement on organisations affected by them. They deny them the resources they need while undermining the confidence of the public. For too long, the defence against such attacks has been poorly organised and unprofessional. In recent years in the United Kingdom, and especially in its National Health Service (NHS) – the third largest organisation in the world, with 1.2 million staff and an annual budget of £70 billion (US $125 billion) – this picture has changed considerably.

The Counter Fraud Service (CFS) was created in 1998 with overall responsibility to protect the NHS and its resources from fraud and corruption. Our starting point is to accurately measure and track losses to fraud and corruption in each area of the NHS budget to an accuracy of within 1 per cent and to have that independently audited. This helps to identify the nature and extent of the problem, which is essential to finding the appropriate solution. Thus we know that losses to patient fraud have been reduced from £171 million (US $305 million) in 1999 to £78 million (US $139 million) in 2004 (a reduction of 54 per cent), and losses to fraud by medical professionals have fallen by about 43–54 per cent over the same period. We are currently measuring losses to payroll fraud involving 'ghost employees', or where people obtain employment by using bogus qualifications and false employment histories. These figures should be available in late 2005.

The CFS has the responsibility not only for 'operational' work to counter corruption (detection, investigation and the seeking of sanctions and redress). It also works to develop a real anti-fraud and corruption culture, to create a strong deterrent effect, and to revise policy and systems to prevent the problem recurring. By integrating these two aspects, we have ensured that we generate not only activity, but also tangible outcomes in terms of reduced losses to fraud and corruption. As a legal requirement, the CFS is staffed by professionally trained and accredited counter-fraud specialists, members of a new profession numbering around 8,500 across the public and private sectors since its formation by the government in 2001.

The CFS has encountered and dealt with many different aspects of corruption. Examples in recent years include:

- We are suing a number of generic drug companies for £152 million (US $271 million) because we believe they formed a cartel to raise prices for the drugs warfarin, penicillin and ranitidine.
- A chief executive of an NHS Trust who falsified his qualifications to obtain the post resigned to avoid dismissal; a criminal prosecution is under way.
- Medical professionals who claimed and pocketed payments for treatments they did not provide are usually prosecuted criminally, with civil legal action to recover losses. Finally, they are suspended or removed from professional bodies.

These and other examples where we have detected and stopped corruption total more than £170 million (US $303 million) since 1999, but this is only part of total financial benefits to the NHS of £675 million (US $1.2 billion), which also includes recovery of monies lost to fraud and reductions in measured losses due to CFS intervention. This amounts to a 13:1 return on its budgetary investment, and the equivalent of what it would cost to build 10 new hospitals.

To achieve this, the CFS has worked to mobilise the honest majority, undertaking more than 1,400 presentations and awareness sessions reaching hundreds of thousands of staff and millions of patients. It also seeks to deter the dishonest minority by publicising the actions taken, with around 400 media articles each year. Detection rates have risen by several hundred per cent, with a 96 per cent success rate in prosecution, alongside extensive use of civil law to freeze and recover assets.

There have been four keys to this success. These are:

- accurate identification of the nature and scale of the problem
- comprehensive action to tackle the problem (not limited to traditional policing)
- professional agency staff with the right skills to reduce losses to corruption permanently
- successful mobilisation of the honest majority and the deterrent effect this has had on the dishonest minority.

The CFS approach is widely recognised as best practice in the UK public sector and increasingly across Europe, with information being shared via the new European Healthcare Fraud and Corruption Network.

It is time that work to counter fraud and corruption moves from its pre-professional period and becomes fully professionalised. No one expects an untrained lawyer to provide good legal advice or an unqualified surgeon to operate on a relative. It is equally unacceptable to take a non-professional approach to the protection of public bodies against fraud and corruption.

Note

1. Jim Gee is chief executive of the National Health Service Counter Fraud Service and director of Counter Fraud Services in the UK Department of Health.

3 Corruption in hospitals

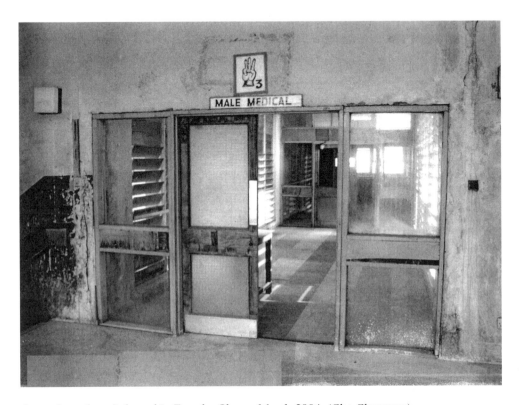

A run-down hospital ward in Tamale, Ghana, March 2004. (Che Chapman)

As the loci of a large proportion of health spending – and given their size and complexity – hospitals provide many opportunities for corruption, as Taryn Vian describes. Money leaks from hospitals through opaque procurement of equipment and supplies, ghost employees, exaggerated construction costs and inflated hospital price tags. In developing countries the result is a depleted budget for other necessary health care services such as primary health care programmes.

Ultimately it is patients that suffer, either because they are asked to pay bribes for treatment that should be free, or because treatment decisions are based on financial motivation rather than medical need. Effects are felt in both the developed and the developing world. Case studies from around the world provide a glimmer of hope by showing how low-cost efforts to increase transparency – of hospital procurement in Kenya and waiting lists in Croatia – can help reduce corruption.

Corruption in hospital administration
Taryn Vian[1]

The hospital sector represents a significant risk for corruption, in both developing and developed countries alike. In the United States alone, fraud and abuse in health care has been estimated to cost US $11.9 to 23.2 billion per year; much of this expense is attributable to hospital-based care.[2]

The size and complexity of hospitals allows the possibility for many kinds of corruption. As many economists have pointed out, corruption is a 'crime of calculation' and is more likely to occur where budgets are large and 'rents' or possibilities for people to gain from decisions made by officials are high. Hospitals meet these criteria for vulnerability. Globally, hospitals account for 30–50 per cent of total health sector spending (public and private); in some regions, such as Eastern Europe, the percentage may be as high as 70 per cent.[3] Hospital spending may also include large investments in building construction and purchase of expensive technologies, areas of procurement that are particularly vulnerable to corruption. The need to manage multiple stakeholders with different interests and asymmetries in information at many levels (between medical personnel and patients, doctors and administrators, and procurement specialists and clinicians, to name just a few) also creates an environment that is susceptible to corruption (see Chapter 1).

Corruption in hospital administration has a direct negative effect on access and quality of patient care. Employee theft of supplies can leave patients without medicines, and extorted, under-the-table payments create anxiety and reduce access to care. As resources are drained from hospital budgets through embezzlement and procurement fraud, less funding is available to pay salaries and fund operations. This in turn leads to demotivated staff and greater absenteeism as medical personnel seek private income from outside jobs, again lowering access and decreasing quality of services. Financial arrangements between hospitals and doctors intended to increase hospitals' and doctors' profits can lead to waste of public money, or medical decisions that are not in the patients' best interests. Persistent corruption in the hospital sector makes it harder to reduce hospital spending as a proportion of overall health expenditures, a goal in many developing countries where needs can be met more cost-effectively in primary care settings, such as health centres and maternal and child health clinics. If officials in power are gaining personally from the current patterns of spending in the hospital sector, why would they favour changes to expand primary care, an area where there is less opportunity for private enrichment?

Table 3.1 provides a typology of corruption in hospital administration. Key areas of concern include the procurement function; embezzlement and theft; payment system fraud; and personnel issues such as absenteeism, informal payments and sale of positions.

Table 3.1: Major types of corruption in hospital administration

Category	Type	Description
Procurement	Overpayment for goods and services	Engaging in collusion, bribes and kickbacks in procurement processes, resulting in overpayment for goods and contracted services; not enforcing contractual standards for quality.
Embezzlement and theft	Embezzlement	Diverting budget or user-fee revenue for personal advantage.
	Theft	Stealing medicines and medical supplies or equipment for personal use, use in private practice or re-sale.
Personnel	Absenteeism	Not showing up for work or working fewer hours than required, while being paid as if full time.
	Informal payments	Extorting or accepting under-the-table payments for services that are supposed to be provided free of charge; soliciting payments in exchange for special privileges or treatment.
	Abuse of hospital resources	Using hospital equipment, space, vehicles or budget for private business, friends or personal advantage.
	Favouritism in billing, spending	Waiving fees or falsifying insurance documents for particular people; using hospital budget to benefit particular favoured individuals.
	Sale of positions and accreditation	Extorting or accepting bribes to influence hiring decisions and decisions on licensing, accreditation or certification of facilities.
Payment systems	Insurance fraud and unauthorised patient billing	Illegally billing insurance companies, government or patients for uncovered services or services that were not actually provided, in order to maximise revenue. May involve falsification of invoice records, receipt books or utilisation records, and/or creation of 'ghost' patients.
	Illegal referral arrangements	Buying business from physicians by creating financial incentives or offering kickbacks for referrals; physicians improperly referring public hospital patients to their private practice.
	Inducement of unnecessary medical procedures	Performing unnecessary medical interventions in order to maximise fee revenue.

Hospital procurement: a hotbed of corruption

Procurement fraud is a large risk in hospitals, as virtually all capital spending involves procurement, and medicines and supplies are often the next largest recurrent expenditure item after salaries. Procurement agents may seek bribes or kickbacks from supply companies, or contractors may engage in collusion or offer bribes to hospital officials in order to win contracts.

Evidence from Argentina, Bolivia, Venezuela and Colombia suggests that these practices drive up the price of supplies purchased. For example, estimated overpayments in 1998 for seven specific medications in 32 public hospitals in Colombia were valued at more than US $2 million per year, an amount that would have paid for health insurance coverage for 24,000 people.[4]

Small hospitals face special challenges in reducing vulnerability to procurement abuse. Where there are only a few doctors in a specialty, they have more power over the decisions made by administrators. The doctors may demand that the hospital purchase certain equipment or supplies for them, or they will move their practice elsewhere. Some may not consider this corruption but merely an economic driver of medical inflation.

In addition, hospitals may be pressured by consultants to buy more technology than the hospital can afford to maintain, because the additional equipment enables the specialist doctors to demand higher fees. This is particularly true in private hospitals, but may also take place in public hospitals where doctors use public facilities for private practice (officially or not), or are able to demand under-the-table payments from patients.

While essential drug lists and hospital formularies can help by restricting procurement to pre-approved drugs meeting efficacy, cost and quality standards, private drug manufacturers or their agents may still try to bribe officials to see that their medicine or formulation appears on the list. For example, in Albania, a Ministry of Health official claimed in 2003 that offers had been made to purchase the not-yet-approved list of new members appointed to the national committees for drug nomenclature and drug reimbursement. Presumably the bribers wanted the list so that they could individually approach the new members to try to influence their selection decisions, perhaps by offering financial incentives for decisions favourable to the bribers. In a similar bid to influence medicines purchasing and use decisions, TAP Pharmaceutical Products was charged with giving inducements directly to Lahey Clinic, a 259-bed US medical centre and primary care practice, allegedly agreeing to pay some US $100,000 for a Christmas party, golf tournaments and seminars if the clinic agreed to continue prescribing its cancer drug Lupron instead of a less expensive rival drug.[5] TAP had already paid a record US $885 million fine in 2001 to settle similar charges.

Procurement agents may also turn a blind eye when vendors substitute lower-quality building materials or deliver goods that do not meet contractual expectations for quality, as in Malaysia, where the Anti-Corruption Agency recently launched a probe into irregular construction of the Sultan Ismail Hospital.[6] Risk of corruption is higher if a hospital lacks systems for documenting and controlling contractor performance. Kenyatta National Hospital in Kenya reportedly lost over US $12 million to procurement fraud between 1999 and 2002.[7] Problems cited by the press included failure to control quality of purchases (obsolete items substituted for the modern equipment described in the bid, or fewer supplies delivered than contracted) and hidden charges or construction overruns not included in the original procurement contract, as well as non-competitive bidding processes resulting in higher prices. Hospitals may not have adequate systems for recording receipt and use of drug orders, leading to situations where they pay for orders that are never received.

Better administrative systems for procurement and inventory control can help to prevent corruption by reducing discretion; however, anti-corruption efforts that rely heavily on administrative controls can be stymied by the problem of collusion. In Venezuela, researchers suspected that collusion between hospital administrators and purchasing officers was feeding the corruption by reducing the probability of detection and punishment.[8]

Transparency and accountability measures must be used to hold hospital administrators accountable. In Argentina, the government adopted a strategy of monitoring how much hospitals were paying for medical supplies and disseminated this information among them. Purchase prices for the monitored items immediately fell by an average of 12 per cent. Prices eventually began to rise again, but stayed below the baseline purchase prices for the entire time the policy was in place.[9] The WHO and Health Action International have also developed a drug-price monitoring tool that could be used for transparency initiatives.[10]

In Bolivia, researchers found that increased citizen health board activism and supervision of personnel played a role in deterring overpayment for drugs by procurement agents,[11] while in Uganda, health unit management committees with community representation began to enforce accountability, particularly in the area of hospital drug management.[12] Of course, if community board members accept kickbacks or collude with hospital officials, the committees will not be effective.

To increase transparency in procurement of medicines, hospitals can channel decision-making through expert pharmacy and therapeutic committees, or procurement committees. The committee structure helps to balance the influence of clinicians with strong personal interests. Pooled procurement decisions for groups of hospitals may help to increase competition and dissipate power of individual physicians. Some countries, like Albania, have moved to centralise hospital procurement as a way to reduce opportunities for corruption. Chile's centralised health procurement agency, CENABAST, has prevented collusion and lowered prices by introducing computerised, auction-style bidding (see 'Corruption in the pharmaceutical sector', Chapter 5, page 76). Centralised procurement may bring other problems, however, if it is poorly designed and controlled. And even with effective centralised procurement systems, the risks of bribery and collusion remain, and must be dealt with through transparency and review.

Embezzlement and theft

Embezzlement involves the theft of cash payments or other revenue from a hospital by employees charged with revenue collection. Hospitals with weak financial systems that are not computerised, or are cash rather than accrual-based, are more vulnerable (see Box 3.1). In developing countries, embezzlement often involves user-fee revenues collected from sale of drugs or diagnostic tests, and registration fees paid by patients. One study found that workers pocketed an estimated 68–77 per cent of revenues from formal user-charges in Uganda's sub-hospital clinics.[13] Researchers compared expected user-fee revenue based on recorded utilisation in 12 facilities, to actual recorded revenue. Although Ministry of Health guidelines allowed some fee exemptions for the poor, the study found that in practice those unable to pay were actually turned away, and estimated that most of the 'gap' in revenue was taken by collectors.

Box 3.1   Cash registers inject transparency – and revenue – into Kenya's Coast Provincial General Hospital

In Coast Provincial General Hospital in Kenya, government staff used information from patient satisfaction surveys to detect fraud in the user-fee collection system.[1] Employees were allegedly pocketing user fees, draining funds from the hospital. Because systems for reporting revenue collection were not computerised, it was hard to determine what the user-fee revenue should have been, and to compare this with actual receipts. Managers lacked the information they needed to take action.

To combat the problem, management installed a network of electronic cash registers. Programme implementers had to replace the fee collectors, who were resistant to the change.

The reform took three months and cost US $42,000. User-fee revenues jumped by almost 50 per cent in three months with no change in utilisation rates. The new system revealed other gaps in hospital systems and accountability, which were also addressed. Within three years, annual user-fee revenues were up 400 per cent. Accountability for spending the windfall in revenue was addressed by introducing more transparency in the planning and budgeting process.

Taryn Vian (Boston University School of Public Health)

Note
1. C. Stover, 'Health Financing and Reform in Kenya: Lessons from the Field. Background document for end-of-project conference for the APHIA Financing and Sustainability Project' (Nairobi: May 2001).

Theft of supplies is another common problem in public hospitals. Although not all theft can be categorised as corruption, the line is crossed when those entrusted with power systematically abuse their position to deplete a hospital's resources. There are indications that the problem is significant. In a study in Venezuela, two-thirds of surveyed medical staff knew of cases where medical supplies had been stolen, while in Costa Rica over 80 per cent of nurses reported 'a lot' or 'some' theft.[14] Uganda has huge problems with drug leakage from hospitals and sub-hospital health facilities, where researchers estimated losses of two-thirds of the purchased drug supply.[15] In interviews with 53 health workers in Mozambique and Cape Verde, about half of whom worked in hospitals, researchers reported frequent misuse of pharmaceutical supply for personal gain.[16]

Misappropriation of drug supply and embezzlement of user-fee revenue in poor countries are seen by some as a personal coping strategy for deteriorating work conditions, including falling salaries and irregular pay. Approaches to prevention and control therefore need to include not only monitoring and control systems for detection and punishment, but also reforms to payment systems and reforms to strengthen professionalism. One suggestion, based on fieldwork in Mozambique and Cape Verde, is to 'introduce legislation that makes the head of an organisation or department legally responsible for the actions of that body' as a way of increasing peer pressure and accountability.[17] Performance contracting is another way to increase accountability and provide incentives for performance.[18]

'Unhealthy' personnel practices

'Stealing time' is another common abuse. A total of 32 per cent of health professionals interviewed in Peru thought absenteeism was common or very common among hospital staff,[19] while in Venezuela respondents reported that doctors and head nurses were absent during 30–37 per cent of contracted hours (see 'A tale of two health systems', Chapter 1, page 14). Absenteeism has been linked to low salaries and dual-job holding,[20] which some consider a 'coping mechanism' rather than corruption. Many doctors are also active in the private sector, driven in part by the inadequate compensation available in the public sector.[21]

To reduce absenteeism, institutional controls must be introduced to increase detection, including personnel supervision, performance measurement systems, and community participation in hospital management. Researchers noted that while control mechanisms can help, 'one size' doesn't fit all. The success of strategies to reduce absenteeism in public facilities will also depend on pay differentials between the public and private sectors, and whether there are barriers to entry into the private sector. Larger reforms to civil service policies and public human resource management systems may be needed, such as shifting from civil service appointments to contractual payment for time and services rendered. If an employee does not perform, the contract would not be renewed. This also permits one to pay a higher hourly rate for hours actually worked.

Informal payments – defined as payments made by patients for services that are supposed to be provided free of charge – are a serious problem in many middle- and low-income countries (see Chapter 4, page 62). Under-the-table remuneration has also been documented in some higher income countries including France and Greece.[22] In addition to causing anxiety and uncertainty among patients, informal payments can cause poor people to forgo or delay seeking care, and can have negative effects on the quality of clinical services. Some patients go into debt or sell assets in order to make informal payments, thus impoverishing themselves. Others seek to keep informal payments low by skipping levels of care – going straight to specialists or the hospital, for example, instead of using primary care services or general practitioners.

Box 3.2 Hospital waiting lists open for scrutiny in Croatia

The Croatian health sector is perceived to be among the most corrupt sectors in the country.[1] It is not surprising then that instances of patients paying bribes to reduce time spent on waiting lists are thought to be commonplace. To curb this problem, the health ministry launched a pilot initiative to publish open waiting lists – a measure obliging hospital executives to disclose lists to patients showing them their position in the line-up to receive medical treatment. Lists are made accessible at hospital and clinic reception desks, and patients that do not want to have their names made public can ask to be listed by number instead. Complaints about irregularities can be made to the head of the hospital or to the Health Ministry.

  With the help of TI Croatia, waiting lists at two major hospitals in Zagreb, Dubrava and Sveti Duh were published in hard copy and on the Internet in late 2004 and 2005. A hotline run by TI Croatia to monitor the effectiveness of the initiative received 90 calls about the Dubrava Hospital waiting list within the first few months starting in October 2004. In one case, a patient had waited two years for heart surgery but, after lodging a complaint with TI Croatia, was operated on within two weeks. The pilot initiative is set to become a precedent in curbing corruption in health care delivery by making it more open and transparent.

Ana First (TI Croatia)

Note
1. Transparency International's Global Corruption Barometer 2004, a public opinion survey, ranked the health services as the second most corrupt institution in Croatia, second only to the legal system/judiciary and equal to political parties and parliament.

Patients report making informal payments to all kinds of health workers, from guards and cleaners, to mortuary attendants and lab technicians, to the doctors and nurses involved in diagnosis and treatment. Some studies have found that patients who are hospitalised are more likely to make informal payments, and to pay higher amounts, than patients seeking ambulatory care.[23] In the foreboding words of one Albanian informant: 'The most important thing is that you should pay the doctor, because he will never forget the face of someone who has not paid him for the rest of his life.'[24]

The fact that it is hard to distinguish informal payments from tips, or gifts given by patients to express gratitude, makes the problem more difficult to address. While informal payments may be seen as a coping mechanism for survival when the salaries of doctors and nurses fall below a living wage, other payments are clearly bribes extorted by workers, a practice detected in a Kenyan mortuary and decried by officials. Mortuary attendants have also been implicated in bribery and other corruption schemes in South Africa and Zimbabwe.[25]

Involving ordinary citizens in oversight or transparency initiatives may be a useful complement to regulatory and bureaucratic reforms to address informal payments. One hospital in Cambodia has had success in reducing informal payments by formalising user fees and promoting professionalism among staff. The hospital created individual contracts with personnel and increased pay scales while enforcing accountability and sanctioning poor performance.[26]

As in other sectors, private interests may also affect the selection and promotion of staff to fill hospital positions, with posts going to the highest bidder or most connected individuals, rather than to candidates with the best qualifications. One study found that auxiliary nurse-midwives pay bribes of six or seven times the monthly salary to obtain positions in Uttar Pradesh state, India.[27] Also in India, the Delhi High Court found that the president of the Indian medical council had accepted bribes to allow medical colleges to 'sell' seats to local students.[28] The cost of this type of corruption can be very serious, affecting both the clinical practice of medicine, and the management of hospital systems and performance. To reduce vulnerability, hospitals can try to open up the hiring and promotion decision-making process, making criteria more transparent. Performance monitoring is also essential to provide accountability.

'Just what the doctor ordered': corruption in payment systems

Other forms of corruption – including insurance reimbursement fraud, treatment decisions based on financial motivation rather than the medical need and improper referral relationships between doctors and hospitals (sometimes involving kickbacks) – can be traced to various forms of payment systems.

Reimbursement-system fraud may occur in countries with social insurance funds or a sizeable private health care insurance market (see Chapter 1). Losses can be substantial: the US government has estimated that improper Medicare fee-for-service payments, including non-hospital services, may be in the range of US $11.9–23.2 billion per year, or 6.8–14 per cent of total payments.[29] This sum must be interpreted with caution as it may include unintentional mistakes or controversial decisions about what is labelled 'necessary' care, but it gives a sense of the magnitude of the problem. Health care fraud includes false billing of insurance funds or governments for medical services that are not supposed to be covered, services that were not actually delivered (sometimes because the person is dead or does not exist, so-called 'ghost patients') or services that were not medically indicated. It also includes the practice of 'upcoding' diagnosis related groups (DRGs), that is, classifying a case as more complicated or as having co-morbidities in order to obtain reimbursement at higher rates.

Whether insurance systems are involved or not, hospitals and doctors may have financial incentives to use increased resources in providing patient care. This is referred to as provider-induced demand. Where services are needed, increased demand can be good; however, financial incentives sometimes cause doctors to provide unnecessary treatments, or marginally useful diagnostic tests. Fee-for-service payment systems have been associated with increased utilisation of resources, sometimes to the point of inappropriate use, as providers try to maximise their revenue by providing more care. For example, researchers in Peru documented excessive caesarean section rates in the Social Security Institute and private hospitals where doctors were paid on a fee-for-service basis.[30] It is important to note that while demand may rise due to financial incentives, it may still fall within the range of normal medical judgement. Where provider-induced demand becomes abuse is when it is excessive and outside the range normally considered medically indicated, yet this is far from simple to determine.

Less recognised but equally harmful from the viewpoint of patients may be the risks introduced by managed care capitation payments, where hospitals and doctors may engage in fraud resulting in underutilisation of care in order to maximise profit (see 'Corruption in health care systems', Chapter 1, page 19). Again, it is hard to determine where underutilisation falls outside the normal range and becomes abuse.

Another area of concern is when hospitals enter into financial relationships with physicians to increase hospital referrals. Where hospitals are reimbursed by the state or private insurers based on patient admissions or days of care delivered, it can be advantageous for them to increase the number of patients admitted and to maintain high occupancy (see the Columbia/HCA case, 'Corruption in health care systems', Chapter 1, page 20). One way to do this is to offer advantages to physicians who refer patients to the hospital. Yet introducing financial incentives for referrals can present a danger: even if the hospital is not best suited to meet a particular patient's medical needs, the physician may still refer the patient there in order to gain the financial advantage.

Financial incentives are sometimes used to promote medically needed care offered at the most appropriate level, so it is not the use of financial incentives per se that creates the danger for corruption. But the situation must be monitored and controlled to prevent abuse. US federal law prohibits physician self-referrals, and a federal statute proscribes kickbacks. Applying these laws in Nebraska, one hospital was charged with underwriting a loan, paying consultants and providing free drugs and medical equipment to a doctor in exchange for referrals.[31]

The definition of corruption in other situations is not so clear, as when a private 231-bed hospital in the United States owned by Tenet, a large for-profit hospital corporation, was charged with using 'relocation agreements' to bribe doctors. Over a period of several years, the hospital paid US $10 million to doctors who agreed to relocate their practices to the area.[32] Although federal law specifically prohibits hospitals from paying or otherwise compensating doctors for referrals, the question was whether the 'relocation agreements' were devised to get around this law. The court case ended in a mistrial as the jury could not agree on whether this was a violation of the law.

Payment system reforms are important to reduce vulnerability to this type of corruption. In northern European countries, such as Finland, Sweden and the United Kingdom, health reforms have shifted health care provision from fixed-budget bureaucratic institutions to contract payments based on performance.[33] While this increased operating efficiency, it also required the state to play a more sophisticated role in regulating services. Because it is difficult to detect and control where utilisation falls outside the range of normal practice, regulators may have more success with approaches that reward providers for quality improvement.[34]

A prescription for reform

Strategies to prevent corruption in hospitals must be tailored to the particular ownership structure, policy environment and health-financing situation in the country. The types of corruption one will find, and the resources available for preventing corruption, are likely to be different in low-income countries, compared with high-income countries.

Yet the range of interventions for reducing vulnerability to corruption does include some standard components. Once the types of corruption have been identified and prioritised, reform strategies such as those below should be considered and adapted. These include strengthening management systems and tools, creating incentives, increasing the likelihood of detecting corruption as well as the consequences of getting caught, and developing better information and transparency initiatives to hold hospital officials and medical personnel to account.

Box 3.3 No bribes for healthy business: India's Transasia Biomedicals[1]

India's leading manufacturer of high-tech diagnostic machines to check for life-threatening blood diseases is Transasia Biomedicals, based in Mumbai. The brainchild of Suresh Vazirani, Transasia began marketing imported diagnostic equipment in 1985, only branching into manufacturing eight years later with the help of international manufacturers, such as Sysmex, Wako and Nittec in Japan, Finland's Biohit and Trace in Australia.

What marks out Transasia is the dogged stance it takes against corruption. Vazirani says he has never paid a paisa in bribes, but that avoiding corruption takes up more of his time than any other issue. When he wanted to install a fountain in the lunch area, two officials demanded a US $100 bribe for a 'licence'. It took four years in court, and US $4,000, to deal with the case.

Vazirani's interest in fighting corruption stems from his nine years as a volunteer with Moral Re-Armament (now Initiatives of Change), running industrial leadership training courses. There he would urge businessmen not to be corrupt, he recalls. '"That's all very well," they would reply, "but you've never run a business. You don't know what it's like."'

He and a friend decided to go into business in 1979 and as the company grew from a modest importer to a global player exporting to over 30 countries, so did the opportunities for corruption. Vazirani risked losing a DM 20 million (US $12.6 million) sales contract to Germany because a customs officer wanted a bribe to release imported components. Rather than pay, Vazirani left the components in the warehouse for three months. He went to the top customs officials and 'appealed to their sense of national pride'. The components were released just in time.

Recently, a politician suggested to Vazirani that it would be 'an opportunity' if they each pocketed part of the World Bank aid the politician had received to improve health care. 'Yes, and is it an opportunity if we land up in hospital needing urgent care ourselves?' replied Vazirani. At this, the politician changed his tune, realising that Vazirani was not to be bought.

In September 2003, Vazirani was a keynote speaker at the launch in Mumbai of Transparency International's new Business Principles for Countering Bribery. 'Corruption is a big road block to progress', he says. 'Because of it everything goes wrong. The intimidation leads to wrong decision-making. Transasia can be an example. But many more companies need to be.'

Michael Smith (For A Change Magazine)

Note
1. Excerpt from *For A Change* Magazine, December 2003/January 2004.

Managerial systems and tools

Important managerial systems and tools for preventing corruption in hospitals include hospital drug formularies, review committees to certify need for new drugs or equipment, competitive bidding and other best-practice procurement procedures, and inventory systems to safeguard supplies. Each management system should have clearly defined levels of responsibility and approval of decision-making, with appropriate checks and balances. In addition to procurement, other management systems include budgeting and planning systems to prevent spending that favours pet projects or people and is not needs-based, and internal financial control systems to prevent theft and embezzlement.

Anti-corruption strategies in the hospital sector need to be one step ahead of different actors trying to abuse entrusted resources, and to penalise corrupt practices. Fraud control programmes have proven effective in reducing corruption; for example, the US federal government gets a return of US $8 on every US $1 spent on fraud control.[35] It recovered US $8 billion over 15 years through enforcement of the False Claims Act, about half of which was health-related.[36] In addition to financial benefits, fraud control efforts can also have health benefits and change patterns of care in desirable ways.[37]

Incentives and consequences

There are conflicts of interest inherent in most hospital payment systems, and the influence of payment systems on health care utilisation is a well-studied topic in health policy literature. It is an area where careful monitoring and continuous analysis is needed to ensure that patient safety and well-being are not being compromised by actions taken to maximise providers' income. A promising new area of research is in performance-based contracting, especially payment systems that reward quality. At the same time, it is important to promote laws and codes of conduct that explicitly regulate hospitals' and hospital administrators' engagement in practices where conflict of interest is likely to be a problem (for example, owning supply companies), and that encourage and reward professionalism.

Transparency and information

Since collusion among hospital personnel can subvert management control reforms, transparency is an essential anti-corruption strategy. In the hospital sector, transparency initiatives that should be considered include public access to procurement bidding results, monitoring of procurement prices paid (as in the Argentinian example discussed above), analysis of procurement bids for evidence of collusion, and setting performance standards for hospitals and suppliers. This type of information, when shared with other hospitals and citizen health boards or oversight committees, can both detect corruption and serve as a deterrent.

Anti-corruption strategies should not target only agents or officials working in hospitals: many forms of hospital corruption are promoted by the producers or dealers of medical equipment and drugs. Laws and codes of conduct for businesses supplying hospitals should also be revised and enforced to prevent offers of bribes. Transparency can also be effective here, through the publication of report cards monitoring the compliance of private companies with these laws and codes of conduct. In addition, in centralised, public health systems the government can create a blacklist of suppliers caught bribing. Alternatively, the government can also share 'whitelists' of suppliers who consistently meet or exceed standards of performance.

Anti-corruption programmes should support health-sector financing and structural reforms to assure that public systems are not over-promising and under-delivering. Hospital systems and the medical personnel who staff them should be organised to provide incentives for improved performance. This is especially important in resource-constrained countries, where pressures to engage in corruption as a survival strategy may be strong. To prevent corruption and promote health, hospitals need management systems that are transparent, accountable and fair to both patients and providers.

Notes

1. Taryn Vian is assistant professor at the Boston University School of Public Health, where she conducts research and teaches courses on health care management and prevention of corruption in the health sector. Carol Karutu assisted in researching this paper and Rich Feeley provided feedback on an earlier draft.
2. D. Becker, D. Kessler and M. McClellan, 'Detecting Medicare Abuse', *Journal of Health Economics* 24(1), January 2005.
3. R. Taylor and S. Blair, 'Public Hospitals: Options for Reform through Public Private Partnerships', (Public Policy for the Private Sector Note Number 241) (Washington, DC: World Bank, 2002); J. Healy and M. McKee, 'Reforming Hospital Systems in Turbulent Times', *Eurohealth* 7(3), 2001.
4. R. Di Tella and W. D. Savedoff, 'Shining Light in Dark Corners' in R. Di Tella and W. D. Savedoff (eds) *Diagnosis Corruption: Fraud in Latin America's Public Hospitals* (Washington, DC: Inter-American Development Bank, 2001).
5. *Boston Globe* (US), 7 April 2004.
6. *Bernama* (Malaysia), 27 September 2004.
7. *The East African* (Kenya), 10 March 2003.
8. M. H. Jaen and D. Paravisini, 'Wages, Capture and Penalties in Venezuela's Public Hospitals', in Di Tella and Savedoff, *Diagnosis Corruption*.
9. E. Schargrodsky, J. Mera and F. Weinschelbaum, 'Transparency and Accountability in Argentina's Hospitals', in Di Tella and Savedoff, *Diagnosis Corruption*.
10. See www.haiweb.org/medicineprices/
11. G. Gray-Molina, E. Perez de Rada and E. Yáñez, 'Does Voice Matter? Participation and Controlling Corruption in Bolivian Hospitals', in Di Tella and Savedoff, *Diagnosis Corruption*.
12. D. Kyaddondo and S. R. Whyte, 'Working in a Decentralised System: A Threat to Health Workers' Respect and Survival in Uganda', *International Journal of Health Planning and Management* 18(4), October–December 2003.
13. B. McPake, D. Asiimwe, F. Mwesigye et al., 'Informal Economic Activities of Public Health Workers in Uganda: Implications for Quality and Accessibility of Care', *Social Science and Medicine* 49(7), 1999.
14. Di Tella and Savedoff, *Diagnosis Corruption*.
15. McPake et al., 'Informal Economic Activities'.
16. P. Ferrinho, C. M. Omar, M. D. Fernandes, P. Blaise, A. M. Bugalho and W. Van Lerberghe, 'Pilfering for Survival: How Health Workers Use Access to Drugs as a Coping Strategy', *Human Resources for Health* 2(1), 2004.
17. Ibid.

18. Management Sciences for Health, 'Using Performance-Based Payments to Improve Health Programmes', *The Manager* 10, 2001.
19. L. Alcazar and R. Andrade, 'Induced Demand and Absenteeism in Peruvian Hospitals', in Di Tella and Savedoff, *Diagnosis Corruption*.
20. Schargrodsky et al., 'Transparency and Accountability', and P. Ferrinho, W. Van Lerberghe, I. Fronteira, F. Hipolito and A. Biscaia, 'Dual Practice in the Health Sector: Review of Evidence', *Human Resources for Health* 2(14), 2004.
21. R. Gruen, R. Anwar, T. Begum, J. R. Killingsworth and C. Normand, 'Dual Job Holding Practitioners in Bangladesh: An Exploration', *Social Science and Medicine* 54(2), 2002.
22. Ferrinho et al., 'Pilfering for Survival'.
23. P. Belli, G. Gotsadze and H. Shahriari, 'Out-of-pocket and Informal Payments in Health Sector: Evidence from Georgia', *Health Policy* 70(1), October 2004; T. Vian, K. Gryboski, Z. Sinoimeri and R. Hall, 'Informal Payments in the Public Health Sector in Albania: A Qualitative Study. Final Report. Partners for Health Reform Plus Project' (Bethesda, US: Abt Associates, Inc., 2004); D. R. Hotchkiss, P. L. Hutchinson, M. Altin and A. A. Berruti, 'Out-of-pocket Payments and Utilization of Health Care Services in Albania: Evidence from Three Districts' (Bethesda, US: Partners for Health Reformplus, 2004).
24. T. Vian, T. Gryboski, Z. Sinoimeri and R. Hall, 'Informal Payments in Government Health Facilities in Albania: Results of a Qualitative Study', forthcoming in *Social Science and Medicine*, 2005.
25. *The Nation* (Kenya), 8 February 2001; *Panafrican News Agency*, 19 July 2003; *African Business* (UK), January 2004.
26. S. Barber, F. Bonnet and H. Bekedam, 'Formalising Under-the-table Payments to Control Out-of-pocket Hospital Expenditures in Cambodia', *Health Policy and Planning*, July 2004.
27. R. Balakrishnan, cited in B. Lee, M. Poutanen, L. Breuning and K. Bradbury, *Siphoning off: Corruption and Waste in Family Planning and Reproductive Health Resources in Developing Countries* (Berkeley: University of California Press, 1999).
28. *The Lancet* (UK), 358, 2001.
29. Becker et al., 'Detecting Medicare Abuse'.
30. Alcazar and Andrade, 'Induced Demand and Absenteeism'.
31. See note 27.
32. *Modern Healthcare* 33, 2003.
33. R. B. Saltman, 'Regulating Incentives: the Past and Present Role of the State in Health Care Systems', *Social Science and Medicine* 54, 2002.
34. *New York Times* (US), 13 March 2005.
35. J. A. Meyer and S. E. Anthony, 'Reducing Health Care Fraud: An Assessment of the Impact of the False Claims Act. Report prepared by New Directions for Policy' (Washington, DC: Taxpayers Against Fraud, 2001).
36. *Pharmaceutical Executive* 21(11), 2001.
37. Becker et al., 'Detecting Medicare Abuse'.

4 Informal payments for health care

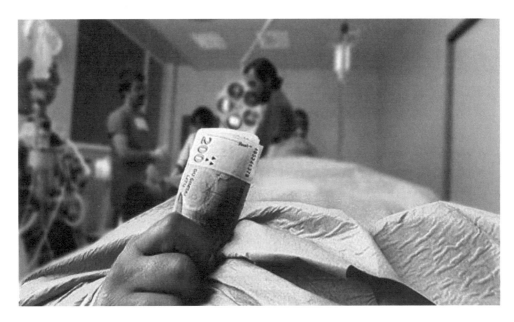

Television spot, autumn 2004, highlighting the problem of informal payments for health care in Lithuania. (TI Lithuania)

Informal payments – charges for services or supplies that are supposed to be free – are common in many parts of the world, especially in developing and transition countries. While it is difficult to draw a line between voluntary gift and mandatory payment, and between payments that should be considered bribes or extortion, and those that are better understood as a coping mechanism for underpaid caregivers, there is less disagreement about the damaging effects these payments have on health systems worldwide.

Sara Allin, Konstantina Davaki and Elias Mossialos look at the causes and consequences of informal payments in Central and Eastern Europe and the Commonwealth of Independent States, where informal financing is a legacy of communist health care systems. They argue that raising the wages of health professionals alone is unlikely to eliminate the problem and point to a number of essential policy measures, such as developing appropriate incentives and suitable information systems to support the accounting and auditing of payments. A case study from Hungary shows that, despite the relatively small sums involved, informal payments can lead to a massive distortion of the health system. The example from Morocco demonstrates that small, under-the-table payments can be a serious obstacle to poor patients accessing medical care.

Paying for 'free' health care: the conundrum of informal payments in post-communist Europe

Sara Allin, Konstantina Davaki and Elias Mossialos[1]

Informal payments for health care in the countries of Central and Eastern Europe (CEE) and the Commonwealth of Independent States (CIS – the former Soviet Union excluding the Baltic states) are widespread. Informal, 'under-the-table' or 'envelope' payments are typically defined as direct payments by patients for services they are entitled to for free, usually in a public health system. Informal payments range from the ex ante cash payment to the ex post gift-in-kind. While the common practice of gift giving as an expression of gratitude is, in principle, benign, informal payments that resemble fee-for-service have potentially serious implications.

They can undermine official payment systems, distort the priorities of the health system, reduce access to health services and impede health reforms. They can also provide undesirable incentives and encourage unprofessional behaviour, including rent-seeking behaviour by health workers. It is difficult to disentangle the specific form of informal payment and decipher what constitutes corruption; the different manifestations of informal payment can be placed on a continuum of gravity ranging from nuisance to obstacle to barrier and, ultimately, to self-exclusion.[2] Reducing the extent of informal charging is far from straightforward and represents an enormous task for policy-makers.

Informal payments exist for several reasons, including economic ones such as a general scarcity of financial resources in the public system; and socio-cultural ones, such as the lack of trust in government and a culture of tipping. Most of the CEE and CIS countries' health systems were modelled on the Soviet *Semashko* system of universal health care coverage, with a virtually exclusive role for the state in financing and delivery. Informal payments became a common feature of these health systems, since the state could not deliver what it promised. Following the economic and social crisis with the fall of communism and the break-up of the Soviet Union, health care suffered even further in terms of resource availability and service quality. Health system characteristics that may help explain the prevalence of informal payments include an excess supply of capital and human resources, low salaries, lack of accountability and government oversight, and an overall lack of transparency. Human resource shortages may also drive informal payments as it may lead to providers giving priority to those patients that can afford to pay. A paucity of private services may also drive informal payments, as wealthier patients have fewer options outside of the public system. Also, the population may not be adequately informed of the health services they are entitled to free of charge.

Some scholars argue that informal payments arose as a reaction by dissatisfied patients and providers to shortcomings within the health system during the communist era.[3] Given the deficiencies regarding quality and availability, there were no opportunities for dissatisfied patients to opt out, as there was no private sector alternative, nor to voice their complaints, as these were regarded as direct criticism of the government. Providers were faced with low salaries and no explicit state-organised rationing mechanisms. Thus informal payments became an established practice and served as an alternative method of enabling patients to pay for better quality.

Throughout the 1990s, staff salaries in CEE countries were, and many continue to be, very low and payments were often delayed. In Lithuania and Ukraine, health care workers are reported to have waited up to three months to be paid, with even longer waiting times in Russia.[4] Money was instead sought directly from patients and provided to staff. While these informal payments allowed health care staff to continue providing services during periods of economic difficulty, the demand for payments also resulted in the exclusion of those unable to pay. Those most severely affected were the poorest and the chronically ill.

The scale of informal payments

The clandestine nature of informal payments makes accurate accounting difficult. By definition, informal payments are made without any record of the transaction and are often illegal, making both patients and providers reluctant to discuss them.[5] Furthermore, interpretation of what constitutes an informal payment differs across regions and countries, making generalisations and cross-country comparisons inappropriate. For example, discrepancies in the perceived nature of informal payments have been shown between providers and the public in Albania, with providers perceiving payments as gifts and the public viewing fees as necessary to receive services.[6] Despite these difficulties, recent surveys and qualitative studies indicate that informal payments have come to represent a large proportion of total health expenditure in CEE and CIS countries.

Informal payments constitute 84 per cent of total health expenditure in Azerbaijan[7] and out-of-pocket payments contribute around 70–80 per cent of total health spending in Georgia, half of which is estimated to be informal.[8] They are also an important form of health care financing in other countries, representing 56 per cent of total health expenditure in the Russian Federation, and 30 per cent in Poland.[9] In Tajikistan, household spending on health averages US $8.58 per person per annum compared to government expenditure of US $3.75.[10] Similarly, the Albanian Living Standards Measurement Survey of 2002 estimated out-of-pocket (both formal and informal) expenditures constituted more than 70 per cent of total health expenditure.[11]

Survey data of the prevalence of informal payments among service users highlight the severity of the problem and identify substantial diversity across countries. Informal payments are mainly associated with in-patient care settings, particularly surgery, and several surveys have found that they tend to be more common in large towns and cities. A 1999 World Bank/USAID survey observed that 71 per cent of GP visits and 59 per cent of specialist visits involved payments in Slovakia.[12] In Latvia, the TI Annual

Report 2000 estimated that approximately 25 per cent of patients made informal payments sometimes, while 5.7 per cent made payments on almost every visit. A regional breakdown showed that Riga had the highest proportion of under-the-table payments, with 46.1 per cent of Riga respondents having made such payments.[13] In Bulgaria, informal payments are more common in the capital city, Sofia, with 51 per cent of survey respondents reporting paying without a receipt for a doctor or dentist.[14] In Romania, informal payments are prevalent and account for 41 per cent of total out-of-pocket expenditure.[15] A recent survey of public perceptions conducted by the Centre for Policies and Health Services revealed that 39 per cent of people with high incomes paid unofficial fees or gifts for medical services in 2001, while 33 per cent of people with below-average income paid unofficial fees or gifts.[16]

There is evidence in some countries of an increasing trend in the proportion of health service visits incurring charges throughout the 1990s. Between 1993 and 1998, the number of patients in Slovakia who paid for hospital admissions grew by approximately 10 per cent.[17] In Bulgaria, out-of-pocket payments (including both formal and informal payments) increased from 9 per cent of total expenditure in 1992 to 21 per cent in 1997.[18] In Kyrgyzstan, while 11 per cent of patients who visited a physician reported paying informally in 1993, 50 per cent did so in 1996.[19] In Kazakhstan, while out-of-pocket payments were, at least officially, virtually non-existent prior to 1991, by 1996, 30 per cent of visits were charged either formally or informally.[20] It is not clear whether these changes reflect a real increase in informal payments or an increase in the willingness of individuals to report them, and surveys have not dealt with this issue.

The role of physicians

The role of physicians in shaping expectations regarding informal payments is crucial. The status of the profession can also shape physicians' attitudes toward accepting payments directly from patients. Evidence on private expenditures in Poland reveals that informal payments nearly double physicians' formal salaries, suggesting overall that managing existing resources poses a more difficult challenge than finding new resources. There is also a direct benefit for hospital physicians, where informal payments constitute 46 per cent of all patient expenditure in hospitals, thereby leading to an increase in physician salaries by 15 per cent.[21]

In Bulgaria, doctors allegedly receive informal payments of up to US $1,100, significantly augmenting the average monthly salary of US $100.[22] Evidence from Bulgaria also suggests that the unofficial cost of an operation accounted for more than 80 per cent of the average monthly wage.[23] With health workers in Tajikistan among the lowest paid in the country, informal payments and gifts-in-kind represent the main source of income for many providers.[24] By contrast, informal payments are not high in the Czech Republic where doctors' salaries have risen above the rate of inflation of average wages. A 2000 survey of health care staff and public officials revealed that 5 per cent of Czech doctors confessed to accepting 'something more' than a small gift.[25]

However, poor pay alone does not seem to explain physicians' readiness to accept informal payments. Doctors in Bulgaria, Slovakia and the Czech Republic were more likely than the average government official to have reported a second income, and were also well above average in their reporting of having a 'family income' that was enough for a 'fair' or 'good' standard of living. More significantly, while poor pay increased the willingness to accept gifts, it was those with the highest salaries and the highest family income who received such payments more frequently, a likely result of the positions of power held by these individuals.[26] It is not enough, therefore, to increase the salaries of doctors in line with or even above general wages or general public sector incomes. For example, in Greece, substantial increases to hospital physician salaries after the introduction of a national health service in the early 1980s had no impact on the prevalence of informal payments.[27]

The impact of informal payments

The impact of informal payments on the health system is difficult to measure. Payments that solely express gratitude in the form of a donation and are given willingly after a service is delivered may not have any adverse impact on efficiency, quality or equity. However, in countries where this gratitude form of payment is common, the fee-for-service type of informal payment that physicians may demand and may determine access to and/or quality of services has serious adverse effects on efficiency and equity.

Informal payments can be viewed either as contributing to the cost of services, or as an abuse of power by the physician since the patient is placed in a situation with little choice of provider and immediate need of service. The two types of informal payment require different policy responses: the former calls for increasing health resources, in part by formalising payments, while the latter necessitates regulating and monitoring providers.[28] However, in either case, it is likely that the practice of informal payments contributes to resource allocation that is distorted away from the social optimum: rather than being allocated to those in most need, health services will instead favour those who are able to pay, or are easily coerced into paying.

The impact of informal payments on quality is uncertain. Some argue that the quality of services is better for those who pay informally, while others contend that payments lead to unnecessary additional services. Using data from a survey of hospital patients in Kazakhstan in 1999, Thompson and Xavier found that informal payment and the amount paid are generally associated with better-quality services. This is evidenced by decreased waiting time, longer length of hospital stay and patients' subjective ratings of quality.[29] But if service quality is improved when payment is made, the benefits are restricted to that individual. Moreover, physicians are likely to keep the payment for their own personal gain rather than improve services by investing it in the facility. As a result, improved medical equipment, more efficient heating systems and infrastructure, raised nursing standards and other necessary elements of a health system are neglected.

There is little evidence on how informal payments affect utilisation, but patients who cannot afford the extra cost are either unable to obtain treatment or they cannot access the same quality of services or have to wait longer for care. Poorer patients have to make significant sacrifices in order to pay for essential health care services, as seen in Romania.[30] In Kyrgyzstan, one in three patients reported borrowing money for in-patient care, and in rural areas, 45 per cent of in-patients sold produce or livestock to cover hospital costs.[31] In Georgia, qualitative evidence highlights several examples of sacrifices people have to make for health services, such as paying 12 lari for treatment for poisoning (compared to the average monthly salary of 15 lari), while others are forced to borrow money or sell household valuables to pay for health services.[32]

Evidence suggests that informal payments are regressive: although poor individuals pay less in absolute terms than the rich, they pay more as a proportion of their income. This is the case in Albania, Bulgaria, Georgia, Kyrgyzstan, Kazakhstan and Moldova. In Kazakhstan, the poor spent 252 per cent of their monthly income on in-patient care, compared to only 54 per cent among the better off for the same type of services.[33] The percentage of household income spent on informal payments in the late 1990s ranges from 4.1 per cent in Romania, 4.4 per cent in Bulgaria, 9.1 per cent in Albania, to 20.6 per cent in Georgia.[34] In Georgia, 94 per cent of survey respondents were unable to seek health care in 1997 due to its high cost, similar to findings from Albania and Tajikistan.[35] Likewise, surveys conducted in 2001 found that in Armenia and Georgia, over 70 per cent of people reporting illness but not seeking care reported not seeking care because they could not afford it.[36] In addition to the financial barriers imposed by fees, patients in some countries are further deterred by the uncertainty about prices caused by informal payments. Nonetheless, there is no evidence as to whether official fees affect equity more strongly than informal payments do.

In some countries, providers may make exemptions for low-income households and engage in price discrimination. Results from a recent study in Georgia suggest that informal payments depend to some extent on the provider's assessment of a patient's ability to pay which, though vague and likely inaccurate, may minimise the financial barrier to access.[37] Nevertheless, the reverse has also been seen, with evidence from Armenia suggesting a refusal to care for people unable to pay informal fees.[38]

One of the most important implications of informal payments is that they undermine governments' efforts to improve accountability and contribute to the growth in corruption endemic in many CEE and CIS countries. The relationship between corruption and informal payments is complex and bidirectional. To simplify, a lack of resources generates the need for additional income, hence informal payments are made and over time become established practice. This, coupled with a lack of regulatory capacity and a lack of monitoring and payment systems that are not linked to output, exacerbates existing corruption in public policy. The existence of informal payments is at odds with transparent public policy and erodes trust in government.

Policy options

In order to reduce informal payments, serious efforts are needed to rebuild lost trust in health care, raise salaries, ensure good quality of care and improve accountability and transparency. Governments should be explicit and reasonable in defining a benefits package of services provided at a sufficiently high standard for everyone within the funding that is available. Efforts should be made to adequately inform the population of the benefits package provided by the state and any services that do incur charges.

One possible policy option is to formalise informal payments and develop appropriate exemption schemes. However, formalising informal payments will not solve the problem since informal payments may continue to exist alongside the formal charges, which has been the case in Georgia and Bulgaria.[39] One difficulty that governments face in converting informal payments into formalised cost-sharing arrangements is securing compliance from providers, many of whom may lose income. Experience from low-income countries suggests that a successful conversion to formal cost-sharing depends on the ability of government to regulate providers and set priorities or limit the services on offer.[40] For example, in Bulgaria, payments were formalised in 1997 with no significant increase in revenue (less than 1 per cent of municipal health expenditure) and there is no evidence that exemptions are being used.[41] While the formalisation of informal payments is one possible option, it is essential that these payments be transparent and monitored in order to ensure they actually replace informal payments. Moreover, funds should remain in the health sector, with decentralised retention of revenue to allow local improvements in quality of care. If payments translate into staff bonuses, these should reflect performance in order to provide incentives to improve quality and productivity.

In addition to formalising informal payments, private sector involvement can take two forms: private provision and private health insurance. Some argue that allowing private sector involvement in health care delivery may help curb the rise in informal payments by allowing wealthier patients an alternative to the public system, and offering providers an alternative or supplementary salary. Private health care organisations have developed significantly in Lithuania, for example, and the number of physicians working in the private sector has increased in recent years. Surveys in that country reveal a decline in informal payments corresponding with the growth of private providers.[42] This trend seems to follow the Czech experience regarding the role and compensation of providers, where there is a clear division in earnings between physicians in private practice and those employed by the state, although average earnings of public physicians have stayed above the average national earnings and informal payments are rare.[43]

However, perverse incentives associated with permitting private practice among public physicians may arise, which may compromise the quality of care and increase waiting times of individuals who cannot afford to pay for private care. It is possible that allowing private practice may boost incomes and lead to a reduction in informal payments but, if public time and facilities are used for private practice, resources are directed to the wealthier individuals and away from those who cannot afford to pay. Also, physicians may make cross-referrals from their public to their private practices, in order to generate more income.

Private insurance may also be an option to formalise informal payments while also pooling risks. However, informal payments and cultural tendencies regarding the financing of medical care may restrict the growth of private insurance. Patients may be more comfortable paying physicians and other providers directly, while paying third-party entities may be viewed as needlessly meddling with the doctor–patient relationship and reducing assurances of quality care.[44] In Slovakia, informal payments are significant and the market for private medical insurance is not substantial. This is despite the fact that a 2001 Agency Markant survey found that one-third of respondents were distrustful of the General Health Insurance Company while almost two-thirds did not trust the Ministry of Health.[45]

At the same time, indiscriminate support of private sector expansion and encouraging individuals to opt out of the public system may not be such a good idea since there is a risk that the majority of quality-conscious patients would leave the public sector, and it is likely to lead to a two-tier system: a poorly performing public and a well performing private one. Enough financial resources should rather be made available to provide the services of a realistic benefit package at a reasonably good standard to everybody, and new innovative methods of accountability should be made available for the transparent handling of local performance problems. The key issue is to ensure a high quality of care.

Although one possible policy approach is to shift toward more decentralised social insurance models of health system organisation, this may not necessarily reduce the extent of informal payments. While surveys conducted before and after the implementation of a national insurance scheme in Lithuania reveal a decline in the extent of informal payments,[46] no decrease was observed after the implementation of a national health insurance system in Romania, despite the fact that monthly contributions under the Romanian system are compulsory regardless of whether any services are actually received.[47]

The ability to improve efficiency and quality without jeopardising equity critically depends on a number of policy measures, including the skills and capacity of staff, the development of appropriate provider incentives, and the existence of suitable information systems to support the accounting and auditing of payments. Health reforms should also target excess capacity, since incentives created by informal payments can lead to overuse of available staff. Reducing the number of physicians, where appropriate, can also help increase wages and the professional status of medical staff, although wages alone are unlikely to have long-term effects. Evidence supporting the view that increased wages reduce informal payments may be found in the Czech Republic, where a reduction in number of Czech physicians was accompanied by salary increases, and in Poland, capitated primary care physicians, who were the highest paid, were the only ones not making additional charges.[48]

The challenges facing CEE and CIS countries regarding informal payments are great. They represent an important source of revenue in countries in which pre-payment systems have collapsed, so phasing them out without developing suitable alternatives may be damaging. It is clear that multiple, concurrent strategies are needed to eliminate informal payments and to convince the population that good-quality health services can be available without paying under the table. The first step is for governments to acknowledge the existence and full impact of informal payments and to develop more appropriate and affordable benefits packages, and information and monitoring systems with genuine penalties for infringement. This is also contingent upon the existence of political will to address corruption and lack of transparency in broader public policy.

Notes

1. Sara Allin is a research officer in health policy at LSE Health and Social Care, London School of Economics and Political Science, and at the European Observatory on Health Systems and Policies. Konstantina Davaki is a research officer in health and social policy at LSE Health and Social Care. Elias Mossialos is a professor of health policy in the Department of Social Policy, London School of Economics and Political Science, co-director of LSE Health and Social Care and research director of the European Observatory on Health Systems and Policies.
2. J. Killingsworth, *Formal and Informal Fees for Health Care* (Manila: WHO Regional Office for the Western Pacific, 2003).
3. P. Gaál and M. McKee, 'Informal Payment for Health Care and the Theory of "INXIT"', *International Journal of Health Planning and Management* 19, 2004.
4. J. Healy and M. McKee, 'Health Sector Reform in Central and Eastern Europe', *Health Policy and Planning* 12(4), 1997.
5. To our knowledge, no country explicitly accepts informal payments in their legislation, though countries vary in the degree to which restrictions are enforced. In Bulgaria, for example, official attitudes to informal payments are ambiguous; between 1989 and 1997 there was no formal ban and a 1997 decree outlining services for which a fee applied left provisions vague and subject to local discretion (D. Balabanova and M. McKee, 'Understanding Informal Payments for Health Care: The Example of Bulgaria', *Health Policy* 62, 2002).
6. T. Vian, K. Gryboski, Z. Sinoimeri and R. H. Clifford, *Informal Payments in the Public Health Sector in Albania: A Qualitative Study* (Bethesda, US: Partners for Health Reformplus Project, Abt Associates, Inc., 2004).
7. M. Lewis, 'Who is Paying for Health Care in Eastern Europe and Central Asia?' (Washington, DC: World Bank, 2000).
8. P. Belli, G. Gotsadze and H. Shahriari, 'Out-of-pocket and Informal Payments in the Health Sector: Evidence from Georgia', *Health Policy* 70, 2004.
9. Lewis, 'Who is Paying for Health Care?'
10. J. Falkingham, 'Poverty, Out-of-pocket Payments and Access to Health Care: Evidence from Tajikistan', *Social Science and Medicine* 58, 2004.
11. M. E. Bonilla-Chacin, *Health and Poverty in Albania: Background Paper for the Albania Poverty Assessment, Europe and Central Asia Sector for Human Development* (Washington, DC: World Bank, 2003).
12. L. Vagac and L. Haulikova, *Study on the Social Protection Systems in the 13 Applicant Countries: Slovak Republic Country Report* (Brussels: Commission of European Communities, 2003).
13. Ibid.
14. D. Balabanova and M. McKee, 'Understanding Informal Payments for Health Care: The Example of Bulgaria', *Health Policy* 62, 2002.
15. P. Belli, *Formal and Informal Household Spending on Health: A Multi-country Study in Central and Eastern Europe* (Cambridge, MA: Harvard School of Public Health, 2003).
16. V. Mihai, *Study on the Social Protection Systems in the 13 Applicant Countries: Romania Country Report* (Brussels: Commission of the European Communities, 2003).
17. Vagac and Haulikova, *Study on the Social Protection Systems: Slovak Republic*.
18. Balabanova and McKee, 'Understanding Informal Payments for Health Care'.
19. J. Falkingham, 'Barriers to Access? The Growth of Private Payments for Health Care in Kyrgyzstan', *EuroHealth* 4, 1998/99.
20. T. Ensor and L. Savelyeva, 'Informal Payments for Health Care in the Former Soviet Union: Some Evidence from Kazakhstan', *Health Policy and Planning* 13(1), 1998.
21. M. Chawla, P. Berman and D. Kawiorska, 'Financing Health Services in Poland: New Evidence on Private Expenditures', *Health Economics* 7, 1998.
22. T. Ensor, 'Informal Payments for Health Care in Transition Economies', *Social Science and Medicine* 58, 2004.
23. E. Delcheva, D. Balabanova and M. McKee, 'Under-the-counter Payments for Health Care: Evidence from Bulgaria', *Health Policy* 42, 1997.

24. Falkingham, 'Barriers to Access?'
25. W. L. Miller, A. B. Grodeland and T. Y. Koshechkina, 'If You Pay, We'll Operate Immediately', *Journal of Medical Ethics* 26, 2000.
26. Ibid.
27. E. Mossialos, S. Allin and K. Davaki, 'Analyzing the Greek Health System: A Story of Fragmentation and Inertia', *Health Economics* 14(51), 2005.
28. Ensor, 'Informal Payments for Health Care in Transition Economies'.
29. R. Thompson and A. Xavier, *Unofficial Payments for Acute State Hospital Care In Kazakhstan. A Model of Physician Behaviour with Price Discrimination and Vertical Service Differentiation.* Discussion Paper 124/2002 (Brussels: LICOS Centre for Transition Economics, 2002).
30. Belli et al., 'Out-of-pocket and Informal Payments'.
31. Lewis, 'Who is Paying for Health Care?'
32. G. Gotsadze, S. Bennett, K. Ranson and D. Gzirishvili 'Health Care-seeking Behaviour and Out-of-pocket Payments in Tbilisi, Georgia', *Health Policy and Planning* 20(4), 2005; Belli et al., 'Out-of-pocket and Informal Payments'.
33. A. Sari, J. Langenbrunner and M. Lewis, 'Affording Out-of-pocket Payments for Health Care Services: Evidence from Kazakhstan', *Eurohealth* 6(2), 2000.
34. Lewis, 'Who is Paying for Health Care?'
35. Ibid.
36. D. Balabanova, M. McKee, J. Pomerleau, R. Rose and C. Haerpfer, 'Health Service Utilisation in the Former Soviet Union: Evidence from Eight Countries', *Health Services Research* 39, 2004.
37. Belli et al., 'Out-of-pocket and Informal Payments'.
38. Lewis, 'Who is Paying for Health Care?'
39. Belli et al., 'Out-of-pocket and Informal Payments'; Balabanova and McKee, 'Understanding Informal Payments for Health Care'.
40. A. Mills and S. Bennett, 'Lessons on Sustainability from Middle to Lower Income Countries' in E. Mossialos, A. Dixon, J. Figueras and J. Kutzin (eds) *Funding Health Care: Options for Europe* (Buckingham: Open University Press, 2002).
41. Balabanova and McKee, 'Understanding Informal Payments for Health Care'.
42. A. Dobravolskas and R. Huivydas, *Study on the Social Protection Systems of the 13 Applicant Countries: Lithuania* (Brussels: Commission of the European Communities, 2003).
43. M. Rokosová, P. Háva, J. Schreyögg and R. Busse, *Health Care Systems in Transition: Czech Republic* (Copenhagen, WHO Regional Office for Europe on behalf of the European Observatory on Health Systems and Policies, 2005).
44. E. Mossialos and S. Thomson, 'Voluntary Health Insurance in the European Union: A Critical Assessment', *International Journal of Health Services* 32(1), 2002.
45. Vagac and Haulikova, *Study on the Social Protection Systems: Slovak Republic.*
46. Dobravolskas and Huivydas, *Study on the Social Protection Systems: Lithuania.*
47. Mihai, *Study on the Social Protection Systems: Romania.*
48. Lewis, 'Who is Paying for Health Care?'

Gift, fee or bribe? Informal payments in Hungary

Péter Gaál[1]

After 15 years of reform, informal payments for health care, a legacy of the socialist health care system, still generate heated debates in Hungary. In 2004, a young father set up a website, halapenz.hu,[2] where parents of newborn babies were invited to share their experiences about the obstetrician that delivered the baby, including how much they paid for the service. What makes this story remarkable is that Hungary has a social insurance system in which virtually everybody is entitled to receive almost all health services, free of charge. The doctors who appeared on the list were quick to react, demanding the website be shut down – which was unsurprising since such payments are subject to income tax and should have been declared. The case attracted strong media attention, especially when the website was shut down after the ombudsman said it violated the doctors' right to privacy. The incident sparked an intense debate about the legality of informal payments, the motivation of the patients and whether or not the practice should be banned. But after a couple of months, interest faded and it was back to business as usual.

How widespread are informal payments?

Research has shown consistently that informal payments are widespread in the health sector in Hungary, but the findings vary widely as to the magnitude. An analysis of available data shows that the share of informal payments was 1.5–4.5 per cent of total health care expenditure in Hungary in 2001.[3] This amounts to 1–3.5 per cent of yearly net income for the average household, even if we take into account that only one-third of households reported expenditures on informal payments in 2001.[4] This does not seem much in comparison with other former communist countries, where the majority of health expenditures are informal payments (see 'Paying for free health care', page 64).

To understand the impact of informal payments, however, the aggregate total of money is less important than its distribution. Surveys in Hungary have shown that 90 per cent of payments go to medical doctors and to particular specialities and services, with deliveries and surgical procedures being the best 'paid'.[5] Using the low estimate and distributing the amount equally among doctors in specialities where informal payments exist, income from informal payments contributes about 60–75 per cent of physicians' official net salary. This suggests that the significance of informal payments stems not from their overall magnitude but from the consequences of their unequal distribution. The case of Hungary shows that policy-makers should not ignore the phenomenon of informal payments, even though the total sums involved are small.

The pressure to pay

Determining whether informal payments are fees, gifts or bribes is important in determining what can be done to curb them but, more importantly, whether they should be eliminated at all.[6] It is not easy to dismiss the donation explanation of informal payments. In Hungary, many surveys found that the majority of patients paid the doctor out of gratitude, or at least the majority said they were motivated by gratitude when they made the payment.[7] On the other hand, a more thorough analysis reveals subtle contradictions, which indicate that surveys are not always the best tool to capture patients' true motivation.

Indeed, in our survey, follow-up interviews with respondents reveal that the motivation behind informal payments is multifaceted and that even in apparently straightforward cases of gratitude payment there is always pressure to pay.[8] For instance, patients take it for granted that a chosen doctor must be paid extra or, in certain cases, patients feel that they must give something, if the doctor pays more than usual attention. These findings suggest that informal payment is rarely motivated by gratitude alone. Yet despite the arguments against it, the gratitude motive has deeply infiltrated the explanation of the phenomenon in Hungary and is stubbornly adhered to by patients, doctors and policy-makers alike.

At the systemic level, informal payments can rather be explained as the response of patients and doctors to the shortages generated by the state's socialist health care system. Though several systemic features contributed to this shortage, the most notable was the low salaries of health care professionals. Low salaries alone created shortage, either because doctors lowered their performance ('No one can expect me to work hard for such a low remuneration!') or because they had to take part-time jobs and made patients suspicious about the quality of the provided service ('Can I be certain that this overworked doctor will provide me with the service I need?'). Taking into account the information asymmetry between patients and doctors, low salaries could also erode trust ('Is it realistic to expect this underpaid doctor to do everything to cure me?'). Hence shortage does not need to be real to generate informal payments.

Lessons from the Hungarian experience

Informal payments in Hungary seem to stem from a reaction by dissatisfied patients and doctors to the shortage generated by the socialist health care system, which was long on promise and short on delivery. Patients and doctors adapted to the situation by reinterpreting the declared but unfulfilled official entitlement to comprehensive high-quality care and a decent salary for honest work. Where the reassessment of patients and doctors coincided, a new, unwritten set of entitlements emerged.

The health sector reforms of the past 15 years have not fundamentally changed this set-up. Informal payments continue to be a challenging problem for health policy since they have the embedded incentives of a fee-for-service policy, without the transparency and control of formal out-of-pocket payments. Neither taxing informal payments nor legally enforcing non-payment are viable policy options since both patients and doctors have seen unrealistic rules flouted. Successful policies have to tackle shortage in the health sector, either by curtailing the generous benefits package and/or incorporating additional funds by formalising informal payments as co-payments.[9]

Mapping informal payments could help in the design of a co-payment system that would be accepted by the population, but it cannot be assumed that the existence of a formal out-of-pocket payment system will necessarily prevent patients from paying extra. Indeed, payment is likely to continue until patients are wholly convinced the system will deliver effective care without additional incentives. Hence attempts to eliminate informal payments require concerted action to rebuild the lost trust in health care. Local initiatives such as the Hungarian care coordination pilot,[10] which builds on partnership and participation, can help to re-establish the trust-based relationship between the public and physicians, and thus provide a different set of expectations for their future encounters.[11] Under this programme, local health care providers (doctors, clinics or hospitals) assume responsibility for the whole spectrum of care for residents in their area, and they are provided with data on their patients by the national health insurance fund to monitor actual service utilisation.

Nevertheless, any reforms have to take into account the political complexities of the current system, as well as the resistance that will inevitably ensue if attempts to eliminate informal payments are made. Though important, recognising that the concept of 'gratitude payment' is no more than a convenient myth that has been used to make an unacceptable phenomenon acceptable is only the first step towards the formulation of more effective policies in this area.

Notes

1. Péter Gaál is assistant professor at the Health Services Management Training Centre, at Semmelweiss University, Hungary.
2. *Hálapénz* is the Hungarian term for informal payment. It literally translates to 'gratitude payment'.
3. Péter Gaál, *Informal Payments for Health Care in Hungary* (London: London School of Hygiene and Tropical Medicine, University of London, 2004).
4. Hungarian Central Statistical Office, *Yearbook of Household Statistics 2001* (Budapest: Hungarian Central Statistical Office, 2002).
5. For a summary of these surveys, see Péter Gaál, Tamas Evetovits and Martin McKee, 'Informal Payment for Health Care: Evidence from Hungary', *Health Policy* (forthcoming).
6. Péter Gaál and Martin McKee, 'Fee-for-service or Donation? Hungarian Perspectives on Informal Payment for Health Care', *Social Science and Medicine* 60, 2005.
7. For a summary of the findings of surveys see Gaál, *Informal Payments for Health Care in Hungary.*
8. Ibid.
9. Péter Gaál and Martin McKee, 'Informal Payments for Health Care and the Theory of "Inxit"', *International Journal of Health Planning and Management* 19, 2004.
10. Péter Gaál, *Health Care Systems in Transition: Hungary* (Copenhagen: WHO Regional Office for Europe on behalf of the European Observatory on Health Systems and Policies, 2004).
11. Gaál and McKee, 'Fee-for-service or Donation?'

Box 4.1   Informal payments take a toll on Moroccan patients

'My husband injured his hand at work and was taken to a public hospital. He had to pay 300 dirhams (US $33) to get an X-ray and 200 to have the injury stitched. He then had to pay another 500 dirhams just to be allowed to stay in the hospital.'

(Woman interviewed in Casablanca)

'When my wife went to the hospital they examined her and prescribed some pills. They said that none were available there, but if we paid 20 or 30 dirhams (US $2–3), someone could provide the "free medication". The problem is, we can't afford the drugs.'

(Man interviewed in Casablanca)

▶

Four out of five people interviewed in a Transparency International (TI) Morocco survey in 2002 described corruption in the public health system as 'common to very common'.[1] Morocco has a system of 'poverty certificates', designed to guarantee the poor access to basic care, but this system has been prone to corruption and a market for obtaining the certificates has developed. The health minister summed up the problem by admitting that '56 per cent of those that have the means to pay are benefiting from public hospitals, while 15 per cent of the country's poorest are paying out of their pockets'.[2]

According to TI Morocco's study, which surveyed 1,000 households,[3] of those who had been in contact with members of the public health service, 40 per cent admitted to making an illicit payment for a service or supply that was supposed to be free. Of those who required hospital treatment, 59 per cent admitted to paying to be examined or admitted into hospital, while 26 per cent paid for treatment. When asked whether the payments had achieved results, 81 per cent said that the expected result had been reached, compared to 3 per cent who claimed that the 'bribe' was ineffectual. This 'success' rate has to be qualified by the fact that 85 per cent of citizens who paid bribes to public health officials were entitled by law to receive the service for free. The average size of the bribe was 140 dirhams (US $15).

While informal payments can be seen as a coping mechanism for poorly paid health workers, everyone pays for corruption in this sector. Citizens who do not consent to making informal payments do not receive access to care. Public hospitals pay because potential revenue is lost, goes unrecorded or is diverted into the hands of medical staff who abuse their position to extort from patients, and equipment and medicines are wasted or are sub-standard. The credibility and perceived integrity of health personnel suffers. The cost for the state is a failed public health policy.

To remedy this situation, hospital staff must be made aware of the duties they have to their patients, and both health system workers and users must be made aware of patients' rights. Pay structures and working conditions in hospitals must be re-evaluated and whistleblowers who denounce corrupt practices need protection.

Azeddine Akesbi, Siham Benchekroun and Kamal El Mesbahi (TI Morocco)

Notes
1. TI Morocco, *La Corruption au Maroc, Synthèse des résultats des enquêtes d'intégrité* (Corruption in Morocco, a summary of the National Integrity System survey) (Rabat: TI Morocco, 2002). The interviews cited here are from a focus group discussion.
2. *La Vie Economique* (Morocco), 4 February 2005.
3. Of the 1,000 interviewed, 80 per cent came from big cities and 20 per cent from rural municipalities. Of those surveyed 79 per cent were men and 21 per cent were women.

5 Corruption in the pharmaceutical sector

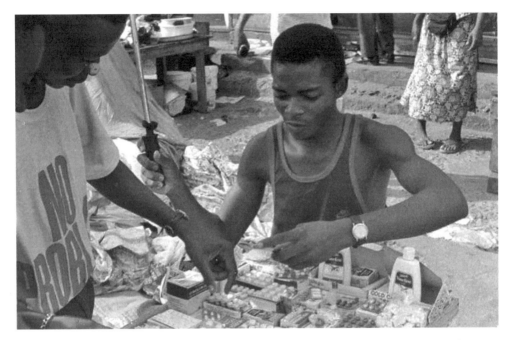

A young medicine vendor from a so-called 'ground pharmacy' offers black market drugs to clients in a street in Libreville, Gabon, 29 August 2003. (Desirey Minkoh/AFP/Getty Images)

The pharmaceutical sector faces many challenges that are not addressed in this volume, including patterns of research and patent systems that do not seem to be meeting all public health needs, particularly in eradicating devastating tropical diseases. Corruption adds a potentially deadly element when patients cannot afford extortion payments for the drugs they need, or they are sold counterfeit medicines.

In this chapter, Jillian Clare Cohen argues that heavy government regulation in the pharmaceutical chain – while essential to safeguard the population against sub-standard drugs and unfairly priced goods – makes this sector particularly prone to corruption. In recent years, much discussion has centred on the close ties between physicians and the pharmaceutical, biotechnology and medical device industries – which, when unchecked, can lead to corrupt practices. Jerome Kassirer highlights the conflicts of interest that may arise when doctors feel indebted to drugs representatives, or when scientists are on the payroll of companies whose drugs they are hired to evaluate.

Efforts are being made to improve the situation. Representatives of the pharmaceutical industry and of physicians describe the voluntary codes set up to reduce potential conflicts of interest. Civil society and concerted efforts by courageous regulators can help curb corruption in the pharmaceutical industries – both legal and counterfeit – as the experiences from India, Thailand and Nigeria show.

Pharmaceuticals and corruption: a risk assessment
Jillian Clare Cohen[1]

Pharmaceuticals are indispensable to health systems. They can complement other types of health care services to reduce morbidity and mortality rates and enhance quality of life for many patients. Because pharmaceuticals have curative and therapeutic qualities, they cannot be regarded simply as ordinary commodities. Access to medicines is often about life and death. This is illustrated most dramatically in sub-Saharan Africa where almost 30 million people are infected with HIV/AIDS and the majority lack access to anti-retroviral therapies.

In a broader context, access to essential medicines has become a central topic at the international policy-making level where it is increasingly viewed as a fundamental right, with human rights law placing obligations on states to ensure access.[2] This includes duties on governments to ensure that pharmaceutical systems are institutionally sound and transparent and that there are appropriate mechanisms to reduce the likelihood of corruption, which can deny medicines to those in greatest need.

A major conundrum in international drug policy is the fact that, despite international aid and a plethora of programmes devoted to improving pharmaceutical access, there is a morally worrying 'drug gap'. The WHO continues to estimate that one-third of the global population lacks regular access to essential medicines.[3] A number of determinants contribute to this drug gap, including market failures, government inefficiencies, poverty and corruption.

For example, OECD countries generally devote US $239 in annual spending on drugs per head, compared to less than US $20 in developing countries and US $6 in sub-Saharan Africa.[4] Pharmaceuticals are the largest public health expenditure after personnel costs in most low-income states, and often the largest household health expenditure of all.[5] One of the most important differences between industrialised and developing countries is that in the latter pharmaceutical expenditures are anywhere from 50–90 per cent of total individual out-of-pocket expenditures.[6] In such countries, illness is a major cause of household poverty. Corruption exacerbates this drug gap: when officials accept kickbacks for purchasing medicines, pharmaceutical expenditure is reduced and fewer of the right drugs get to the right people when they need them.

Many determinants are responsible for disparities in access to medicines, but little research has been devoted to just how corruption impacts on drug availability. Fortunately, this area is gaining interest and a number of studies have begun to address this issue.[7] The pharmaceutical system is susceptible to corruption for a variety of reasons. One of the most significant is the degree of government involvement in its regulation: studies from other sectors have found that the incidence of corruption is noticeably higher when the state retains a major involvement in the economy and its bureaucracy is pervasive.[8] Without robust institutional checks, government regulators can make discretionary decisions rather than decisions based on uniform criteria. In addition, wide information asymmetries exist between patient and physician (see Chapter 1). Patients trust their doctor to prescribe the most effective drug for their condition, but the doctor's decision as to which drugs to prescribe may be influenced by pressure from pharmaceutical companies. There are often poorly documented processes in the quality control system that can lead to the manufacture of sub-standard drugs. This occurred in Brazil when a well known pharmaceutical manufacturer was found to

---

Box 5.1 US pharmaceutical company fined for payments to charity headed by Polish health official[1]

In June 2004, the pharmaceutical company Schering-Plough agreed with the Securities and Exchange Commission (SEC) to pay a fine of US $500,000 for violations of the books and records and internal controls provisions of the Foreign Corrupt Practices Act (FCPA).

According to the SEC's findings, the Polish subsidiary of the New Jersey-based company, Schering-Plough Poland (S-P Poland), made payments amounting to approximately US $76,000 between February 1999 and March 2002 to a foundation for the restoration of Silesian castles, the Chudow Castle Foundation. The foundation was run by the director of the Silesian Health Fund,[2] one of 16 regional state-run Polish health authorities which provides funding for the purchase of pharmaceutical products by hospitals and other medical centres.

The SEC alleged that these payments were made to induce the director to buy S-P Poland's products for his health fund. It alleged that, in order to conceal the nature of the payments, the S-P Poland manager deliberately set them at or below his approval limit and provided false medical justifications for them in documents submitted to the parent company's finance department.

Although the SEC conceded that the foundation was a bona fide charity and that the donations were made without the knowledge or approval of the US parent company, it charged that the parent's internal controls were inadequate to detect and prevent the financial irregularities committed by its Polish subsidiary. Although the SEC did not go so far as to state that the payments were bribes, it did find that the manager viewed them as necessary, in order to influence the action of the government official.

This case highlights that companies should not only have clear policies covering charitable donations, their permitted amount and approval procedures, but should conduct due diligence across their organisation. The case also underscores the aggressive stance of the SEC in holding suppliers accountable for the actions of their subsidiaries.

Transparency International

Notes
1. This text is based on Wilmer Cutler Pickering Hale and Dorr LLP, *Foreign Corrupt Practices Update*, 30 June 2004, www.wilmerhale.com
2. *Rzeczpospolita* (Poland), 11 June 2004.

---

have manufactured sub-standard contraceptives.[9] Finally, the pharmaceutical market is so lucrative that it attracts entrepreneurs who are both honest and, more perplexingly, dishonest. All of these factors expose the pharmaceutical system to the possibility of corruption.

This essay focuses primarily on the role of government, since state intervention, particularly through regulation, is vital to the pharmaceutical sector. There are two central reasons why governments regulate the pharmaceutical market: first, to ensure that health policy and other governmental interventions, such as quality assurance of drugs and fair drug pricing, enhance the health of the population; and second, to ensure that industrial policies strengthen economic competitiveness of the pharmaceutical sector and improve innovation and efficiency. These two objectives can sometimes lie at cross-purposes. If regulators are subject to pressure from commercial groups, health objectives can be compromised.

Key decision points

The pharmaceutical system is technically complex and replete with a number of 'core decision points'.[10] Each decision point needs to function optimally so that the system as a whole offers good-quality, cost-effective, safe and efficacious medicines. Figure 5.1 shows key processes in the selection and delivery of pharmaceutical products and illustrates the potential for corruption that exists at any one of its decision points (post-manufacturing) unless there are solid institutional checks and balances in place. For example, procurement is particularly susceptible to corruption unless there are open bidding processes, good technical specifications, and consistent and transparent

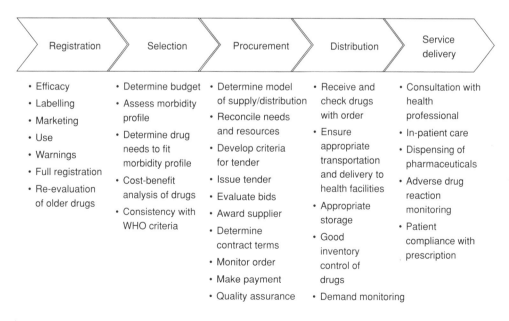

Figure 5.1: Key processes in the selection and delivery of pharmaceutical products

procedures for redress if needed. While the design of good institutions with oversight is crucial for the reduction of corruption, there is also a significant role for civil society. If community groups closely monitor pharmaceutical companies and regulators, there is a greater likelihood that corruption can be caught or even prevented out of fear of disclosure (see Boxes 5.2 and 5.3).

Registration

The first decision point in the pharmaceutical chain is registration, which was originally introduced to protect patients from catastrophes like the thalidomide cases in the 1950s, and evaluates a drug's efficacy against a specific disease and its possible side-effects. The process regulates the labelling, marketing, usage, warning and prescription requirements for a drug. Registration procedures need to be transparent and applied uniformly, and should leave no room for individual discretion. The registration process should guarantee drug safety and efficacy, but these guarantees risk being eroded by the pharmaceutical industry lobby. A high-profile inquiry into risks posed by the pain pills Vioxx, Bextra and Celbrex in 2004 highlighted already existing concerns regarding the US Food and Drug Administration's (FDA's) capacity as an unbiased regulatory body (see 'The corrupting influence of money in medicine', page 88). Critics point to the fact that between 1997 and 2004, 12 major prescription drugs, with a market value of billions of dollars, were recalled by the FDA or withdrawn by companies. According to Sheldon Krimsky of Tufts University, the rise in for-profit clinical trials, fast-tracking of drug approvals, government–industry partnerships, direct consumer advertising and industry-funded salaries for FDA regulators has contributed to degrading the institutional integrity of the FDA, suggests 'regulatory capture' of the FDA by the pharmaceutical industry to some degree and also illuminates the need for the institution to demonstrate more independence from its stakeholders.[11] Meanwhile, in low-income countries, regulatory agencies are often weak or non-existent due to lack of resources.

Selection

Drug selection processes should ensure that the most cost-effective and appropriate drugs for a population's health needs are chosen fairly. The WHO Model List of Essential Medicines is a helpful framework in this regard for most developing countries because it establishes priority areas of treatment and covers the most common diseases.[12] But this can open a new avenue for corruption since manufacturers have a strong interest in getting their products selected as essential medicines. If institutions are weak and individuals have incentives to engage in corrupt activities, the selection process can be replete with kickbacks and payoffs so that drugs on a national drug list may not necessarily reflect appropriate and cost-effective drugs (see 'Corruption in hospital administration', Chapter 3, page 51).

However, there are methods that can reduce the likelihood of corruption in the selection process and promote sound, evidence-based decision-making. The pharmaco-economic techniques used by Australia and the Canadian province of British Columbia have proved helpful in ensuring that objective decision-making takes place if the correct models and techniques are employed. Pharmaco-economics, or outcomes research, uses cost-benefit, cost-effectiveness and cost-utility analyses to compare the economics of different pharmaceutical products, or to compare drug therapies with other medical treatments.

Drug selection committees must be composed of impartial persons with the appropriate technical skills. Their members must be obliged to declare any conflicts of interest, and meetings should be regular and well publicised so that the public can observe proceedings. Minutes of meetings should be posted on the Internet and decisions clearly justified. In the event of a potential breach, an appeal process must be in place that ensures due process.

Final selection criteria should be based on discussions and acceptance by key prescribers, and the WHO criteria for selection should be used as a basis for decision-making. These are: relevance to the pattern of prevalent diseases; proven efficacy and safety; evidence of performance in a variety of settings; adequate quality, including bio-availability and stability; favourable cost-benefit ratio in terms of total treatment cost; and preferences for drugs that are well known to have good pharmaco-kinetic properties. Lastly, all drugs listed on a government essential medicines list should be identified by generic name.

Procurement

Procurement is the principal interface between the public system and drug suppliers, and its goal is to acquire the right quantity of drugs in the most cost-effective manner. This involves inventory management, aggregate purchasing, public bidding contests, technical analysis of offers, proper allocation of resources, payments, receipts of drugs purchased and quality control checks.

Procurement is often poorly documented and processed, which makes it an easy target for corruption. Drug procurement is even more vulnerable to corruption than contracting in other sectors. This is due to several factors, including: the method to determine the volume of drugs needed is often subjective; there are difficulties in monitoring quality standards in drug provision; suppliers use different prices for the same pharmaceutical products and can artificially inflate prices; some marketing practices by pharmaceutical companies induce demand for products; and an additional challenge is posed by emergency situations, which call for speedy and adequate intervention.

The best protection against corruption is open, competitive procurement that prevents personal discretion in the selection of suppliers, and requires clear criteria for the selection and process of winning bids. However, procurement procedures require ongoing monitoring, including reviews from the inspector general's office.[13]

Strong oversight mechanisms can drastically reduce corruption. A World Bank study from 2001 examined the use of an electronic bidding system for pharmaceutical purchases in Chile.[14] Contrasting the innovative Chilean system to other procurement practices, the authors argued that outcomes are greatly improved by the adoption of good incentive structures for public officials and the reduction of informational asymmetries through the posting of drug prices on the Internet.

A comprehensive study of corruption in the pharmaceutical system in Costa Rica found that in many cases competition was reduced, or procedures were followed incorrectly.[15] Some health care professionals and pharmaceutical company executives alleged that participants in public tenders had on occasion colluded to extend the purchasing cycle as long as possible. This was done by submitting frivolous appeals, which were then extensively contested by both sides, or by delaying the delivery of drugs for unfounded reasons. The effect of these long delays was the eventual depletion of the social security system's inventory resulting in direct purchases from private suppliers. These purchases were then made at much higher unit prices than would be obtained through formal bidding processes. Studies from Argentina and Bolivia show that increased transparency and citizen participation in the procurement process can reduce corruption and cut costs considerably (see 'Corruption in hospital administration', page 52).

Distribution

Distribution in the pharmaceutical system ensures drugs are allocated, transported and stored appropriately at all points where they are to be dispensed. This involves central and regional warehouses, pharmacies and service floors. Information must flow easily through every level of the system to control inventory movements and deliveries. In addition, the system requires storage facilities, including refrigeration units, to guarantee the integrity of the drugs and good security to minimise the risk of theft. The electronic monitoring of transport vehicles and careful checking of delivery orders against inventories of products delivered are some of the methods that can reduce this likelihood.

In one Central American country, inventory records showed that stocks of oral antibiotic eye treatment and other products were intentionally oversupplied because government purchasers received commissions for their orders.[16] This demonstrates one way that corruption can drain public expenditure on pharmaceuticals and have the greatest impact on the poor.

Service delivery

Service delivery involves the participation of physicians, pharmacists, nurses and other health care providers who diagnose patients and identify what drugs a patient should consume to treat a particular disease. This is the decision point at which patients should experience the benefits of the entire system. Here physicians prescribe, pharmacists dispense and nurses administer drugs to treat patients. Health providers ideally utilise evidence-based practice to provide effective therapy to their patients.

The interface between the pharmaceutical industry and physicians is an area that is particularly susceptible to corruption, as service delivery can be influenced by the marketing practices of the pharmaceutical industry (see 'The corrupting influence of money in medicine', page 86).

Some physician–industry interaction is necessary to educate doctors about the therapeutic qualities of new drugs. However, there is compelling evidence that suggests that the motivation is often not health education, but profit maximisation. A 2000 study by Wazana found that physician interaction with the pharmaceutical industry was associated with increased requests for additional drugs on hospital formularies and changes in prescribing practice.[17] The influence of industry on physicians is an issue of concern in both developed and developing countries. But it can be particularly dangerous in developing and transition countries where doctors make paltry salaries and may rely heavily on gifts (both monetary and material) from the pharmaceutical industry to supplement their livelihood.

The US authorities have recently demonstrated concerted efforts to address inappropriate marketing practices by some pharmaceutical companies. In 2001, TAP Pharmaceutical Products was required to pay one of the largest fines in the industry's history, with the government demanding US $875 million for civil liabilities and criminal charges.[18] Other governments are introducing stricter laws and regulations. For example, in April 2005 a report by the UK's House of Commons Health Select Committee on 'The Influence of the Pharmaceutical Industry' recommended greater transparency in drug regulation processes, reduction in the excessive promotion of medicines, tougher restrictions on physicians to avoid inappropriate prescribing and an end to Department of Health relationships with the drugs industry in favour of the Department of Trade and Industry.[19] Following press accounts of the free trips pharmaceutical companies offer medical doctors and the lavish parties thrown for them, the Deputy Mayor of Social Affairs and Public Health of Helsinki, Paula Kokkonen, banned all trips funded by the pharmaceutical industry for the capital's medical doctors.[20]

In view of the potential for undue influence on prescribing behaviour, global standards have been developed and a number of professional bodies, including pharmaceutical industry associations, have enacted codes of conduct that detail best practice in minimising corruption (see 'Promoting trust and transparency in pharmaceutical companies', page 92, and 'Fighting corruption: the role of the medical profession', page 94). Whether such guidelines have made an impact is questionable. The WHO issued its Ethical Criteria for Medicinal Drug Promotion in 1988, but a 1997 WHO roundtable discussion concluded that inappropriate drug promotion is still a problem in developing and industrialised countries.[21] Even though the criteria have been disseminated widely, their effective implementation is a major problem, as governments need to revise legislation and regulation, and to promote them forcefully in medical schools and associations.

While self-regulatory codes of conduct may be beneficial, they should not delay meaningful reform in terms of external, enforceable regulations. Current voluntary codes are not audited or enforced with meaningful penalties, or overseen by independent and objective observers.[22] More robust policies are needed to address the serious conflicts of interest that arise in the service delivery segment of the pharmaceutical system.

Counterfeit medicines: the bad and the ugly

When institutions are weak and unable to regulate the pharmaceutical sector accurately, they increase the opportunities for corruption, including the manufacture of counterfeit drugs, a problem that precedes the first decision point in the pharmaceutical chain in Figure 5.1. For example, regulators may receive kickbacks to ignore makers of counterfeit products, or customs agents may be paid to turn a blind eye to their import or export.

In 2001, China had roughly 500 illegal medicine manufacturers and Laos around 2,100 illegal medicine sellers. In Thailand, sub-standard medicines account for 8.5 per cent of those on the market.[23] India plans to introduce the death penalty for the manufacture or sale of counterfeit medicines that cause grievous harm. 'Profiting from spurious drugs that might harm or kill innocent people is equivalent to mass murder', said Health Minister Sushma Swaraj recently.[24] Meanwhile, an estimated 192,000 people died last year in China because of fake drugs.[25] Regulatory bodies in the South need resources to root out corruption and stem the flow of counterfeit drugs. The success of Nigeria's National Agency for Food and Drug Administration and Control is one example of what can be achieved through strong leadership (see page 96).

Moving forward: how to do better?

Corruption in any one of the critical decision points in the pharmaceutical system can be harmful to a country's ability to improve the health of its population by limiting access to high-quality medicines and reducing the gains associated with their proper usage. While corruption affects the entire population, it is typically the poor who are most susceptible when officials hoard drugs, or waste resources on the wrong kind of medicines. Good governance is therefore a sine qua non for ensuring better access to essential medicines.

Greater transparency in the pharmaceutical system will help to improve drug access. Honest assessment of the institutional robustness at all core decision points in the pharmaceutical system is the first necessity. Governments need to know what areas of the system are less than optimal and vulnerable to corruption. There is a need for more monitoring of how pharmacies, hospitals and health care providers are reimbursed for drugs. Further research is needed to determine what systems offer the best incentives for providers to behave honestly and control fraud. Second, consumer groups and other third parties need to be vigilant about monitoring both the public and private pharmaceutical systems to ensure they are directed towards the public interest.

While international statements and professional guidelines on best practice are well intentioned, they are meaningless unless they are properly enforced. Individual governments must have the courage to enact and, most importantly, to implement policies and processes which encourage ethical behaviour and punish firms and individuals for corrupt actions. If this happens, hopefully we will see a change for the better in terms of ensuring that people in need get the right drugs at the right time.

Notes

1. Jillian Clare Cohen is assistant professor in the Leslie Dan Faculty of Pharmacy at the University of Toronto and Director of the Comparative Program on Health and Society at the University of Toronto's Munk Centre for International Studies.

2. Philippe Cullet, 'Patents and Medicines: the Relationship between TRIPS and the Human Right to Health', *International Affairs* 79(1), 2003.
3. Michael R. Reich, 'The Global Drug Gap', *Science* 287(5460), 1979–81, 17 March 2000.
4. *WHO Medicines Strategy: Framework for Action in Essential Drugs and Medicines Policy 2002–2003.* (Geneva: WHO, 2000), www.who.int/medicines/strategy/strategy.pdf
5. Ramesh Govindaraj, Michael Reich and Jillian Clare Cohen, 'World Bank Pharmaceuticals Discussion Paper' (Washington DC: World Bank, 2000).
6. Ibid.
7. For example, the World Bank, the WHO and USAID have all commissioned studies in recent years on the issue of corruption in the pharmaceutical system.
8. Ian E. Marshall, 'A Survey of Corruption Issues in the Mining and Mineral Sector', Mining, Minerals and Sustainable Development Project (London: International Institute for Environment and Development, 2001).
9. Jillian Clare Cohen, 'Public Policies in the Pharmaceutical System: The Case of Brazil', (Washington DC: World Bank, 2000).
10. This section borrows heavily from Jillian Clare Cohen, James Cercone and Roman Mayaca, 'Improving Transparency in the Pharmaceutical System: The Case of Costa Rica', internal study, World Bank, October 2002.
11. Sheldon Krimsky, 'A Dose of Reform: But Do the FDA's Actions Go Far Enough?' *The Star Ledger*, 20 February 2005.
12. See www.who.int/medicines/publications/essentialmedicines/en/
13. USAID, 'A Handbook on Fighting Corruption', Center for Democracy and Governance (Washington, DC: USAID, 1999).
14. Jillian Clare Cohen and Jorge Carikeo Montoya, 'Using Technology to Fight Corruption in Pharmaceutical Purchasing: Lessons Learned from the Chilean Experience' (Washington, DC: World Bank Institute, 2001).
15. Cohen et al., 'Improving Transparency in the Pharmaceutical System'.
16. Management Sciences for Health, with the WHO, *Managing Drug Supply* (West Hartford, US: Kumarian Press, 1997).
17. Ashley Wazana, 'Physicians and the Pharmaceutical Industry: Is a Gift Ever Just a Gift?', *Journal of the American Medical Association* 283(3), 19 January 2000.
18. US Department of Justice, press release, 1 October 2001. Available at: www.usdoj.gov/opa/pr/2001/October/513civ.htm See also 'Corruption in hospital administration', Chapter 3, page 51.
19. The UK parliamentary report is available at www.parliament.the-stationery-office.co.uk/pa/cm200405/cmselect/cmhealth/42/42.pdf
20. *Kauppalehti Presso* (Finland), 11 December 2004.
21. See the Drug Promotion Database website at www.drugpromo.info/about.asp#1
22. The Code of Marketing Practices of Canada's Research-Based Pharmaceutical Companies from January 2005 is a case in point. See www.canadapharma.org/Industry_Publications/Code/code_e05Jan.html (accessed 15 March 2005).
23. *British Medical Journal* 327(1126), November 2003.
24. *British Medical Journal* 327(414), August 2003.
25. PharmaBiz.com, 18 March 2005.

The corrupting influence of money in medicine

Jerome P. Kassirer[1]

Pharmaceutical, device and biotechnology companies have created new drugs and devices that have prolonged the lives and improved the health of millions of people. Many interactions between academic scientists and industry have been responsible for such advances, and these collaborative research projects should be encouraged. Yet the collaborations sometimes go beyond research and merge into marketing by physicians who become paid company consultants or speakers. The financial relationships between the pharmaceutical industry and physicians yield a subtle form of corruption, one that escapes legal supervision and challenges.

My comments apply principally to the United States, but the manifestations are similar in countries all over the world. In recent years, the pharmaceutical, device and biotechnology industries have spent some US $16 billion annually in the United States on marketing to physicians.[2] Of this, more than US $2 billion was spent on meals, meetings and events alone.[3] Companies seek to influence doctors with US $ 1,000–5,000 honoraria (or more) to participate in their speaker's bureaus and hire them as well paid consultants and members of their advisory boards. They also bombard doctors with journal ads, and almost 90,000 friendly drug salesmen.[4] They pay academic physicians to help them develop educational materials and befriend medical students and doctors with gifts of textbooks, stethoscopes, and free lunches and dinners. Such payments can lead some physicians to act in their own best interests rather than in the interests of their patients. There can be a fine line between legitimate marketing outlays by a pharmaceutical company and an unethical practice. But when compensation to salespeople and medical professionals translates into higher sales revenues, the temptation to cross the line becomes especially great.

The enticements on offer by pharmaceutical companies

The attempt to seduce young people is particularly worrisome. Some years ago, I witnessed a typical drug company-sponsored lunch at an academic medical centre. Two well dressed pharmaceutical representatives had brought food for a regular teaching conference for the house staff. One by one, house officers and medical students arrived to join a buffet line and were greeted warmly by the male 'drug rep' with 'How was your weekend?' or 'How're you doing?' These reps were obviously a familiar presence. The line moved slowly because it took some time to scoop up the food, and the two drug reps used the opportunity to make a sales pitch. One was stationed strategically at the beginning of the line, and the other at the end. The reps were describing two of the company's popular new (and expensive) products, as well as recommendations for dosages.[5] The seduction moves on to the dinner hour as well. One evening in a pizza parlour, I observed a resident with his team of interns and students enjoying pizza and beer with a drug representative. There were two 'costs' for the free food and drinks. The resident had to listen to the drug rep's sales pitch during the meal, and at the end of the party he was given a pile of reprints to take back to the rest of his team.

These trinkets and meals are simply marketing ploys, intended at minimum to ingratiate the drug rep to the doctor, perhaps to raise awareness of certain products and, at the other extreme, to create a sense of indebtedness. Such indebtedness is problematic, however, because the physician's obligation to the drug salesman or his company often conflicts with his obligation to his patients. The prescribing practices of physicians have been examined in a few studies in relation to some kind of exposure to a drug company promotion.

In one, 40 physicians who requested additions to their hospital's drug formularies were compared to 80 who had not requested any new drugs.[6] Statistically, doctors who requested the additions were 9 to 21 times more likely to have eaten free meals provided by the companies, to have accepted drug company money to attend or speak at a company-sponsored symposium, or to have received research support from the companies. An independent review (in the same study) indicated that the newly requested drugs had little or no advantage over the drugs already available.

Another study of the prescribing practices of 10 physicians who had attended company-supported symposia in resort locations showed a two- to threefold increase in the physicians' use of the drugs in the months after their trip.[7] Interestingly, a majority of physicians attending the symposia claimed that they would not be influenced by the enticements; most dismissed the possibility – defying common sense – that all of these efforts by industry could affect them.

Financial conflicts of interest in medical research

Fundamentally, big business and physicians alike are involved in a charade. The drug companies say that marketing helps to educate doctors so they can prescribe drugs more appropriately. At the same time, the companies press their drug salesmen to push the newest products, and they allow their surrogate intermediaries, the medical education companies, to advertise their services as 'persuasive' education. And the physician-recipients of drug company largesse act as if they were immune to its influence.

Physician–industry involvement is widespread. A 1996 survey showed that half of full professors and lesser fractions of more junior faculty who conduct life science research have substantial financial arrangements with industry, and disclosures at medical meetings and in published journal articles confirm the widespread involvement.[8] During my tenure as editor-in-chief of the *New England Journal of Medicine*, we only allowed physicians to write review articles and editorials if they had no financial conflicts with a company whose products (or their competitors) were featured in the article. Finding authors without such conflicts became progressively more difficult during the 1990s and, by the end of the decade, we often had to reject several prominent potential authors before we found one who had no conflicts. Finally, an industry-connected legal group admitted the extent of involvement. It wrote: 'It is widely acknowledged that most of the top medical authorities in this country, and virtually all of the top speakers on medical topics, are employed in some capacity by one or more of the country's pharmaceutical companies.'[9]

Several specific examples will illustrate the problem: one involving practice guidelines; the second, a human research study; a third involving radiological diagnosis; and the fourth, a decision by the Food and Drug Administration (FDA).

Four case studies from the United States

The National Cholesterol Education Program at the National Institutes of Health regularly updates its practice guidelines when new data become available. The latest, reported in July 2004, was a combined effort of the American Heart Association, the American College of Cardiology and the National Institutes of Health. These three organisations selected nine individuals to analyse all the clinical trials that had been published since the previous guidelines and come up with new recommendations. The group was impressive. It consisted of a nutritionist, the chief of the molecular disease branch at the National Institutes of Health, a well known pharmacologist, a former president of the American Heart Association and other well regarded cardiologists. Their recommendations included greater lowering of low-density lipoprotein (LDL) with diet, exercise and treatment with statins. Later, it was revealed that seven of the nine participants had financial arrangements as paid speakers or consultants for companies that make statins. They had these arrangements not with just one company, but three to five of them. These connections made it difficult to know whether the relations of these high-level physicians with the statin manufacturers may have influenced their recommendations.[10]

In 1999, a 17-year-old boy died at the University of Pennsylvania four days after receiving genes imbedded in a common cold virus. The boy had only a mild deficiency of a particular enzyme, but was participating in the research because he thought the results might help others. Neither he nor his parents had been told that the experiment had previously shown some toxicity; nor were they told that both the principal investigator and the university had financial stakes in a company that might have benefited from the outcome of the work. The principal investigator denied that money had anything to do with his decision or the institution's decision to move ahead with these studies.[11]

An interesting study was reported in the journal *Academic Radiology* in 2004. It was a re-analysis of 492 chest X-rays read by 30 radiologists employed by law firms who were suing companies for people exposed to agents that damage the lungs. To explain the findings, I will call these 30 the 'hired' hands. The authors of the study had the same chest X-rays re-read by six radiologists who were not paid by lawyers. I will call these radiologists the 'independents'. All 36, the hired hands and the independents, were certified 'B' readers by a federal agency, meaning that they all had undergone the same training to interpret chest X-rays. The results are interesting: the hired hands diagnosed 96–97 per cent of films as abnormal, whereas the independents said only 4–6 per cent were abnormal. The hired hands said none of the films were completely normal, whereas the independents said 38 per cent were normal. One does not need a chi square test to appreciate the gross discrepancy in these interpretations.[12]

In mid-February 2005, an advisory panel of the FDA met to assess whether the risk-benefit profile of various Cox-2 inhibitors made by Merck and Pfizer warranted removing the drugs from the market. This was a highly visible decision because of the increased risk of cardiovascular complications of some of the drugs, especially Vioxx, and because of Merck's decision only weeks before to take Vioxx off the market. The 32-person panel voted 31:1 to keep Celebrex on the market; there seemed to be little controversy about this decision. However, the votes on Bextra and Vioxx were much closer. The panel voted 17:13 to keep Bextra on the market, and 17:15 to allow Vioxx to return to the market. But there was a hitch: it was later learned that 10 of the panel members had financial ties to both companies that made these two drugs, and that these company-paid physicians had voted 9:1 in favour of keeping both drugs on the market. If none of these conflicted panel members had voted, the recommendation would have been not to allow either on the market. The votes would have been 12:8 opposed for Bextra and 14:8 opposed for Vioxx. Bextra has since been removed from the market, but both Vioxx and Bextra could return if the FDA follows the advisory board's recommendations.[13] The FDA decision will affect millions of people as well as the enormous profits of two major pharmaceutical companies.[14]

Though these examples are worrisome with respect to their effect on patient care, and cannot be condoned from an ethical construct, none constitutes either fraud or overt corruption. None is punishable by legal means and any sanction would have to come from state or professional organisations, but these bodies rarely impose any (see below). Each example strongly suggests a pattern of overt bias, but the problem with each is trying to assess an individual's motivation. One possibility is that none of the tilt towards company products was intentional, yet the close ties between physicians and companies yielded biased recommendations in some subconscious way. It is even possible that the recommendations these physicians made were completely objective, and that anyone else with the same expertise would have come up with exactly the same conclusions. Finally, it is possible that some doctors on industry payrolls are knowingly greedy and that they are intentionally profiting at the expense of the validity of information that doctors use in their daily practices. In the latter case, we must assume that they perceive the consequences of their actions on patient care to be negligible. These examples illustrate the essential problem with financial conflicts of interest: we don't know what to believe.[15]

A threat to the public's trust

Extensive analyses of the effects of financial conflicts of interest have documented its corrosive influences on patient care, medical information and the public's trust in the profession.[16] These huge financial subsidies can influence the validity of the information that doctors use every day in their practices. It tends to distract faculty into emphasising profitable research and to neglect their teaching duties. It replaces openness with secrecy, 'privatises' knowledge and replaces part of the social commons by commercialising discovery. It has also created a culture in which the design of studies is sometimes jiggered to create positive results; in which unfavourable results are sometimes buried; in which communication of results is sometimes hindered for commercial reasons; and in which bias in publications and educational materials has sometimes gone unchecked.[17] All of this amounts to a serious threat to public trust in medicine. These financial conflicts can undermine the faith of the public in medical research, threaten government funding, reduce enrolment in clinical trials and damage the trust between patients and their doctors.

In the United States, some progress has been achieved in dealing with financial conflicts. The Association of American Medical Colleges has issued new guidelines for individuals and institutions,[18] while many medical schools are now in the process of revising their conflict-of-interest policies. The National Institutes of Health, in response to a public outcry about important financial connections of several of its senior scientists, issued strict guidelines in 2005 that effectively limit investigators from having these associations.[19] The United States Congress has also expressed an interest in the concerns raised here.[20] The pharmaceutical companies and the American Medical Association have both issued guidelines about physician engagement in company programmes, but neither has precluded marketing of products by physician-consultants or speakers.

Far more work on this is needed. All gifts from the industry should be prohibited, even items that might be considered useful in a doctor's practice or education. Consultations with industry for anything except scientific matters should also be prohibited, while marketing by physicians of drugs or devices in which they have a financial interest should be outlawed. Physician participation in company-sponsored speaker's bureaus should be excluded. Clinical practice guideline committees and FDA advisory panels must contain a minority of individuals with financial conflicts of interest. Positions of journal editors, officers of major professional organisations and leaders of medical centres and academic institutions should be preserved only for individuals without conflicts. Given that complete elimination of all financial conflicts of interest is unlikely, the full disclosure of relevant financial conflicts on an easily searchable website should be introduced.

It is difficult to understand why the standards on conflicts of interest in medicine should be lower than those of other professions, such as the media. Reporters for the most ethical media outlets such as the *New York Times* and CNN are not allowed to accept any gifts, meals, honoraria or paid consulting arrangements.[21] This is an exceptionally high standard, but one medicine must adopt. The bar must be raised if we are to maintain the public's trust in medicine.

Notes

1. Jerome P. Kassirer is distinguished professor at Tufts University School of Medicine and adjunct professor of medicine and bioethics at Case Western Reserve University. He was editor-in-chief of the *New England Journal of Medicine* from 1991 to 1999.
2. *Boston Globe* (US), 10 March 2004.
3. Jerome P. Kassirer, *On The Take: How Medicine's Complicity With Big Business Can Endanger Your Health* (New York: Oxford University Press, 2004).
4. B. Darves, 'Too Close for Comfort? How Some Physicians are Re-examining their Dealings with Drug Retailers', *ACP Observer*, July/August 2003.
5. *Journal of the American Medical Association* (US), 284(2156–7), 2000.
6. *Journal of the American Medical Association* (US), 271(684–9), 1994.
7. *Chest* (US), 102(270–73), 1992.
8. *New England Journal of Medicine* (US), 335(1734–9), 1996.
9. D. J. Popeo and R. A. Samp, comments of the Washington Legal Foundation to the Accreditation Council for Continuing Medical Education concerning request for comments on the 14 January 2003 draft: 'Standards to Ensure the Separation of Promotion From Education Within the CME Activities of ACCME Accredited Providers', Washington Legal Foundation, 2003.
10. *Washington Post* (US), 1 August 2004.
11. *Washington Post* (US), 30 December 2001.
12. J. N. Gitlin, L. L. Cook, O. W. Linton and E. Garrett-Mayer, 'Comparison of "B" Readers' Interpretations of Chest Radiographs for Asbestos-related Changes', *Academic Radiology* 11(843–56), 2004.

13. Despite the FDA ruling in February 2005 in favour of allowing Vioxx back on the market, at this writing Merck had decided against its return.
14. *New York Times* (US), 25 February 2005.
15. Kassirer, *On The Take*.
16. Ibid., and Sheldon Krimsky, *Science in the Private Interest: Has the Lure of Profits Corrupted Medical Research?* (Lantham: Rowman and Littlefield, 2003).
17. Ibid.
18. Association of American Medical Colleges (AAMC), 'Protecting Subjects, Preserving Trust, Promoting Progress I: Policy and Guidelines for the Oversight of Individual Financial Interests in Human Subjects Research', AAMC Task Force on Financial Conflicts of Interest in Clinical Research, December 2001; 'Protecting Subjects, Preserving Trust, Promoting Progress II: Principles and Recommendations for Oversight of an Institution's Financial Interests in Human Subjects Research', AAMC Task Force on Financial Conflicts of Interest in Clinical Research, October 2002.
19. www.nih.gov/about/ethics_COI.htm
20. waysandmeans.house.gov/hearings.asp?formmode=view&id=2933
21. 'Ethical Journalism: Code of Conduct for the News and Editorial Departments', *New York Times* (US), January 2003.

Promoting trust and transparency in pharmaceutical companies: an industry perspective
Harvey Bale[1]

The twentieth century saw enormous improvements in overall health care standards in the developed world. Yet in both the developed and developing worlds, patients are still in need and are waiting for treatments, cures and vaccines for AIDS, cancer, diabetes, heart disease, Alzheimer's disease and many hundreds of other debilitating and life-threatening conditions. Even older diseases, once thought conquered or controlled, such as tuberculosis, malaria and polio, are re-emerging as clear and present dangers because of resistance to existing treatments or failings in immunisation programmes. Biological resistance to current treatments for HIV/AIDS infections is on the rise, making it imperative that industry and governments continue to fund heavily research into this as well as other diseases.

According to surveys by member associations of the International Federation of Pharmaceutical Manufacturers Associations (IFPMA), industry currently spends more than US $50 billion in research and development into finding drugs and vaccines annually worldwide. The industry is subject to a high degree of government regulation at every nearly stage of its activity. The large interface between industry and government throughout the life cycle of medicinal products poses continuous risks of corruption. Before clinical trial tests can begin, government must approve them. Before a drug is approved after such trials, another formal approval is needed in every country where the drug or vaccine is to be used by patients, physicians and nurses. Many countries set prices – another government decision. Before companies invest they need to have their ideas and innovation protected against copiers – another government function. Furthermore, where poor countries are concerned about certain epidemic threats, like

HIV/AIDS or malaria, companies work with governments and NGOs to find ways to get medicines to those who cannot afford them. Governments must be involved, from customs authorities to regulators to health ministry and local officials, to ensure the medicines get to intended patient groups. All of these points of governmental intervention raise the possibility of corrupt practices entering to distort and damage the development and delivery of new drugs and vaccines to patients.

Corruption in the pharmaceutical supply chain can take many forms: products can be diverted or stolen at various points in the distribution system; officials may demand 'fees' for approving products or facilities, for clearing customs procedures, or for setting prices; violations of industry marketing code practices may distort medical professionals' prescribing practices; demands for favours may be placed on suppliers as a condition for prescribing medicines; and counterfeit or other forms of sub-standard medicines may be allowed to circulate. While corruption carries economic costs, corruption adds further costs to the end goal of patient well-being.

Given the impact of corruption, the IFPMA and other industry bodies have taken significant steps to address the dangers of corruption. But the industry and other stakeholders must intensify efforts to prevent and avoid abuses.

The need to minimise the chances of corruption in the distribution chain is well illustrated by the diversion of heavily discounted GlaxoSmithKline (GSK) anti-retroviral (ARV) HIV/AIDS drugs from Africa to Europe unearthed in the summer of 2002. GSK had committed to providing its full range of ARVs at not-for-profit prices to the world's poorest countries. These prices were, on average, 70 per cent less than developed world prices. Registration of special 'access' packs in target countries would have taken between 6 and 18 months. With the HIV/AIDS epidemic spreading quickly, GSK was anxious to respond to the global crisis as quickly as possible. GSK's initial consignments to Africa were therefore dispatched in European packaging. The medicines had originally been sold by GSK at not-for-profit prices to an NGO and the procurement arm of a ministry of health, for distribution to African HIV patients. In the beginning of the sales programme, the company had not received approval for box designs to differentiate the countries to which they were destined – as such approvals take time; and some of the ARVs were diverted by West African public officials, almost undetected, back into the European market, with traders making substantial profits and patients in Africa being denied access to the medicines they desperately needed. Prosecution is under way for those involved in this scheme, which should help send the signal that this behaviour cannot be tolerated. In the meantime, GSK has developed 'access' packages for its main ARVs that are differentiated from developed country packs.

Another area where the industry has been active in recent years is in strengthening its product-promotion practices. The prescribing behaviour of medical professionals, who are frequently paid poorly under national health care systems, may be affected by the compensation offered by suppliers for administering their products or services, rather than by the interests of their patients. Though the direct evidence is thin that prescribing behaviour is directly and significantly affected by trips and gifts from the industry, there are cases that involve travel including coverage for spouses, despite the fact that the IFPMA Code and various national codes forbid spousal travel to be sponsored by companies to educational symposia. Companies belonging to the IFPMA adhere to a marketing and promotion code that requires that companies refrain from offering inappropriate hospitality or gifts to medical professionals that would tend to 'influence them in the prescription of pharmaceutical products'. The IFPMA Code is supplemented by its national member associations, by individual company ethical marketing codes and by a variety of measures that seek to redress the situation when violations of the codes occur. The code is based on self-regulation, but its application is obligatory. These codes are activated by complaints that are made to IFPMA or its member associations by physicians, other medical professionals or other interested parties, and violations are accompanied by publicity or fines paid in some countries.

Transparency is important in many other areas. Significant new initiatives have been introduced over the past two years regarding the pharmaceutical industry's approach to clinical trials. In a few cases, companies have been accused of disclosing and publishing only favourable clinical results. To increase the transparency of companies' clinical trials undertaken to develop new drugs and vaccines – and recognising that there are important public health benefits associated with making clinical trial information more widely available to health care practitioners, patients and others – easily accessible web-based clinical trial registers have been set up by companies to publicly record relevant details of the trials they are conducting. Beginning in summer 2005, the industry is making public the results of all clinical trials that have taken place and also information on those just being initiated, from the first stage of patient registration and enrolment through to final outcomes. At the same time, to make trial information easily accessible to those seeking information, the IFPMA is establishing a web-based search portal, linking the various clinical trial registries for information on ongoing clinical trials and databases for the summary results of completed clinical trials. This one-stop location will simplify and ease access for patients and medical professionals to the company registries and data.

Health care expenditures, and spending on innovative pharmaceuticals, will inevitably increase throughout the world. Whereas the past 20 years have seen an informatics revolution, the next quarter-century will witness major advances in the biosciences. Public confidence in the pharmaceutical industry is crucial and companies are taking significant steps through their member associations to maintain and improve public trust. To ensure that patients are able to benefit from medical advances, it is also important to ensure that access be addressed, and one way will be to help prevent the selective allocation of health care – by those in the public or private sector – on the basis of bribery and corruption.

Note

1. Harvey Bale is director-general of the International Federation of Pharmaceutical Manufacturers and Associations.

Fighting corruption: the role of the medical profession

John R. Williams[1]

Physicians are human beings and, like everyone else, are subject to the temptation to put their own interests above those of others. As self-regulating professionals, they have less oversight than many other individuals and consequently more opportunity to conceal unethical behaviour. On the other hand, they belong to a profession that has high ethical standards and that encourages and expects its members to uphold these standards.

Physicians encounter corruption in health care at all levels: in government, hospitals and other health care institutions, and in their own practice. For the most part, they are among the victims of corruption, seeing resources that should go to patient care or professional development siphoned off for other purposes. In some cases, however, they may be beneficiaries of corruption, insofar as they personally receive part or all of the resources that have been designated for other legitimate purposes.

The extensive guidance for physician behaviour provided by their professional associations seldom includes a responsibility for dealing with corrupt practices by non-physicians. It is quite a different matter when it comes to themselves and their colleagues. The World Medical Association (WMA) International Code of Medical Ethics exhorts physicians to 'always maintain the highest standards of professional conduct ...; not permit motives of profit to influence the free and independent exercise of professional judgement on behalf of patients ...; deal honestly with patients and colleagues, and strive to expose those physicians deficient in character or competence, or who engage in fraud or deception'.[2] These general principles have been elaborated in detail in policy statements from the WMA and its national medical association members.

It should be noted that the word 'corruption' seldom appears in medical association policy statements. These deal with 'unethical' or 'unprofessional' behaviour and practices that cover a wide spectrum from impoliteness to various degrees of conflict of interest to euthanasia. 'Corruption' would be considered an extreme form of conflict of interest whereby physicians receive substantial personal benefit at the expense of others, whether individuals, institutions or society in general. Most professional guidance deals with 'softer' forms of conflict of interest where it is not immediately obvious that wrongdoing is involved.

In what follows, I describe activities designed to prevent or deal with such conflicts of interest between physicians and the pharmaceutical industry.

The conflicts of interest inherent in the relationships of physicians and industry are described elsewhere in this volume (see 'The corrupting influence of money in medicine', page 87). Beginning in the late 1980s, the World Health Organization (WHO), industry groups and national medical associations began to produce guidelines for such relationships. In 1988, the WHO Assembly adopted a resolution endorsing a set of ethical criteria for medicinal drug promotion.[3] In 1991 the Canadian Medical Association adopted guidelines for physician–pharmaceutical industry relationships,[4] followed by many other professional organisations, including the American Medical

Association in 1992,[5] the Finnish Medical Association in 1993,[6] the Australian Medical Association in 1994,[7] the Israeli Medical Association in 2004[8] and the World Medical Association in 2004.[9] These guidelines deal with gifts to physicians, continuing medical education/professional development, industry-sponsored research and drug samples. Though their primary concern is to avoid conflicts of interest between physicians and patients, they are equally applicable to conflicts between the interests of physicians and those of society in general, for example regarding cost-effectiveness in prescribing drugs that are paid from public sources.

The principal reason why the WMA took so long to produce its guidelines is the great variation in access of physicians to continuing professional development activities throughout the world. In less developed countries, the pharmaceutical industry is often the only source of funding for physicians to attend conferences, whereas in wealthier countries such a relationship would be considered an unacceptable conflict of interest for physicians.

These guidance documents are directed to individual physicians, organisers of educational events and medical associations. Though they are ethical rather than legal in nature and therefore not generally binding, various mechanisms exist for turning them into enforceable rules, whether for those who offer conflict-of-interest incentives (for example, the pharmaceutical industry) or for those to whom they are offered (physicians and other health professionals). The pharmaceutical industry is increasingly subject to laws and regulations regarding its educational and promotional activities with physicians.[10] In some countries medical conferences are not eligible for continuing professional development credits unless they follow strict rules for industry sponsorship.[11] Some physician licensing bodies are beginning to define acceptable limits for industry–physician relationships and warning physicians that overstepping these limits will result in disciplinary action. Progress in this area has been slow for several reasons; for example, the difficulty of monitoring physician relationships with industry and the need to address more serious instances of physician misconduct, such as murder and the sexual abuse of patients. Unless the medical licensing authorities define more precisely the rules for physician behaviour regarding conflicts of interest and can obtain extra resources to enforce them, the individual consciences of physicians will have to be the principal resource for identifying and dealing with conflicts of interest.

Several educational programmes are available to inform physicians how to avoid conflict-of-interest situations with industry. The American Medical Association has developed an on-line resource for self-study by physicians,[12] and a group of health care providers has developed the 'No Free Lunch' website[13] to encourage their colleagues to maintain complete independence from industry in their clinical and educational activities. In the field of medical research, where there have been many reports of unethical conduct in recent years, educational resources for the responsible conduct of research are plentiful and many institutions now require researchers to demonstrate familiarity with the basic principles of responsible conduct of research.

The effectiveness of educational measures in this area is difficult to measure. Enforcement mechanisms may be somewhat more effective but are expensive to implement. The best hope for improving physician behaviour is a combination of reasonable and well publicised standards; continuing education about the standards and their foundations (beginning in medical school and continuing at all other levels); peer pressure from colleagues and medical associations; stricter government regulation of industry involvement in medical research and practice; and the threat of disciplinary action for egregious breaches of the standards. However, unless all interested parties cooperate to address conflicts of interest in health care, it is unlikely that progress will ever be achieved.

Notes

1. John R. Williams is director of ethics at the World Medical Association. The views expressed in this article are his own, not those of the World Medical Association.
2. www.wma.net/e/policy/c8.htm
3. World Health Organization, *Ethical Criteria for Medicinal Drug Promotion* (Geneva: WHO, 1988).
4. www.cma.ca//multimedia/staticContent/HTML/N0/l2/where_we_stand/physicians_and_the_pharmaceutical_industry.pdf
5. www.ama-assn.org/ama/pub/category/4001.html
6. www.laakariliitto.fi/e/ethics/industry.html
7. www.ama.com.au/web.nsf/doc/WEEN-5GJ7MH
8. www.pharma-israel.org.il/eng/htmls/article.aspx?C1004=578&BSP=4
9. www.wma.net/e/policy/r2.htm
10. See Susan Chimonas and David J. Rothman, 'New Federal Guidelines For Physician–Pharmaceutical Industry Relations: The Politics Of Policy Formation', *Health Affairs* 24(4), 2005 and House of Commons Health Committee, 'The Influence of the Pharmaceutical Industry', 22 March 2005, www.parliament.the-stationery-office.co.uk/pa/cm200405/cmselect/cmhealth/42/42.pdf
11. For example, the Standards for Commercial Support of the US Accreditation Council for Continuing Medical Education, available at www.accme.org/dir_docs/doc_upload/68b2902a-fb73-44d1-8725-80a1504e520c_uploaddocument.pdf
12. www.ama-assn.org/ama/pub/category/8405.html
13. www.nofreelunch.org/

The fight against counterfeit drugs in Nigeria
Dora Akunyili[1]

The presence of sub-standard and counterfeit drugs on Nigeria's streets escalated after the distribution of pharmaceuticals was denationalised in 1968. The lack of proper regulation and monitoring meant that import licences were readily issued to non-professional companies and drug regulations were flouted with impunity. Companies producing quality drugs found it difficult to compete with those who skimped on active ingredients, or relabelled expired drugs for resale. The result for the user of the fake pharmaceuticals was often prolonged illness, organ damage or death.

Though counterfeit drugs remain a serious problem in Nigeria, the situation has changed since 2001 thanks to a combination of mass education campaigns targeted as potential users of counterfeit drugs, and a more rigorous testing and enforcement regime. Nigeria's National Agency for Food and Drug Administration and Control (NAFDAC) has been at the centre of these efforts. A baseline study conducted in April 2001, as the current NAFDAC directors took office, showed that 68 per cent of the drugs available in Nigeria were not registered with NAFDAC, which is taken as an indication of counterfeiting.[2] A repeat of the study in 2004 revealed an 80 per cent reduction in the level of counterfeit drugs in the country.

The manufacture of counterfeit drugs is a global problem, but opinions as to what constitutes counterfeiting vary from country to country, making it difficult to control. The WHO describes counterfeit medicine as one 'that is deliberately and fraudulently mislabelled with respect to identity and/or source. Counterfeiting can apply to both branded and generic products, and counterfeit products may include products with the correct ingredients or with the wrong ingredients, without active ingredients, with insufficient active ingredients or with fake packaging.'[3]

In Nigeria NAFDAC has identified each form of counterfeit drug. These include drugs that contain no active ingredient but are made up merely of lactose, chalk or olive oil; herbal preparations that are toxic, ineffective or mixed with orthodox medicine; expired drugs that have been relabelled; drugs that are issued without publishing the full name and address of manufacturer; and drugs that have not been certified and registered by NAFDAC.

Corrupt officials protect counterfeiters

The counterfeiting of medicine is financially lucrative, as several organised crime syndicates have discovered. Moreover, it entails relatively low risks compared to narcotics or gun trafficking. The low risk may be deliberate: according to the WHO, corruption and conflict of interests are the driving forces behind poor regulation which, in turn, encourages drug counterfeiting. Corruption and conflicts of interests result in laws not being enforced and criminals not being arrested, prosecuted and convicted.[4]

An example of how authorities collude with organisations that fake or sell counterfeit drugs is the falsification of shipping manifests. In 2002, a 20-foot container of Napfen (ibuprofen tablets) imported through Apapa Port was falsely declared as containing motorcycle spare parts in order to evade NAFDAC regulations. The consignment was released by custom officials but later intercepted by NAFDAC officials. Similar-sized containers intercepted later that year contained hidden Gentamycin injections and Seven Seas Cod Liver Oil in one case, and Tramal capsules imported from Pakistan in a second. The drugs were discovered by the Port Inspection Directorate, which was established by the present NAFDAC administration.

Early on in the current administration, NAFDAC agents were themselves discovered to have engaged in corrupt practices in a series of high-profile cases. Two NAFDAC officials at Port Harcourt were dismissed and publicly reproached for releasing imported products without inspection in 2002. In Akwa Ibom state, two NAFDAC staff members were caught extorting money from the Nigerian Association of Patent Medicine Dealers and were dismissed in 2003.

Until recently, NAFDAC staff were allowed to collect cartons of expensive products as samples, which they could then sell off. This led to the practice of deliberate oversampling and sparked industry complaints. NAFDAC subsequently adopted clear sampling guidelines and disseminated information about correct sampling sizes to employees and the industry. New guidelines also prohibit NAFDAC staff from accepting free transportation, lunch or gifts from the companies they are inspecting. Instead, inspectors are provided with all the necessary resources to carry out their tasks.

The registration process produces another opportunity for corruption by NAFDAC staff. It is still common for it to take two years or more to register a product, although recent streamlining and automation of the process have shortened the process to two or three months in most cases. The lengthy exceptions are partly due to inefficiency, but corruption also plays a role, with NAFDAC staff dragging their heels and extorting bribes from applicants to speed up the process. Staff guidelines have been disseminated among industry members so that manufacturers might be less vulnerable to extortion. NAFDAC officers face suspension, demotion or dismissal if they are found to be corrupt.

Inadequate legislation contributes to the problem

Nigeria has a multiplicity of drug control laws that have become unwieldy, overlapping and sometimes conflicting. The result is a legal framework that fails to deter counterfeiters or that moves so slowly once allegations of wrongdoing have been identified that the suspect is rarely brought to trial.

Penalties for some offences related to counterfeiting are not commensurate with the severity of the crime. For example, the maximum punishment for contravening the decree on counterfeit or fake drugs and unwholesome processed food is less than N500,000 (US $3,600), or a prison sentence of between 5 and 15 years. NAFDAC does not believe that this level of punishment deters offenders and is calling for amendments to the law.

Judicial authorities have on occasion failed to act against counterfeiters or importers of fake drugs, even when NAFDAC has provided evidence of wrongdoing. For example, a well known importer of fake drugs, Marcel Nnakwe, was arrested three times in 1997 for importing more than N19 million worth (around US $137,700), but was protected by a judge who issued an interlocutory injunction restraining NAFDAC from taking any further action without court clearance.

One month after the present NAFDAC administration took office, a team of regulatory consultants and legal experts were invited to review existing obsolete laws and recommended detailed amendments. These have been reviewed and at the time of writing were before the National Assembly.

Discriminatory regulation by exporting countries

In many countries more lenient control of drugs for export has compromised the quality of drugs on the international market. A case that came to light in Nigeria recently involved the importation of poorly packaged, fake paracetamol tablets labelled 'not for use in Southeast Asia'. The poor regulation of exports from manufacturing countries exposes those countries with non-existent or weak regulations to the dumping of counterfeit pharmaceuticals.

There are 84 pharmaceutical manufacturing companies in Nigeria, which together produce less than 30 per cent of the country's drug requirements: the rest is imported. Most counterfeit drugs are imported from Asia, more than 98 per cent from China and India. Nineteen pharmaceutical companies, mainly Indian and Chinese, were blacklisted and banned from exporting drugs to Nigeria in 2001, and a further 12 were debarred in 2004. NAFDAC recently prohibited the importation of products marked 'for export only'.

Other factors that militate against effective regulation and encourage counterfeiting include: ignorance and poor public awareness of the problem; the chaotic drug distribution system; misleading advertising; the demand for drugs exceeding supply; inadequate funding of regulatory authorities; lack of cooperation between government agencies; false declarations by importers; the sophistication of clandestine drug manufacturing; and the irrational use of drugs, making demand difficult to control.

NAFDAC's role and future

NAFDAC's dual strategy of creating a strong regulatory environment, while encouraging intolerance of counterfeit drugs through public enlightenment campaigns, seems to be working. Jingles, media interviews, public alerts and notices in the national press publicising drugs identified as fakes are helping to lift the shroud of secrecy from the problem.[5] Efforts have been made to stop fake drug imports at source; surveillance at all ports of entry has been beefed up; many counterfeit drugs already in circulation have been mopped up by the agency; good manufacturing practices of local manufacturers are being monitored; and registration guidelines have been streamlined and are being strictly enforced.

But success comes at a cost. Testament to NAFDAC's achievements over the past few years is the vehemence with which corrupt manufacturers have sought to block our work. During my time as head of NAFDAC, my family and I have been the victims of numerous death threats and in December 2003 we narrowly escaped an assassination attempt.

Efforts to tackle counterfeit medicines must be redoubled. While national measures are working, the international community must realise that poor nations lack the funds, manpower and technology to fully address the problem. NAFDAC strongly advocates for harmonised regulation of pharmaceutical products on the international market and the establishment of an international convention for the control of counterfeit drugs similar to the one on psychotropic substances. The international community should recognise the control of counterfeit drugs as an international health emergency.

Notes

1. Dora Akunyili is director general of the National Agency for Food and Drug Administration and Control (NAFDAC), Nigeria. Her five-year mandate expires in April 2006. She was the winner of TI's Integrity Award in 2003.
2. Ijeoma Nnani et al., Baseline Study to Ascertain the Level and Quality of Unregistered Drugs on the Market (NAFDAC, 2001).

3. *WHO Drug Information* 6(2), 1992.
4. WHO (1999) *Counterfeit Drugs. Guidelines for the Development of Measures to Combat Counterfeit Drugs* (Geneva: WHO, 1999).
5. Ibid., and D. N. Akunyili, 'Understanding the Problem: The African Perspective with Special Emphasis on Nigeria', Global Forum on Pharmaceutical Anti-Counterfeiting (22–25 September 2002), Geneva Switzerland.

Box 5.2   Corruption in the Ministry of Public Health, Thailand[1]

The Rural Doctors Forum (RDF)[2] of Thailand traces its origins to the student demonstrations of 1973 and an ideological commitment to serving the rural public. This political commitment initially placed it in a difficult position in relation to the government. Towards the end of the 1970s, however, the head of the RDF was given a position in the Ministry of Health, which increasingly came to accept the Forum as a means of resolving the problems involved in decentralising health services to the rural areas.[3]

In 1998, the RDF departed from its role of supporting the ministry's work to expose corruption in the procurement of medicines and medical supplies. It claimed that its members had been ordered by the central authorities to procure supplies from some companies, rather than others, at prices two to three times higher than normal. It also alleged that senior administrators had put in place a regime that fostered corruption by cancelling medicine price ceilings and changing budgeting arrangements so as to make provincial-level officials, rather than officials in individual hospitals, responsible for procurement. The latter move made it easier for administrators in central government to interfere with the procurement process for personal gain.

The RDF's chairman wrote an open letter to the prime minister asking for an investigation. The RDF and another professional association, the Rural Pharmacists Forum (RPF), began to collect evidence on corruption and encouraged their members to step forward as witnesses. They also approached existing networks of NGOs, including the Drug Study Group and Consumers Protection Group, to form a coalition of 30 organisations against medical supplies corruption. The coalition provided information to the media and the public, and petitioned the court to force the country's National Counter Corruption Commission to release information on the case. The court decided in its favour and the information was released.

The committee set up to investigate the case confirmed that there was indeed corruption among politicians and civil servants in the ministry.[4] It recommended that the procurement system be reformed to promote transparency and accountability, and that those guilty of corruption be punished through a free and neutral committee. Two ministers resigned as a result,[5] and several senior and mid-level officials were dismissed or reprimanded. Rakkiat Sukthana, Public Health Minister at the time of the scandal, was later found guilty of accepting bribes from drug companies, and began serving a 15-year prison sentence in November 2004.[6]

Despite this victory, there continue to be calls for other politicians and high-level officials to face legal sanctions.[7] It was widely felt that the committee's recommendations for reforming the procurement system to prevent corruption were ignored.[8] But the improved coordination among civic organisations, which previously knew little about each other's work, is likely to help them to promote transparency and exert pressure on government in future.[9]

▶

The role of the RDF and RPF in the case was particularly important because of the position of members of the associations in the Ministry of Public Health. Most were medical professionals and had privileged access to information, such as changes in budget allocations, yet were able to maintain their independence, rather than being drawn into the corruption.[10] This degree of independence can be attributed both to the fact that many rural doctors were involved in public health NGOs, and to the RDF's history as a force for public health reform.[11]

Stuart Cameron (Institute of Development Studies, UK)

Notes

1. This essay draws from N. Trirat, 'Two Case Studies of Corruption in Medicine and Medicine Supplies Procurement in the Ministry of Public Health: Civil Society and Movement Against Corruption', Institute of Development Studies, UK: Civil Society and Governance Programme Working Paper, 2000; S. Wongchanglaw, 'Case Study: Citizen Mobilisation in the Fight Against Corruption: The Case of Health-Care Funding in Thailand', paper written for the Open Government Forum held in Seoul, February 2003, see www.thinkcentreasia.org/documents/healthcarecorruptionthailand.html; U. Tumkosit, 'Two Case Studies of Corruption in Medicine and Medicine Supplies Procurement in the Ministry of Public Health: A Framework of Relationships between Civil Society and Good Governance', Institute of Development Studies, UK: Civil Society and Governance Programme Working Paper, 2000.
2. Sometimes referred to as the Rural Doctors Society.
3. Trirat, 'Two Case Studies of Corruption'.
4. Wongchanglaw, 'Case Study'.
5. Dr Rakkiat (alternative spelling, Rakkied) Sukthana resigned on 15 September 1998 and Deputy Public Health Minister Teerawat Siriwanasarn resigned on 20 September 1998.
6. *The Nation* (Thailand), 2 November 2004.
7. Pasuk Phongpaichit, 'Corruption, Governance and Globalisation: Lessons from the New Thailand', Corner House Briefing 29, 2003, www.thecornerhouse.org.uk/item.shtml?x=51987
8. Trirat, 'Two Cases of Corruption'.
9. Wongchanglaw, 'Case Study', and Tumkosit, 'Two Case Studies'.
10. 'In one sense, it [the RDF] is inside the ministry it is attacking ... But in another sense, the Rural Doctors Society is not an official part of the ministry structure. It is just a *chomrom* (club).' See C. Noi, 'Six Rules for Fighting Corruption', *The Nation* (Thailand), 15 November 1998. Available at www.geocities.com/changnoi2/ruraldoc.htm
11. Trirat, 'Two Cases of Corruption'.

Box 5.3   Malpractice in the Office of the Drug Controller in Karnataka, India[1]

The Karnataka *Lokayukta* (KLA) is a statutory judicial body charged with improving standards of public administration in the state of Karnataka, India. Although other Indian states also have *lokayuktas*, the KLA is exceptional in that it is better funded – its annual budget for 2002–03 was around Rs72 million (around US $1.7 million) – and is proactively led by a high-profile retired judge, Justice Venkatachala. It is able to investigate grievances and complaints against public bodies through the police, and direct the relevant authorities to take corrective action when a grievance is justified. Its actions in the health sector have included paying unannounced visits to hospitals to check for bribes being paid, and requesting hospitals to display citizens' charters detailing which drugs are available, the fees for services, and what kind of facilities and services are offered.

NGOs occasionally make vital contributions to the KLA's investigations. A medical doctor and activist from Drug Action Forum (DAF), a group aiming to raise awareness about

▶

drugs promotion and policy, made a complaint to the KLA in 2003, alleging malpractice in the Office of the Drug Controller (ODC). A preliminary investigation revealed a number of irregularities. The office's mandate is to ensure that only authorised drugs of specific quality are sold. Many drugs were found to be sub-standard, but the test results were only available after several months and no action had been taken to withdraw them. Nor had any action been taken against the companies manufacturing the drugs. In this way, sufficient time had passed for all of the sub-standard drugs to be sold to the public.

It was discovered that companies that paid bribes were allowed to circumvent drugs standards, and those that refused to pay were harassed. Other irregularities included non-enforcement of price controls and accepting kickbacks. The ODC's remit also included granting licences to blood banks, but it did this with little regard for enforcement of standards or monitoring. The investigation found that a complaint had been filed about a blood bank in the district of Gulbarga that had provided HIV-positive blood; no action was taken in response.

The KLA responded to these findings by calling a meeting of over 50 officers from the ODC. It was claimed at the meeting that each drugs inspector was required to give Rs20,000 (around US $460) every six months to the Drugs Controller, who then passed it on to the Minister of Health.[2] Hearings were open to the media, with politically damaging consequences for former ministers who had also been implicated. In a bid to limit the damage, the ODC suspended the three officers who were cooperating with the inquiry, but the KLA threatened to hold the government in contempt of court for obstruction of justice if it did not reinstate the men and protect them from further harassment.

The KLA's final report of the investigation called on the government to suspend the ODC's top three officials, but did not implicate the Minister of Health.[3] The three officials were duly suspended on grounds of misconduct and dereliction of duty in October 2004.[4] The *Lokayukta*'s powers have limitations: it is not able to remove someone from office without the permission of central or state government, or of a senior official in the same department as the accused. It therefore depended on pressure from the public, via media exposure, to push the government into acting on its recommendations. It is not yet clear whether this pressure has been sufficient to bring about sustainable reform in the ODC.

DAF's involvement in the case was instrumental. There are obvious difficulties for ordinary individuals who make a complaint to a judicial body like the KLA. The judicial process is slow and cumbersome, and can seem daunting. Patients may lack information about their entitlements or health standards, and may fear losing access to services if they file a formal complaint. Moreover, expert pressure groups like DAF can provide the detailed information that may be necessary in order to proceed with an investigation.

Stuart Cameron (Institute of Development Studies, UK)

Notes

1. This essay draws from two articles by Asha George, 'We Need to Fix This Leaky Vessel' and 'Small Steps Ahead' published in *Humanscape Magazine* 10(9) 2003, and 10(10) 2003, respectively. See www.humanscape.org/Humanscape/new/sept03/weneedto.htm and www.humanscape.org/Humanscape/new/october03/smallsteps.htm The issues were uncovered by Anuradha Rao, in 'Karnataka Lokayukta: Initiatives in the Public Health Sector: A review', Mimeo, Bangalore: Public Affairs Centre, 2003.
2. *Humanscape Magazine* 10(10), 2003.
3. *Deccan Herald* (India), 1 October 2003; *The Hindu* (India), 1 October 2003.
4. *Deccan Herald* (India), 3 October 2004. The officials were the Drugs Controller, Anand Rajashekar, the Additional Drugs Controller, H. Jayaram, and the Deputy Drugs Controller, B. G. Prabhakumar.

6 Corruption and HIV/AIDS

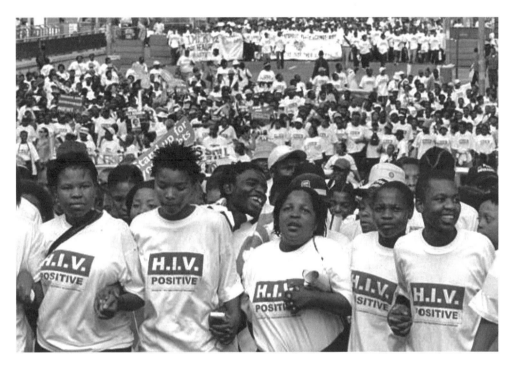

Some 5,000 demonstrators take part in a protest march to the Constitutional Court in Johannesburg on 2 May 2002 to protest the government's appeal of a court ruling forcing it to provide a key AIDS drug to HIV-positive pregnant women. (Themba Hadebe/AP)

While the corruption that affects HIV/AIDS prevention and treatment does not look very different from corruption found in other areas of the health sector, the scale of the pandemic, the stigma attached to the disease and the high costs of drugs to treat it magnify the problem. The response to HIV/AIDS must involve an increase in funds available to purchase drugs. But scaling up budgets without paying due regard to the anti-corruption mechanisms needed to ensure their proper use provides further opportunity for corruption. A case study from Kenya shows a worst-case scenario, of corruption and profligacy at the national AIDS body set up to coordinate prevention programmes. An examination of the Global Fund finds that including all stakeholders in the design of programmes, from governments and NGOs to the sufferers themselves, could help provide a safeguard against corruption.

The link between corruption and HIV/AIDS

Liz Tayler and Clare Dickinson[1]

While it is difficult to draw a causal link between corruption and the spread of HIV, there is ample evidence that corruption impedes efforts to prevent infection and treat people living with AIDS in many parts of the world. The mechanics of corruption affecting the prevention and treatment of HIV/AIDS are not substantively different from those affecting the health sector more generally: opaque procurement processes, the misappropriation of funds earmarked for health expenditure and informal payments demanded for services that are supposed to be delivered free. What are different are the scale of the problem and the nature of the disease – a chronic, usually fatal and often-stigmatised disease that can be contained only with expensive drugs. Moreover, the individuals responsible for tackling corruption may themselves be severely affected by AIDS. These factors create particular vulnerabilities to corruption.

There are multiple opportunities for corruption in the prevention and treatment of AIDS. In prevention programmes, corruption occurs when false claims are presented for awareness-raising activities that never took place, or for materials that were never purchased. Corruption occurs in programmes aimed at alleviating the socio-economic effects of the disease on victims and their families, such as feeding programmes or support for school fees. Corruption can also contribute directly to infection when relatively low-cost measures, such as the use of sterile needles and the screening of blood donations, are ignored because a corrupt procurement or distribution process holds up supplies. Alternatively, health workers may use non-sterile equipment as an additional source of income by extorting illicit payments from patients who demand clean equipment.

But it is treatment programmes that are most vulnerable. Money for high-value drugs can be embezzled at any number of points in the procurement and distribution chain. At the grand end of the scale is theft by ministries and national AIDS councils of funds allocated for treatment, and the misappropriation or counterfeiting of medicine. At the petty end are doctors who extort 'tips' for medicines and patients who sell their own medication because it is the only valuable commodity they have.

The international response to the epidemic has increased in recent years and there is pressure to spend large sums of money in countries with limited capacity to oversee their proper usage. The IMF reports that HIV/AIDS resources flows were US $5 billion in 2003 and US $8 billion in 2004. With this much money in play, and with donors insisting that disbursement be the standard metric for judging programme success, recipient nations will find ways to absorb the funds, whether legally or illegally. The prime requirement for recipient nations seems to be 'spend it or lose it'.

The numbers of people infected with HIV are high and rising. In sub-Saharan Africa overall, 7 per cent of women and 2 per cent of men aged 15–24 are infected.[2] In Botswana, Swaziland and Zimbabwe, over 25 per cent of the adult population is now HIV infected. In Asian countries the rates are generally lower, but they are rising fast. The impact of a large proportion of a community becoming sick and dying is unclear.

Some have suggested that more widespread corruption might be a result of increased 'short-termism' as those infected seek financial security by any means possible for the families they will leave behind, and informal structures emerge to meet the vast needs that formal health systems are failing to meet.[3]

Corruption in the treatment of HIV/AIDS

Relatively effective drug treatment has changed the nature of HIV/AIDS in the West. Increasingly, it is seen as a condition people can live with. Hospitalisation and death rates have fallen, and anti-retroviral drugs (ARVs), when properly administered, offer people with HIV many extra years of productive life, depending on when treatment begins.

In Africa, it is estimated that people live an average six and a half years after infection. If ARV treatment is started at the appropriate time, life expectancy is doubled or tripled. Over the past decade, ARV treatment has gone from being something that even people in developed countries could not afford to a treatment that over 700,000 people in developing countries now receive. The WHO is attempting to get 3 million people onto treatment by 2005 under its '3 by 5' initiative.

Even with this massive and rapid scaling-up, treatment is not available to all who need it. This is no different from other health services in Africa and the rest of the developing world where many are excluded through financial or cultural constraints, or because of the distance to health facilities. Access to ARV sharpens these issues, however. Demand frequently exceeds supply even when there is an official policy to determine who gets treatment, such as a cut-off point based on blood test results (the CD4 count). Those whose result is 'not quite bad enough' may try to use financial, political or other inducements to get onto treatment programmes. A 29-year-old Nigerian father of three spoke for many across the continent in the 2005 civil society organisation statement to the African Union Summit of Heads of States: 'The ARVs that come to the centre are not given to those of us who have come out to declare our status, but to those "big men" who bribe their way through, and we are left to suffer and scout round for the drug.'[4]

Where ARVs are provided for free or at heavily subsidised rates through donor-funded programmes, requests for 'top-up payments' are common. The Malawi Network of People Living with HIV/AIDS (PLWHA) reported instances of abuse from hospital workers demanding sexual, monetary or material favours in return for proper medication and care. Those who refuse are either neglected or receive sub-standard care. In cases where PLWHA do report receiving high-quality care, it is followed by suspicion by other care providers and patients that those who furnish it are receiving bribes.[5]

Those that get onto programmes offering free or highly subsidised drugs receive a valuable commodity. They and their family will have other needs as well, and many elect to share or trade their drugs to meet these needs. There is a ready market for ARVs. In Tsavo Road, Nairobi, huge quantities are traded every day.[6] Some come from patients, others leak out of the health system, and a large proportion is counterfeit. The drugs are often cheap and there are fewer stigmas, no hassle and no waiting. Some vendors sell their own treatment drugs; some are registered on multiple programmes and have ARVs to spare; and others have access to the supply chain through central and hospital pharmacies.

People buy drugs from informal sources like Tsavo Road because it is convenient and anonymous. The problem with doing so is that ARVs are effective only when there is rigid adherence to the treatment protocol. Buying treatment from those who know little about the appropriate combinations, side-effects or dosage, and substituting one drug for another depending upon availability, means treatment is likely to become ineffective and result in the development of resistance to ARVs. Moreover, the product may be expired or fake.

The WHO estimates that the global market in fake and sub-standard drugs is worth US $32 billion – or around a quarter of all drugs used in developing countries.[7] Well substantiated reports from Ethiopia,[8] DRC[9] and Cote d'Ivoire[10] indicate that the problem may be even greater and is increasing. Given the demand for, and value of the drugs, faking ARVs is potentially much more profitable than faking other drugs. Corruption contributes to the extent of the problem when regulatory authorities turn a blind eye to counterfeiting or public officials receive inducements to procure from less reputable suppliers, as Dora Akunyili describes (see 'The fight against counterfeit drugs in Nigeria', Chapter 5, page 97).

Concerted advocacy by civil society groups and governments, and competition from generic and research-based companies have been extremely effective in lowering the price of ARVs in the developing world, resulting in a system of differential pricing between OECD countries and developing countries. A month's supply of GlaxoSmithKline's Combivir, for example, costs around US $610 in Britain and US $20 in Uganda, Tanzania and Kenya. The potential profit from re-importation or smuggling is large for vendors in developing countries and drugs brokers in developed countries. How much of a problem this is in reality is controversial, however, and there have been allegations that the pharmaceutical countries are exaggerating the scale of the problem in order to dampen pressure for differential pricing.[11]

Competition in the supply of ARVs has not stopped corruption in national procurement processes. For example, the Romanian government has launched an investigation following allegations by US Ambassador Michael Guest that ARVs were being sold at prices 50 per cent higher than in the United States and that the health ministry had engaged in corrupt dealings with drug suppliers. A government watchdog agency reported in April 2003 that the ministry had ignored an agreement with GlaxoSmithKline to reduce the price of its ARVs by up to 87 per cent[12] and denied drug importation contracts to foreign companies, granting them instead to four local ones. These levied 'taxes and commissions' were worth up to 55 per cent of the drugs' value.

National programmes: new approaches and roles

Where systems are weak and corruption endemic, it is difficult to disentangle corruption from mismanagement and system failure as the root cause of poor HIV/AIDS responses. Nigeria's ARV programme attracted much criticism in 2003 when treatment centres began handing out expired drugs and rejecting patients.[13] But it is not yet clear whether the prime cause was corruption or a weak drug procurement, supply and distribution service that was unable to respond to the demands that the rapid scaling-up of the programme had placed upon them.

Fresh approaches have developed involving new actors and sectors not traditionally involved in health programmes, such as education, security, agriculture and social services. National AIDS commissions have been established to coordinate the response in many countries. They are often seen as a donor construct, however, and the extent to which they have been assimilated into domestic governance systems is variable. Kenya provides an example of the worst-case scenario: its agency was discredited when it was discovered that senior staff had paid themselves inflated salaries and allowances (see 'Corruption in Kenya's National AIDS Control Council', page 112).

In Zimbabwe the government has imposed an 'AIDS levy' since 2000 whereby employees contribute 3 per cent of their gross salaries towards a fund administered by the National AIDS Council (NAC). It is estimated that the government collects about US $20 million per year through this mechanism, but no information about how the fund is used and who benefits from it has ever been made public. In March 2005, the health ministry ordered an audit of the NAC, but at the time of writing it had not yet been published.

Civil society organisations (CSOs) are increasingly seen as important providers of services and receive substantial grants to do so, but the transaction costs of processing and monitoring CSO applications are very high. An attendant risk is that CSO directors will siphon off their funding. For example, the director and senior staff at the Zimbabwe National Network for People Living with HIV/AIDS were suspended after allegations of corruption.[14] The network received more than US $1.8 million from the NAC between 2003 and 2004.

The international response: more money

The sums now being disbursed to tackle HIV/AIDS are huge compared to the existing budgets of many countries.[15] In Ethiopia, Liberia and Malawi, the money allocated by global health partnerships such as the Global Fund to Fight AIDS, Tuberculosis and Malaria represents more than a doubling of the health budget. Funds from the World Bank and the US President's Emergency Project for AIDS Relief (PEPFAR) are also massive.

While the need for money is undisputable, the systems to use these funds appropriately are poorly developed. The fact that the 'performance' of a grant or loan is assessed by how rapidly it is disbursed gives incentives to donor and recipient to allocate the money carelessly. For corrupt officials, rapidly expanding budgets offer greater scope to siphon off significant volumes without anyone noticing. This is especially true where health systems are fragile, where there is a lack of monitoring and oversight, and where the capacity to channel the money effectively is limited.

Beyond the immediate risk of money being squandered by corruption, commentators such as Stephen Knack[16] suggest that development assistance may actually reduce

Box 6.1 Accountability in a time of crisis: corruption and the Global Fund

The Global Fund to Fight AIDS, Tuberculosis and Malaria was established in January 2002. At the time, international efforts were failing to dent a death toll of 6 million people each year who die of illnesses that in rich countries are controlled or cured. Its foundation coincided with growing concern that corruption was lessening the impact of development aid.

The Global Fund's mandate was simple: to provide a massive infusion of financing for efforts to combat these three diseases in developing countries. Its role would be limited to supplying funding rather than, as has classically been the case in development assistance, bundling financing with technical support to prepare and implement programmes. This model was developed out of a recognition that adequate capacity existed at local level to scale up disease control interventions, should sufficient financing be made available. No country offices would be established, and instead the Global Fund would be created with a small board supported by a small Secretariat in Geneva.[1]

To date, the Global Fund has approved proposals totalling almost US $3.5 billion for combating the three diseases in nearly 130 countries. More than US $1.41 billion was disbursed as grants in the organisation's first three years, and the figures are growing rapidly. The countries being financed are among the most corrupt in the world: 23 of the 25 lowest-ranked countries in Transparency International's 2004 Corruption Perceptions Index have received money from the Global Fund.[2]

Working in countries where corruption is endemic, and under pressure to work fast, the Global Fund's approach has been to include parties from government, civil society, the private sector, UN and donor agencies, and people affected by the diseases in Country Coordinating Mechanisms that have responsibility for submitting proposals and overseeing the use of funds. The idea is that the different stakeholders will exert peer pressure to promote more effective implementation and reduce the likelihood of money disappearing.

But the experience to date with this approach to ensuring accountability has been mixed.[3] In Armenia, Cambodia, Ghana and Rwanda, the country bodies have taken on active roles in overseeing implementation, including developing monitoring tools and operating procedures. In other countries, however, they have been appropriated by a single constituency – typically the government – particularly in Eastern Europe and central Asia; have fallen prey to competing political agendas; or simply have not met regularly enough to ensure any adequate oversight role.

A second aspect of the Global Fund's accountability system is that ongoing funding is performance-based. Global Fund resources are provided as advances and the financial reporting requirements are generally quite streamlined. But expenditure reporting is required to be linked with programme monitoring and evaluation, shifting the focus from inputs (whether or not a computer was bought or a shipment of drugs arrived at the port, for example) to outputs (such as whether the financing was used to scale up interventions against AIDS, tuberculosis or malaria). If expenditures occur without demonstrable results, it is an immediate red flag that corruption may be diverting resources away from their intended purposes. This enables the Global Fund's Local Fund Agent (LFA)[4] to pay increased attention to the recipient's financial records.

However, LFAs are more familiar with financial data than health outcomes and have not always adequately addressed this weakness by bringing in outside expertise. Adding to

▶

the problem, the contracting system does not systematically ensure that an LFA working in a very corrupt country has more resources at its disposal than one working in a country with robust accountability systems. The Global Fund has terminated grant agreements because of corruption concerns in two cases, Ukraine and Uganda. In both cases, the corruption was detected as a result of a combination of the work of the LFA and that of partners in the country.

A third innovation of the Global Fund is its transparency. The Global Fund makes information about the dates and amounts of every disbursement available on its website and in its publications. The ideal is that the government and non-government partners with a stake in the programme will use this information to ensure that resources are not diverted.

There are concerns that this vision is losing some of its clarity, however, as the Global Fund Secretariat grows in size and slowly takes on more responsibility for doing the work that its partners were originally expected to be able to assume. This has arisen both because of pressure on the new organisation to prove itself and because partners have tended to view the Global Fund as yet another external body coming in to finance its own projects, rather than one that simply provides additional resources to a national response that all parties would support.

Given the Global Fund's short history, it is difficult to assess fairly how well these various accountability and transparency mechanisms are working. What speaks in the organisation's favour is that it has been willing to amend its processes as corruption concerns emerged; for example, in deciding in mid-2005 to set up an Office of the Inspector General to tackle suspected fraud and abuse. It has also begun to introduce risk management principles into its operations, both to allocate staff resources appropriately and to tailor procedures and responses to varying contexts.

Toby Kasper[5]

Notes
1. Of the 19 board members, 14 are from national governments or regional groups, generally represented by health ministries, HIV/AIDS committees, and development cooperation ministries. Three are from non-governmental organisations and two are from the private sector. Two of the NGO members were from developing country NGOs, while the 14 governmental representatives were evenly divided between developing and developed countries.
2. Transparency International, *Global Corruption Report 2004*, available at www.transparency.org/cpi/2004/cpi2004.en.html#cpi2004
3. See www.theglobalfund.org/en/apply/mechanisms/casestudies/default.asp
4. The Global Fund Secretariat does not have any offices outside Geneva, so it contracts independent firms to assess the capacity of the principal recipients of the funds to handle the large volume of resources and to monitor implementation. The LFAs are generally accountancy firms (particularly PricewaterhouseCoopers and KPMG), selected through a competitive tendering process.
5. The author worked at the Global Fund to Fight AIDS, Tuberculosis and Malaria from August 2002 until March 2004, initially responsible for the management of a portfolio of countries and later as policy manager.

the quality of governance in recipient countries. Donors may set up parallel systems to avoid the risk of corruption, but this means taking talent and capacity away from the official government system, with the concomitant that governments and officials become more accountable to the donor than to their own constituents. PEPFAR is an example of an approach that combines a political imperative to spend money rapidly within narrow political constraints.

In an attempt to prevent this, some donors – mainly European, but also the Global Fund (see page 108) – are moving towards 'budget support', essentially putting their money through government channels. While recognising the fiduciary risk, they believe that the benefits – improved efficiency, legitimacy in focusing on public financial management and support to domestic accountability – outweigh the disadvantages in many countries.

Could more be done to minimise corruption?

As with attempts to tackle corruption in the health sector generally, the terms and conditions of health workers should be improved in parallel with the introduction of mechanisms to increase their accountability to the communities they serve. However, though paying health workers and civil servants more is necessary, it is not enough to limit corruption, as the Nigerian experience in 2000 illustrated. And minimising the opportunities for corruption without providing alternative sources of income may induce health workers to give up, resulting in an escalation of the human resource crisis in the health sector.

Increasing transparency is vitally important in health services. The public needs to be more aware of the eligibility criteria for ARV programmes, which should ideally become more consistent within and across countries. They need to be aware of what they have to pay and what they will receive. The quantities and values of drugs supplied at each level of the system should be well publicised, and health workers should have to account for them. There also needs to be a mechanism whereby people can complain without fear of victimisation.

Pharmaceutical companies also need to take action. To minimise the risk of drugs for developing countries being reimported, GlaxoSmithKline is rebranding and changing the colour of ARVs sold in developing countries. An alternative approach is to develop different branding and packaging for products designed for use in developing countries.

The EU employs a system of registration whereby products are given a number and bar code, and can be identified by customs or drug brokers if reimported. Tight monitoring of pharmaceutical sales within the United States and Europe is an important disincentive to reimportation, and needs to be maintained. However, implementation of the recent WTO agreement regarding compulsory licences, and the export and import of generic varieties of drugs may restrict the availability of cheap generic varieties of drugs, providing additional scope for bureaucratic corruption.

Donors have an important role to play in minimising corruption, one that is not specific to HIV/AIDS treatment or prevention programmes. With vast resources flowing in for HIV/AIDS, however, a new paradigm has been created that distorts the donor–recipient relationship. What rich nations view as the provision of funds to purchase AIDS medicines, many in poor nations have monetised upwards as a currency of street trade.

Donors need to find a choke point to reduce corruption. One step towards making recipient governments more transparent would be for donors to be open and explicit about what they are giving, when and to whom. This requirement is included in international recommendations, but the reality is far from ideal. Donors should ensure that aid is used in line with good procurement guidelines, and work with pharmaceutical companies to encourage and ensure responsible behaviour.

Ultimately, it is the responsibility of national governments to deal with corruption. Given the associated sensitivities about international action, regional pressure may be more appropriate; in Africa, the New Partnership for African Development (NEPAD) peer review system could become an important tool. Finance and health ministers control the foreign exchange that is used to purchase medicines and need to be aware of the long-term effects of their misuse. When medicines are sub-standard or distributed inadequately, the onset of drugs resistance is accelerated, leading to a growing burden of chronically ill people. The cost of medical care to treat them will be far greater than the price of the legitimate medicines in the first instance.

HIV/AIDS is going to be a major problem for the next two decades at least. Experience gained in other areas of development, and the need for transparency and strong domestic accountability, should not be ignored if sustainable and effective approaches to tackling the disease are developed.

Notes

1. Liz Tayler is a UK public health physician, who worked for several years as the DFID health adviser in Nigeria before joining the HLSP institute as an adviser. Clare Dickinson is an HIV/AIDS specialist with HLSP and formerly worked in Indonesia on a health policy project based in the Ministry of Health.
2. UNAIDS, 2004 situation report, www.unaids.org/wad2004/EPI_1204_pdf_en/Chapter3_ subsaharan_africa_en.pdf
3. Alex de Waal, 'HIV and the Security Threat to Africa'. Evidence submitted to the high-level forum panel on security threats and challenges, Justice Africa, May 2004.
4. Statement by CSO at the fourth ordinary African Union Summit of Heads of States, January 2005 Nigeria.
5. Malawi Network of People Living with HIV/AIDS (Manet), 'Voices for Equality and Dignity: Qualitative Research on Stigma and Discrimination Issues as they Affect PLWHA in Malawi', July 2003, www.synergyaids.com/documents/Malawi-MANET.pdf
6. *The Nation* (Kenya), 22 January 2004.
7. 'Fake and Counterfeit Drugs', WHO Fact Sheet 275, November 2003.
8. www.addistribune.com/Archives/2003/10/10-10-03/Black.htm
9. www.essentialdrugs.org/edrug/archive/200402/msg00028.php
10. www.essentialdrugs.org/edrug/archive/200401/msg00004.php
11. *Financial Times* (Britain), 23 May 2005.
12. Agence France-Presse (France), 22 April 2003.
13. Associated Press, 4 February 2004.
14. *The Chronicle* (Zimbabwe), 3 February 2004, 23 April 2004 and 19 July 2004.
15. In 2001, US $2.1 billion was spent on HIV and AIDS; within three years this almost tripled to US $6.1 billion, with an expectation that needs will triple again by 2008. See 'Resource Needs for an Expanded Response to HIV/AIDS in Lower and Middle Income Countries' (UNAIDS, 2005).
16. Stephen Knack, *Aid Dependence and the Quality of Governance: A Cross-Country Analysis* (Washington DC: World Bank, 2001).

Corruption in Kenya's National AIDS Control Council

Kipkoech Tanui and Nixon Ng'ang'a[1]

HIV/AIDS is one of the biggest challenges facing the health sector in Kenya, and was declared a national disaster in 1999. The National AIDS Control Council (NACC) was set up later that year to coordinate the prevention and control of HIV/AIDS. Its role became even more critical when the current government placed at the centre of its 2003–07 development plan the goal of achieving 90 per cent awareness of the disease and its effects across society.

The NACC was given control over funds pooled under the Kenya HIV/AIDS Disaster Response Project (KHADREP), financed by the World Bank, the UNDP, and the UK and US development agencies. In the 2004–05 financial year, the NACC was allocated just under KSh4 billion (US $41 million). The most significant portion of its budget is channelled into community-based organisations. It claims to have channelled KSh1.8 billion (US $24 million) to community-based organisations during 2000–03.

The NACC was set up under the Office of the President (OP). However, a more natural home for it is the health ministry, which is also a recipient of large amounts of bilateral funding and runs the National AIDS and STD Control Programme (NASCOP). The choice of the OP as home for the NACC was made ostensibly out of the government's desire to control the sizeable budget it manages. The OP's record belies the wisdom of this decision, however. It has been the focus of some of Kenya's most egregious acts of corruption, often perpetrated by well-connected officials who have proved almost impossible for prosecutors to touch.

In April 2003, the OP was enveloped in scandal when it was revealed that the head of the NACC, Margaret Gachara, had been receiving a salary seven times what she should have been entitled to as a senior civil servant. She had negotiated the salary based on a fraudulent letter from her previous employer that exaggerated her earnings there. Once in office, she raised her salary even higher than the already inflated amount she had been offered. In August 2003 she was ordered to refund US $340,000 to the NACC.

Fears that the corruption did not end with her high salary were confirmed in April 2005 when a report by the Efficiency Monitoring Unit (EMU), also based in the OP, revealed that for years high-level public servants had used the NACC as their personal cash cow. There had been a number of early warning signals. An internal audit in June 2002 found irregularities in procurement procedures and in June 2003 the Global Fund to Fight HIV/AIDS, Tuberculosis and Malaria withheld a US $15 million AIDS grant until the government addressed corruption in the NACC.

The 300-page EMU report revealed that Kenya could not account for KSh3.64 billion (US $48 million) donated by the United Kingdom over five years since 2001. It put a figure of more than KSh37.3 million (US $490,000) on the amount used by NACC employees to pay themselves inflated salaries and fraudulent allowances, such as the payment of private water, electricity, telephone and home security bills. The largest sum was the money embezzled by Gachara, but others were also involved, including eight permanent secretaries or their representatives, and NACC Chairman Mohammed Abdallah, who was charged with embezzlement but later acquitted due to 'lack of evidence'.

Even where money did find its way out of NACC to the community organisations it was intended to support, the report into its use was damning. The EMU found that on a sample examination of the community-based organisations funded by the NACC, at least half of the money allocated has been squandered.

Investigators probed three of the 10 national NGOs funded by NACC and several provincial, district and constituency-level organisations. They found wanton theft of the NACC money granted to noble-sounding projects that turned out to be sham. The worst cases involved shell organisations purposely formed to cash in on the NACC windfall. The NACC itself had cracked down on some of the so-called 'briefcase' NGOs cited in the report, including the Neema Children's Centre in Nairobi. The NACC awarded Neema US $14,000 out of a World Bank grant to finance grassroots work on HIV/AIDS. It was closed down in mid-2003 after inspectors could not find a single Neema worker or a single orphan who had benefited from the children's centre.

Money was squandered by almost all the AIDS Control Units (ACUs) formed in each ministry to sensitise staff to the disease. Grants were spent on needless seminars, usually involving the same participants. Of the US $205,000 given to the Ministry of Agriculture, for example, more than 75 per cent was spent on staff accommodation, allowances and participation fees at various awareness-raising shows, the EMU report noted. Almost one-third of the amount spent was not accounted for and was presumed wasted.

Investigations into the three national NGOs revealed similar misdeeds. Par Aid, a well-connected organisation based in Eldoret, received US $100,000 for a proposal to study the efficacy of Par Aid herbal medicine in the treatment of HIV/AIDS infection. The chairman of the Institutional Research and Ethics Committee at Moi Teaching Referral Hospital, which is part of Moi University, withdrew a letter approving the project because he was concerned that Par Aid was not serious about the study, but his decision was quickly overturned with no explanation given by the hospital's director. The study went ahead, and the EMU report found that most of the money was spent on trips to collect the medicine, or on fuel. The medicine that should have been used in free trials was sold to desperate patients, leading the EMU to conclude that Par Aid was conducting a profitable business with NACC funds.

Corruption in the case of the AIDS Prevention Forum of Kenya (APFK) is even more blatant. Also given US $100,000 in NACC funds, its directors appear to have gone on a spending binge under the guise of organising seminars and workshops.

EMU noted a claim by the organisation that it spent US $16,000 hosting school pupils at a seminar in the Chania Tourist Hotel. The schools said to have been involved denied any knowledge of the activity and said some of the pupils alleged to have participated did not even exist. Similarly, hotels refuted several account entries, saying they were either paid considerably less, or did not host the seminars at all. For example, the Hotel Big Five in Homa Bay, which was said to have hosted 150 students at a cost of US $6,200, consists of just 12 rooms and denied ever accommodating the group.

A number of APFK directors were simultaneously directors of the third NGO investigated, Technologies and Action for Integrated Development (Techno Aid), where similar practices were uncovered. Techno Aid claimed to have organised seminars and workshops for the same people as APFK, consulted academic experts who denied ever working for the NGO, and paid large bills to non-existent hotels. Both Techno Aid and APFK presented receipts for stationery from the University of Nairobi bookshop, which has disowned them as frauds.

The report points the finger of blame at the lax implementation of the NACC's own funding rules and, in the worst cases, outright collusion between crooked NGOs and NACC staff. In some cases the NACC continued to finance organisations even when its own officers had expressed concerns over the accounting for previous allocations.

As isolated cases, the funds may seem petty especially when juxtaposed with the huge sums that HIV/AIDS attracts. But in their consolidated amounts, and if spent on effective prevention programmes, life-prolonging anti-retroviral drugs (ARVs) or income-generating activities for the affected and infected, the sums are significant.

The fight against HIV/AIDS in Kenya attracts massive funding. The Global Fund has promised US $129 million over five years while the United States has pledged US $115 million. Other donors who have responded to Kenya's appeal for more funds include UNAIDS (US $15 million) for disease mitigation initiatives and the World Bank (around US $658,000 on top of a 2004 grant of US $4 million). The bulk of these funds go to NASCOP, which has also fallen under suspicion for failing to deliver results commensurate with its budget. If there were no leakage or inefficiencies in the use of NASCOP funds, they should be enough to provide ARVs to 200,000 of the 1.4 million Kenyans who are estimated to be infected with HIV. The real figures are scandalously small. By November 2004 only 24,000 people were reported to be on ARVs.

The EMU is based in the OP, and was created in response to donor pressure to contain corruption in the institutions they support. Every state institution is liable to be investigated by the unit, but given its scant resources – staffed by just 50 people – it opts to probe those with sizeable budgets, often guided to them by rumours of sleaze. The EMU is reputed to conduct thorough and impartial investigations. Its report, 'Financial Management Audit of the National AIDS Control Council (NACC) in the Office of the President' is the culmination of a two-year investigation.

The EMU has called on the Anti-Corruption Commission to investigate all the cases of fraud and abuse of office listed in the report. Gachara, the former NACC director, was sentenced in August 2004 to one year in prison on three counts of fraud and misuse of office. She was granted a presidential pardon in December 2004, along with 7,000 'petty offenders' who had stolen from various government offices. Her release was publicly decried.

In response to the report, the NACC claims to have hired auditors to probe the accounts of the NGOs it funds. It says it will release funds in tranches, conditional on proof that the previous allocation was properly utilised. It ordered 20 NGOs to refund money that was misappropriated, or face prosecution. At the time of writing none had refunded the money and none had been taken to court.

The role of constituency-based AIDS councils has also been bolstered in response to the scandals. These had already been given a larger role in resolving the Global Fund's concerns and now have responsibility to scrutinise the expenditure of NACC money. Many MPs – who are the patrons of their respective constituency councils – have welcomed moves in this direction and some have called for the NACC to be disbanded in favour of constituency-based AIDS management committees, citing bias in NACC decisions over which NGOs to fund. Whether this will help curb corruption is questionable, however. Civil society groups and the media have levelled accusations of favouritism in appointments to the constituency councils and in their decisions over the disbursements of funds.

Note

1. Kipkoech Tanui is deputy managing editor and Nixon Ng'ang'a is a journalist with *The Standard*, Kenya.

Part two
Country reports

7 Lessons learned from anti-corruption campaigns around the world

Cobus de Swardt[1]

The past year saw the unfolding of several dramatic corruption scandals, including the removal of the vice-president in South Africa after corruption allegations; investigations of heads of state or former political leaders in Israel and Costa Rica; and major corruption trials in France, Nepal and Venezuela. No country is immune to graft. As New Zealand and Finland demonstrate in the *Global Corruption Report 2006*, even countries that are consistently ranked in the top 10 in Transparency International's Corruption Perceptions Index experience lapses in accountability. Corruption affects all sectors of society, from construction (France and Malaysia in this book), education (Uganda) and police (Malaysia, Nepal, Papua New Guinea), to parliament (Japan), the judiciary (Brazil, Burkina Faso, Ecuador, Israel and Nepal) and even the church (Greece). As highlighted by the Algeria report, corruption continues to be an obstacle to investment. It impedes effective management of natural resource revenues (Cameroon and Venezuela) and can lead to misappropriation of disaster relief funds (Sri Lanka).

But the news is not all bad. These scandals highlight the increasing role played by civil society and the media in monitoring public funds and holding public officials to account. Corruption is no longer taboo in some countries, including Kuwait, and in Morocco and Uganda the media has played a key role in exposing it. Civil society is developing new ways to collaborate with reform-minded governments. South Korea witnessed the signing of a nationwide, anti-corruption 'compact' involving the private sector, civil society and government.

Corruption and new governments

We have witnessed a dramatic turnaround in many countries, sparked by concerns over corruption. After Georgia's 'rose revolution' in 2003, Ukraine followed suit with the electoral victory of opposition leader Viktor Yushchenko in January 2005, and then Kyrgyzstan with its 'tulip revolution' in March 2005. The new governments were quick to commit themselves to fighting corruption. A principal driving force behind these changes was public outrage at the extreme methods used by previous regimes to stay in power, and the realisation of the potential of civil society involvement. Across the globe in Latin America, two presidents were forced to step down because of events that were perceived to be related to corruption: the independence of the judiciary in Ecuador and conflict of interest in Bolivia's oil and gas sector.

New leaders face huge challenges in meeting the expectations of their electorates. The example of Kenya shows how difficult it can be for a leader to maintain the mantle of an anti-corruption reformist. Prosecuting past and new cases of corruption has proved daunting for governments in Kenya, Kyrgyzstan, Morocco and elsewhere.

International pressure is often a motor for change: efforts by Romania and Croatia to pass anti-corruption measures are driven less by domestic demand than the pull of becoming members of the EU. Peer pressure is also evident in Asia-Pacific where the ADB-OECD Anti-Corruption Initiative has brought 25 countries together to tackle corruption. In Latin America, the OAS Anti-Corruption review mechanism is providing a valuable opportunity for independent groups to assess corruption-related developments.

Reforms at country level

Reform of the judiciary is one of the most powerful anti-corruption measures. Georgia passed a law to increase the independence of the courts in February 2005, strengthening the government's capacity to prosecute corrupt judges. A series of high-profile corruption scandals involving judges forced change in Greece and Kenya, while in Brazil, recent reforms have focused on increasing transparency in what is already a very independent institution. Other countries, including Burkina Faso, Ecuador and Venezuela, have seen a reversal of this trend: the judiciary's capacity to tackle corruption cases has been seriously called into question in these states.

Notable progress has been made in adopting reforms in other areas, including the drafting, passing and implementation of laws that are at the heart of efforts to curb corruption. Examples from the *Global Corruption Report 2006* include:

- increasing transparency in public procurement (Cameroon, Finland, France, Guatemala, Malaysia, South Korea and the United States)

- reducing corruption in politics (Croatia and Slovakia)

- increasing access to information (Slovakia, Switzerland and Panama)

- ensuring the independence and transparency of the judiciary (Brazil, Georgia, Greece, Poland and Romania)

- enhancing public sector integrity through codes of conduct and conflict of interest rules (Croatia, New Zealand and Panama)

- protecting whistleblowers (Japan, Papua New Guinea and Romania)

- improving transparency in financial services (Ireland, Malaysia and South Africa)

Signing up to international conventions

Another positive trend is the increased attention governments give to ratifying anti-corruption conventions. Every country report indicates which conventions a country has signed and ratified.

The UN Convention against Corruption, signed in Mexico in December 2003, has now attained the minimum 30 ratifications required and is expected to enter into force in early 2006. All OECD countries have ratified the 1997 OECD Anti-Bribery Convention, which makes overseas bribery a criminal offence for companies in their home countries, but its enforcement has been weak in many countries (including Japan and the United Kingdom). A further problem, highlighted in the New Zealand report, is the astonishingly low level of awareness of the Convention among the business community.

Reducing poverty by tackling corruption

There is a growing consensus that progress on reaching the Millennium Development Goal (MDG) of halving the number of people living in extreme poverty by 2015 is dependent on tackling corruption. Poverty and corruption are clearly linked: corruption leads to poverty when money to cover basic needs such as health and education ends up in the pockets of corrupt officials; when the private sector is harmed, leading to lower investment; and when the environment is damaged through corrupt infrastructure projects. Poverty can also exacerbate corruption because funds are not available to properly finance the institutions that keep corruption in check. The G8 summit of leaders in July 2005 confirmed that anti-corruption measures in the poorest countries of Africa must be a priority to reduce poverty. But it is not enough to combat corruption at country level. Foreign companies are often the source of big-ticket bribes in the developing world. It is just as important that wealthy governments publicise and enforce their anti-corruption laws to ensure that companies no longer view bribery as an acceptable way to win business. The multifaceted nature of corruption makes it difficult to tackle, and for this reason it is crucial that anti-corruption initiatives are initiated, monitored and enforced at government, civil society and private sector levels.

About the country reports

As in previous editions of the *Global Corruption Report*, the country reports reflect the unique combination of historical context, political, socio-economic, legal and cultural climates that present a country with particular challenges in its efforts to combat corruption. Mostly written by TI's national chapters, the reports are intended to provide an overview of key developments in fighting corruption across the world. The number of countries covered has expanded steadily over the years: from 34 in 2004, to 40 in 2005, and 45 this year. Special attention has been given to ensure a balance of information from developed and developing countries of various sizes. The absence of a particular country in this section does not reflect a high or low level of corruption in that country.

The country reports do not cover the same issues; topics of particular importance to individual countries are presented instead. Nevertheless, the structure is consistent across reports. Each begins with a list of which anti-corruption conventions the country has signed or ratified, followed by a list of key legal and institutional changes of July

2004–April 2005. The reports then delve into an analysis of the main corruption-related issues that arose during the period under review.

Note

1. Cobus de Swardt is director of global programmes at the Transparency International Secretariat.

8 Country reports

Algeria

Conventions:
AU Convention on Preventing and Combating Corruption (signed December 2003; not yet ratified)
UN Convention against Corruption (ratified August 2004)
UN Convention against Transnational Organized Crime (ratified October 2002)

Legal and institutional changes

- A **unit to process financial information**, appointed by presidential decree in April 2004, became operational in the Ministry of Finance in December 2004. The unit is an independent body with responsibility for receiving, analysing and dealing with suspicions relating to banking or financial operations that may constitute money laundering or the financing of terrorism.

- A **draft anti-corruption law** that brings legislation into line with the UN Convention against Corruption had its first reading in January 2005 and was adopted by the Council of Ministers in April 2005, pending presentation in parliament. The draft provides for the creation of a national body vested with the widest powers in terms of preventing and combating corruption. More particularly it will have responsibility for the drafting and implementation of a national anti-corruption strategy. This body will have the status of an independent administrative authority. Critics question the seriousness of the government's will, given the recent crackdown on the media (see below). Similar initiatives have been scuppered in the past: in 1996, the government set up a National Anti-Corruption Observatory that was dissolved by President Abdelaziz Bouteflika in 2000.

Crackdown on corruption – or on the press?

The state of emergency that has existed in Algeria from 1992 to the present has had many consequences, notably restrictions on civil liberties, opposition parties and civil society organisations. Public demonstrations are frequently banned and the right to strike has effectively disappeared. Journalists often find themselves at the sharp end of these restrictions. In June 2004, Mohamed Benchicou, managing editor of the daily *Le Matin*, was sentenced to two years in prison for writing a book critical of the president. The newspaper was forced to cease publication in July 2004 when the state-owned printing company suddenly demanded payment of debts; its website suffered the same fate; and its offices were sold at auction by the tax authorities. *Le Matin* was noted for publishing investigations into allegations of corruption involving senior officials.[1]

In the past year the authorities issued a stream of statements reiterating their commitment to uprooting corruption in response to increasing pressure for action from international financial institutions, foreign trading partners and the public. While the government claims to be working overtime on the problem, no concrete actions have actually resulted. The rhetoric strikes the right note, as did the ratification of the UN Convention against Corruption in August 2004, but there are fears they will both be used as excuses for doing nothing.

To take one example, the auditor general's department (Cour des comptes) was created in 1980 and is required under the constitution to publish annual reports, but only two have been submitted in the entire quarter century of its existence. In spite of an order in July 1995 that set out its mandate, the status of its investigators has still not been clearly defined. Its association of officers has repeatedly protested against the department's marginalisation, most recently at a public meeting attended by the press in August 2005, but the authorities have never deigned to give an explanation of their behaviour towards it.

Though sanctioned under the constitution, access to information held by the government is more likely to be denied than granted. Despite the pledge to eliminate corruption, no law facilitating access to information has been promulgated or included in any legislative programme. On the contrary, departments are more likely to restrict access to information, whether for use by the public or by the press. The latter finds it difficult to conduct investigations, particularly into corruption, when the authorities systematically refuse to collaborate with information or sources. This seriously inhibits media activity, as do the numerous libel actions taken against them.

Public procurement is also tainted by irregularities, including the excessive use of private agreements. President Bouteflika referred to this in a televised speech in April 2005 when he said such agreements would henceforth be prohibited in the public procurement process. Algeria is set to invest US $55 billion in infrastructure and other public works over the next five years, but the IMF expressed reservations on how public money is utilised in a report on Algeria's budgetary policy published in March. It concluded that Algeria only partially observes the norms on fiscal transparency. It went on to say that the distribution of data on the execution of the budget is 'severely restricted and sporadic' and the transparency measures laid down by law are not fully respected.[2] Capital flight is also a serious problem with an estimated €500 million (around US $612 million) leaving the country annually, according to government figures.[3]

Despite government efforts to the contrary, the limited amount of foreign investment Algeria receives can be principally explained by the corruption prevailing among public departments and officials. According to the World Bank, which surveyed more than 1,400 investors and companies in 2003, 'corruption is a major constraint for investment in Algeria with 75 per cent of firms reporting bribes are paid'.[4] The World Bank estimated that companies in Algeria spend an average 6 per cent of their turnover on corruption, while the OECD and the African Development Bank called corruption 'endemic' in a recent joint report.[5]

The state is the main shareholder in Algeria's wealthy oil and gas sector through the company Sonatrach, which rarely publishes details about its activities or the payments it receives from foreign investment partners. The only information it does make available relates to export revenues. It is a difficult company for journalists to investigate and any attempt to do so is quickly halted. The procurement process is also obscure. In April 2005, following the lead of the president, energy and mines minister Chakib Khelil expressed his own concerns at the growing number of public contracts being replaced by private agreement. He observed that 'more and more procurement contracts are being placed privately. This is a source of many abuses. The top priority is, in consequence, to exclude private agreements from public procurement processes.'[6] This same minister, however, filed a writ for libel against four journalists at *Le Matin* for an article published in August 2003 that questioned the legality of a sale of Sonatrach buildings and denounced the business interests of a number of politicians. Editor Youcef Rezzoug and journalists Yasmine Ferroukhi, Abla Cherif and Hassan Zerrouky were sentenced to two- and three-month jail terms, while Mohamed Benchicou, who had already spent 10 months in jail, saw his two-year sentence increased by five months. The International Federation of Journalists complained of a campaign of 'systematic judicial harassment' against reporters in Algeria.[7]

Since 2004, the government has announced a number of initiatives to combat corruption, particularly in the wake of the Khalifa affair (see below). It has also launched criminal proceedings against elected representatives and senior civil servants implicated in cases involving the misappropriation of funds. One case involved the former prefect of Oran, who was sentenced to a prison term, and in May 2005 the spotlight fell on the prefect of Blida, who was forced to resign. The latter's son was also charged with corruption in which his father may have been involved.[8] The case led to the arrest of, or charges against, several magistrates and senior officials from the justice ministry and the president's office. In May, the minister for religious affairs sent a note to *imams* asking them to stress the need to fight corruption in their Friday sermons through references to *sharia* law.

These gestures leave Algerians perplexed as to whether, behind all the apparent activity, there is any true commitment to combating corruption. Past anti-corruption campaigns rarely produced effective action and were widely viewed as power struggles in the higher reaches of government. It is now up to the authorities to demonstrate that their latest effort is more than another empty exercise.

The Khalifa affair

Revelations continue to tumble out about this enormous corruption case, reported in detail in the *Global Corruption Report 2004*. According to documents submitted to the French courts in July 2004 by the liquidators of El Khalifa Bank, the group owned by Algerian businessman Rafik Khalifa improperly transferred €689 million (US $843 million) to other countries between 1998 and 2002.[9] Khalifa, who has refused to comment on the collapse of his group, was sentenced in absentia to five years' imprisonment and a fine of 6 billion dinars (US $85 million) for banking violations in March 2004.

Financed by local investors, El Khalifa Bank provided cash for the group's subsidiaries in air transport and the media, which subsequently failed. The bank received sums from numerous companies because it offered an interest rate of 17 per cent and a high commission to new business providers. The French courts are particularly interested in Khalifa Airways' purchase of real estate in Paris for persons close to President Bouteflika. The police have drafted an investigative memorandum referring to the acquisition of two apartments. The first was acquired for someone close to the president and the second was transferred to Abdelghani Bouteflika, the president's brother, who also worked as the Khalifa group's lawyer. The authorities do not deny these allegations.

Candidates showed little interest in the Khalifa affair during the presidential campaign in April 2004 which returned Bouteflika for a second five-year term, but this hardly surprised analysts. Resolving the affair risks opening a Pandora's box so explosive that nobody could expect to derive benefit. None of the subsequent inquiries has reported on the generous facilities that Algeria's political, economic and financial elites extended to Khalifa, nor examined the factors that led the authorities to ignore the warning signs until it was too late. Algeria's courts routinely say they are continuing their investigations into this matter, but a trial originally set for March 2005 was postponed without any new date being set. They have issued an international arrest warrant for Rafik Khalifa, who remains at large. French investigations have focused on Khalifa's business dealings in France, including some financial transactions and his generous gifts to celebrities in the cinema and media.

According to the chief prosecutor in Blida, the court dealing with the Khalifa affair, the investigation is 'well under way'. 'It is a case which has caused considerable damage to the national economy', he said. 'All those who contributed to this fraud, from near or far, will be severely punished.'[10] His predecessor, who died in December 2004, had expected the trial to be held in March 2005, but judicial sources said in late October the investigation would only conclude in June 2005.[11] The same source said more than 800 people were involved in the Khalifa affair, of whom 600 had been interrogated and 20 charged.

Djilali Hadjadj (Association algérienne de lutte contre la corruption)

Further reading

Lounis Aggoun and Jean-Baptiste Rivoire, *Françalgérie: crimes et mensonges d'Etats* (French Algeria, Crimes and Lies of States) (Paris: La Découverte, 2004)
Djilali Hadjadj, *Corruption et démocratie en Algérie* (Corruption and Democracy in Algeria) (Paris: La Dispute, 2001)
Reporters Sans Frontières, *Algérie, livre noir* (Algeria: The Black Book) (Paris: La Découverte, 2003)
'Soir Corruption', a page devoted to news about corruption, has appeared in the evening newspaper *Le Soir d'Algérie* every Monday since 2000. See www.lesoirdalgerie.com

Association algérienne de lutte contre la corruption (Algerian Anti-Corruption Association) (AACC): www.chafafia.new.fr

Notes

1. Reporters Sans Frontières, press release, 2 February 2005, available at www.rsf.org/article.php3?id_article=12443
2. *Liberté* (Algeria), 3 March 2005.
3. *El Watan* (Algeria), 12 March 2005.
4. World Bank, *World Development Report 2005* (Washington, DC: World Bank, 2004).
5. OECD and African Development Bank, *African Economic Outlook*, May 2005.
6. *Liberté* (Algeria), 17 April 2005.
7. Agence France-Presse (France), 19 April 2005.
8. *Jeune Afrique L'Intelligent* (France), 5 June 2005, and *El Watan* (Algeria), 22 May 2005.
9. *Le Monde* (France), 8 February 2005.
10. *Liberté* (Algeria), 24 March 2005.
11. *El Watan* (Algeria), 31 October 2004.

Bangladesh

Conventions:
UN Convention against Corruption (not yet signed)
UN Convention against Transnational Organized Crime (not yet signed)

ADB-OECD Action Plan for Asia-Pacific (endorsed November 2001)

- The long-awaited **Anti-Corruption Commission** was set up in November 2004, allowing the government to claim credit for meeting its electoral commitments, as well as responding to the demands of civil society and international donors (see *Global Corruption Report 2005*). But a troublesome takeoff, questionable staff policies and curbed financial independence led TI Bangladesh and other NGOs to question the commission's potential to curb graft (see below).

- A cabinet meeting in December 2004 approved the appointment of a **Tax Ombudsman** (passed into law in July 2005), whose main tasks will be to receive taxpayers' complaints, to call the National Board of Revenue (NBR) to account and to suggest measures to redress injustices or malpractices. Widespread corruption in the NBR is partly responsible for the extremely low level of internal revenue collection,[1] while many tax officials are believed to aid tax evaders upon receipt of a bribe. At the time of writing, the appointment of the Tax Ombudsman was still awaiting approval from the Ministry of Law, Justice and Parliamentary Affairs. Civil society and the business community have long called for the foundation of such a post. In the absence of information about its independence, investigative powers and resources, however, it is still questionable whether it will prove an adequate response to corruption in the NBR (see below).

New anti-corruption commission disappoints expectations

When the Anti-Corruption Commission (ACC) was set up in November 2004, it was viewed as a timely institutional reform, and a strong signal that the government was committed to fighting corruption. Hardly a day has passed since then without the publication of media reports highlighting the scepticism that surrounds the ACC's lofty goals.[2] Indeed, since the key stimulus to set up the commission came from a combination of civil society demands and pressure from international donors, it could be argued that the government made the concession reluctantly, rather than out of genuine political will.[3]

The lack of impartiality in the procedures used to select the ACC's three commissioners, one of whom was appointed chairman, drew fire from the outset. Under the Anti-Corruption Commission Act of February 2004, commissioners were supposed to be approved by the president following recommendations by a selection panel of judges. As soon as the appointments were announced, however, critics cried foul saying

that political considerations had prevailed over the panel's recommendations. The eligibility of the chairman was also queried since he had formerly served as Chief Election Commissioner (CEC) and Supreme Court judge. Constitutional experts and some former election commissioners claimed that the new appointment was in violation of the constitution, which does not allow former CECs or judges to take up other public posts.[4] Public interest litigation challenging the legal validity of the appointment was filed in the High Court in March 2005. Irrespective of the case's outcome and the constitutional debate surrounding it, such events do not bode well for the ACC's future.

Disputes over staffing ensued, with the ACC following no clear rules of appointment. More controversially, it decided to rehire the former staff of the defunct Bureau of Anti-Corruption, which was dissolved due to its ineffectiveness and lack of independence.[5] The commission subsequently annulled the hiring decision, but the damage to its credibility had been done. Furthermore, contrary to the provisions of the Anti-Corruption Commission Act, decisions on personnel appointments and transfers were taken without consultation between the three commission members, leading to serious doubts as to their capacity to provide the leadership needed for the challenging tasks ahead. Most problematic of all, however, is the issue of the ACC's independence since the government retains authority over key policy issues, such as budget, staff recruitment and organisational structure. Indeed, the commission currently requires cabinet approval before implementing any of its decisions.[6]

Despite the powers bestowed on it, the commission has failed to take specific policy measures in the past five months, or to convey to the public any sense of its strategy for fighting corruption. Instead, it has limited its mandate to a number of ad hoc decisions that demonstrate lack of vision and poor performance. For instance, the ACC framed charges against a number of transfer orders for government officials, but failed to follow them up.[7] Similarly, it announced it was going to investigate the unauthorised use of government vehicles, the misappropriation of public land (belonging to the railways) and the importation of rotten rice.[8] No concrete measures were taken apart from issuing letters to the relevant departments.

Corruption in the customs department

According to a study published by TI Bangladesh in September 2004, corruption is rife in the customs department, which comes under the jurisdiction of the National Board of Revenue. The study was conducted in Chittagong port, which handles about 75 per cent of the country's imports and exports. Shipping companies have to submit descriptions of their goods, either in an Import General Manifesto (IGM) or Export General Manifesto (EGM), in accordance with regulations. The study found that 'tipping' for permissions went without objection for so long that it had become institutionalised, with bribes paid in 100 per cent of cases for both the IGMs and EGMs. Bribes were also demanded in 100 per cent of cases to amend IGMs or EGMs for various reasons.[9]

Under the regulations, if a container with imported goods has not been released within 45 days, it must be auctioned. Researchers found that importers bribed customs officials to delay the auctions in order to take advantage of price fluctuations in the market. To obtain release orders from the customs authority for imported goods, moreover, clearing and forwarding agents have to pay bribes at a minimum of 16 and up to 37 different customs personnel levels. The study estimates the amount of bribes paid by importers and exporters to officials at Chittagong port at around 8 billion takas (US $130 million) annually.[10]

In the wake of the TI Bangladesh report, the Parliamentary Standing Committee on the Ministry of Finance demanded in October 2004 that customs reduce the number of steps importers and exporters have to pass through to release their goods. The Chittagong Port Authority (CPA) formed a five-member inquiry team to investigate the cases of corruption revealed in the report. In January 2005, it launched a 'one-stop' service for importers and exporters in a bid to minimise corruption. It is too soon to evaluate the impact these initiatives may have on curbing corruption, but the business community has embraced them.

Other recommendations emerged, including the privatisation of port management, the restructuring of the CPA, the introduction of more flexible clearance procedures and the privatisation of goods handling and labour management, to facilitate a system of incentives to reduce the undue influence of vested interests. Steps could be taken, for example, to include representatives of port users on the CPA's board of directors, so beginning the process of transforming it into a fully autonomous organisation.

Professionalism in the police force questioned

Concern has grown in recent years over the role of the police force as a law enforcement agency. Indeed, it has not only failed to enforce the law, but violations have often taken place with the passive connivance, if not active participation of its members.

A survey by TI Bangladesh, conducted in September/October 2004 and released in April 2005, revealed that 92 per cent of all respondents who filed complaints to the police administration had to pay bribes, while 80 per cent paid bribes to obtain police clearance certificates for various purposes. The survey estimated the amount of bribes paid by households to the police at 15.3 billion takas (US $260 million) a year.[11]

Members of the police have been implicated in cases of extortion, bribery, arbitrary arrest and even custodial torture and murder in some cases. In one case, an officer killed a man in Badda thana (police station) after he refused to pay a bribe. A case against the officer has now been filed in the magistrate's court.[12]

In July 2003, the government formed the Rapid Action Battalion (RAB), a mixed force of police, army, air force and paramilitary personnel, with the special task of curbing crime. Nine months later, the government claimed the controversial unit had succeeded in improving law and order. Although it recovered a total of 718 arms, over 200 people were killed in questionable circumstances that were officially described as crossfire.[13] In May 2005 alone, police killed 24 people and the RAB a further 21.[14] The deaths sparked a flood of criticism from civil society, human rights organisations, opposition parties and donors. The RAB was also reportedly engaged in extortion, robbery and bribe-taking.[15]

Given that professionalism in the police force and in other law enforcement agencies is crucial to the fight against corruption, developments like these are scarcely conducive to ensuring better governance in Bangladesh.

Iftekhar Zaman, Sydur Rahman and Abdul Alim (TI Bangladesh)

Further reading

Asian Development Bank, *Controlling Corruption in Asia and the Pacific* (Manila: ADB, 2004)
Centre for Policy Dialogue, *Reforming Governance in Bangladesh* (Dhaka: CPD, 2002)
Centre for Policy Dialogue, *Business Competitiveness Environment Report* (Dhaka: CPD, 2004)
Transparency International Bangladesh, *Corruption Database* (Dhaka: TI Bangladesh, 2004)
Transparency International Bangladesh, *Parliament Watch* (Dhaka: TI Bangladesh, 2005)

TI Bangladesh: www.ti-bangladesh.org

Notes

1. In a country of 140 million people, there are only around 1.5 million registered taxpayers, of whom perhaps half actually pay any taxes. See *Daily Banglabazar* (Bangladesh), 17 January 2002.
2. *New Nation* (Bangladesh), 6 March 2005.
3. One sign of Bangladesh's lack of commitment to the anti-corruption drive was its failure to send any representatives to the 6th Steering Group Meeting of the ADB-OECD Anti-Corruption Initiative held in Hanoi, Vietnam, in April 2005, although it is one of 25 Asia-Pacific countries to have endorsed the initiative.
4. *Daily Star* (Bangladesh), 13 March 2005.
5. *Independent* (Bangladesh), 15 March 2005; *Daily Star* (Bangladesh), 18 February 2005; see also *Global Corruption Report 2005*.
6. *Global Corruption Report 2005*; *Daily Jugantor* (Bangladesh), 13 April 2005.

7. *New Nation* (Bangladesh), 7 April 2005.
8. *New Nation* (Bangladesh), 27 March 2005.
9. TI Bangladesh, *Chittagong Port: A Diagnostic Study* (Dhaka: TI Bangladesh, 2004).
10. Ibid.
11. TI Bangladesh, *Household Corruption Survey* (Dhaka: TI Bangladesh, 2005).
12. *Daily Prothom Alo* (Bangladesh, in Bengali), 20 May 2005.
13. *Daily Star* (Bangladesh), 29 March 2005.
14. *Daily Jugantor* (Bangladesh, in Bengali), 1 June 2005.
15. Asian Human Rights Commission, Urgent Appeals Programme, 25 July 2005, www.ahrchk. net/ua/mainfile.php/2005/1182/

Bolivia

Conventions:

OAS Inter-American Convention against Corruption (ratified February 1997)
UN Convention against Corruption (signed December 2003; not yet ratified)
UN Convention against Transnational Organized Crime (signed December 2000; not yet ratified)

Legal and institutional changes

- Members of the justice department and presidential anti-corruption delegation are drafting a **conflict of interest law** that is expected to be approved in 2005. The law is aimed at bringing Bolivian legislation on the issue into line with the Inter-American Anti-corruption Convention and is being drafted with the support of a US-funded anti-corruption programme.

- An **amendment to the penal code** is being drafted under the same process as above, and is also expected to be approved in 2005 if the full congressional agenda allows for the changes to be debated. The aim is to incorporate new corruption-related crimes into the criminal code in order to make it easier to prosecute acts of corruption.

Conflicts of interest: relationships between the public and private sectors

The debate over the future role of multinational companies in Bolivia's large natural resources sector has led to the uncovering of a number of events that allowed foreign natural resources companies to obtain very favourable contracts, to the detriment of the government. Questions have since arisen about the need for conflict of interest mechanisms to safeguard decision-takers against undue influence from the private sector or other interest groups.

A practice that has become commonplace is for public officials to cross over into private sector positions – or vice versa – in the same sphere of work. Employees in state-owned companies, the energy minister or the state regulator might cross the revolving door to private sector companies, for example, where they are required to negotiate with the government on issues that were their direct responsibility when public servants. This means that they have an unfair advantage of information and experience when it comes to negotiating favourable contracts.

In April 2005, *El Diario* newspaper reported that the civil society Committee to Defend National Heritage (CODEPANAL) had complained that Jaime Barrenechea, the former president of the Bolivian state oil company Yacimientos Petrolíferos Fiscales

Bolivianos (YPFB), is now a manager for Repsol-YPF Argentina, while former YPFB executives Hugo Peredo and Arturo Castaños have moved to Repsol-YPF and the Bolivian branch of the Brazilian state-owned company Petrobras, respectively.[1] Another recent scandal involved Eduardo Baldivieso, a former regulator of the industry, who moved to GAS del Sur to become managing director. He was able to negotiate a favourable contract to export liquefied petroleum gas for GAS del Sur.[2]

Similar situations have arisen in the water sector. Aguas del Illimani and Aguas del Tunari, two companies with potable water and sewage concessions, have profited from staff that moved from public sector roles directly connected to the contracts they subsequently negotiated on behalf of their private sector companies. The government, in 2005 and 2000, respectively, rescinded both contracts in response to protests.

These and other cases have highlighted the need for a law regulating conflicts of interest. The use of privileged information and contacts by people switching between public and private sector posts in the same area of work has undermined the credibility of both sectors and led to protests.

President Gonzalo Sánchez de Lozada was forced to step down in October 2003 in response to protests demanding the nationalisation of Bolivia's natural gas reserves, the second largest in Latin America. His successor, Carlos Mesa, resigned in June 2005. While protests centred on the question of privatisation, the fact that private companies were seen to be profiting unduly from contracts thanks to government connections probably contributed to the protest movements.

Unlawful enrichment at local government level highlights need for new law

Over the past few years, cases of unlawful enrichment at municipal government level have increased, highlighting the need for greater powers to investigate acquisition of wealth by public office holders.

Cases of illicit enrichment by authorities at national policy bodies and in central government continue to arise, but official records point to municipal authorities as the perpetrators of corruption in a surprising number of cases. Many cases against mayors and local councillors are currently going through the courts.

Examples are the mayor of Achocalla, a small municipality near the cities of La Paz and El Alto, who faces charges of misusing public funds. Also implicated in cases of abuse of public funds are representatives of local authorities in Tiquina, Viacha, Caranavi, Ayoayo, Yanacachi, Copacabana and Uyuni.[3]

Nepotism, influence peddling and abuse of authority all exist at local and central government level, and there are laws aimed at curbing some of these practices. One missing piece of the legislative puzzle, which makes it difficult to tackle such forms of corruption, is a law allowing authorities to probe assets of public officials. Draft laws setting out the ways and means in which authorities might be able to scrutinise the assets and earnings of public officials have been presented to Congress, but have been rejected.

There is, however, a Financial Investigations Unit within the bank regulator with the capacity to probe transactions of people within the banking system. This unit could identify possible cases of illegal enrichment for further investigation.

Reforms at the national highways authority aimed at reducing corruption by its staff proved successful in reducing cases of unlawful enrichment by staff, and could provide a useful model for possible reforms at other government bodies. Among the key pieces of reform were a move to more competitive recruitment; decisive action against employees accused of corruption; and the introduction of transparent and open contracting processes.

In the final analysis, the political will of the authority is key to any successful reform process, and pressure from civil society can help keep the issue on their agenda. Over the past few years a number of civil society organisations have developed to monitor public authorities, in particular local authorities. The development is not positive a priori, however, and needs to be monitored as well to ensure that civil society organisations do not participate in corrupt acts themselves, or are not co-opted by private interest groups.

Public contracting processes still provide opportunities for corruption

Public contracts are regulated by very detailed legislation and mechanisms such as Internet-based information systems that allow contracts to be placed and bid for on-line, in order to reduce the risk of corruption. Nevertheless, while instances of corruption in public procurement appear to have decreased in the past few years, they continue to arise.

In 2003 the government planned to promote a law to regulate once and for all problems associated with purchasing processes. The draft law was rejected and converted into a presidential decree, which attempted to incorporate the main details of the law, but lacked the weight and support of a law. The decree also contained an ethics code for public officials responsible for procurement.

There remains a need, therefore, for a reform to streamline and simplify the resulting morass of laws, norms and decrees. There are several loopholes and areas of corruption that fall between the gaps where laws do not knit together well. It is still not practice across the board, for example, for contracting authorities to present transparent terms of reference to bidders.

While it is true that important steps still have to be taken to increase the transparency of contracts offered by government, comparable steps by the private sector have yet to be taken. There are too few good examples of integrity mechanisms, such as codes of conduct preventing attempts to exert undue influence over government decision-makers, which could be disseminated across private sector companies.

Guillermo Pou Munt Serrano
(Centro de Desarrollo de Éticas Aplicadas y Promoción de Capital Social)

Further reading

Andean Commission of Jurists, 'Informe anual sobre la región Andina' (Annual Report on the Andean Region, January 2002)
Fundación Etica y Democracia, 'Informe de evaluación ciudadana de implementación de la Convención Interamericana contra la corrupción' (Report of Citizen Evaluation of the Implementation of the Inter-American Convention against Corruption, 2004)

Notes

1. *El Diario* (Bolivia), 24 April 2005.
2. *CA$H* (Bolivia), 15 April 2005.
3. Presidential Anti-corruption Delegation, 'Registro de seguimiento de casos de corrupción' (Register of follow-up of cases), 2005.

Brazil

Conventions:
OAS Inter-American Convention against Corruption (ratified July 2002)
OECD Anti-Bribery Convention (ratified August 2000)
UN Convention against Corruption (ratified June 2005)
UN Convention against Transnational Organized Crime (ratified January 2004)

Legal and institutional changes

- New legislation regulating **public–private partnerships** (PPPs) was approved in December 2004. The PPP is a relatively new method of financing and developing infrastructure in Brazil. Mechanisms were introduced into the new law to curtail opportunities for private sector companies to unduly influence the terms of a PPP tender.

- After 13 years of discussions and negotiations, congress passed a constitutional amendment in December 2004 aimed at **streamlining the judiciary** and speeding up judicial process. The amendment introduced the concept of 'binding precedent', conceived as a means of guaranteeing uniformity of jurisprudence and restricting recurrent appeals, and established a National Council of Justice as an external control mechanism over the judiciary (see below).

- A **parliamentary front against corruption** was created in the lower house of Congress in July 2004 to address matters on corruption.

The judiciary: who guards the guardian?

In contrast to a number of other Latin American countries, where strengthening judicial independence against political pressure is the main challenge to anti-corruption campaigners, the calls for judicial reform in Brazil paradoxically derive from its excessive independence. Once defined by President Lula da Silva as a 'black box',[1] the judiciary lacks transparency and is often accused of being isolated, dedicated to preserving corporate privileges and unaccountable to society.

Understandably, there was concern to strengthen the independence of the judiciary when the current constitution was drafted after two decades of military rule, though it was granted extremely wide latitude. The constitution gave the judiciary broad functional and structural autonomy. At the same time, in order to guarantee the protection of a number of social rights, it allowed for almost endless rights of appeal at different levels of the legal system – besides rejecting the binding nature of superior court decisions on lower courts.

This constitutional architecture has fatal results insofar as accountability and performance are concerned. The judiciary is slow and inaccessible to the poor. One example of how these characteristics can be abused was the decision by José Serra, the new mayor of São Paulo, in early 2005 to suspend payments to suppliers even as he acknowledged that R2 billion (US$ 851 million) was owing, since he knew a judicial decision was likely to take 10 years or more due to the sluggish pace of justice.

Inefficiencies in the judiciary lead to impunity. According to a survey by Congresso em Foco (Congress in Focus), an Internet site specialising in legislative news, 102 out of 595 MPs currently face criminal, administrative or electoral accusations in protracted lawsuits. Corruption, such as the 'Anaconda scandal' in 2003 that involved a judge selling favourable sentences to criminals, completes the picture of a dysfunctional judiciary.[2]

These factors led to calls for change in the judicial structure and procedures as a way to broaden access to juridical services, to make justice more expeditious, to simplify the system of appeals, to allow for a faster solution of conflicts and to put an end to self-interested practices by judges. Judicial reform proved hard to push through, given the resistance from judges themselves. Finally, after 13 years of discussion, Congress approved an amendment to the constitution in December 2004.

A key measure is the provision of 'binding precedent', conceived as a means of guaranteeing uniformity of jurisprudence and restricting the recurrent appeals in similar cases. Another important development, the National Council of Justice, was praised in some quarters, including the government, as a promising initiative to introduce an 'external control mechanism' over the judiciary.

Given that the council is part of the judiciary and is composed largely of judges (nine of its fifteen members are judges; two are lawyers; two are public prosecutors; two are citizens appointed by Congress), its independence will be in question. Moreover, it has been given only limited powers, since its decisions can be contested and annulled by the judiciary. Many see the council as a cosmetic move, rather than one that will make the institution more accountable and efficient.

As approved, the reform does not tackle the gravest problem afflicting the Brazilian judiciary: the absence of aggregated and comparative information on its workings. Although every judicial decision is public (and is published on the Internet), the judiciary does not collect or publish statistics about its workings, making it impossible for external observers to effectively monitor it. The 'black box' of the Brazilian judiciary remains to be opened.

Lula's anti-graft platform is shaken by corruption scandals

A series of corruption scandals in 2004 and the first half of 2005 has shaken the ruling Workers' Party (PT), and cast doubts over its ability to make good on its campaign pledge to tackle corruption. In its winning campaign, the PT had championed fiscal and ethical probity.

The scandals date back to February 2004 when news broke that chief of staff José Dirceu's closest aide, Waldimiro Diniz, had taken kickbacks from the operators of bingo parlours (see *Global Corruption Report 2005* for an analysis of corruption in Brazil's gambling industry). The government blocked efforts to launch a congressional inquiry into the case. Diniz was director of the lottery sector of Rio de Janeiro at the time and he had allegedly offered contract privileges for on-line and over-the-phone lotteries in exchange for campaign donations to fund certain PT candidates' campaigns during the 2002 election. The report of a congressional investigation into the fraud was approved by the Rio de Janeiro State Assembly in October 2004.

In June 2004, 'Operation Vampire' was launched into possible illegalities at the Health Ministry and four other ministries connecting officials to the illegal sale of blood supplies worth more than US $660 million from 1990 to 2002.[3] Government auditors launched an investigation into the high prices paid for blood; the suspicion was that public officials were buying blood at one price and invoicing the government at a higher rate.

Later, in August 2004, the weekly magazine, *IstoÉ*, published that the Central Bank president and a director hid overseas assets from tax authorities. The article led to the downfall of the director of monetary policy at the Central Bank, Luiz Augusto de Oliveira Candiota, and tarnished the reputation of the Bank's president, Henrique Meirelles. As soon as the accusations were made public, a presidential decree was issued giving Meirelles (and all future central bank presidents) the status of cabinet minister, so that he could be better protected against accusations of improbity. The Supreme Court is currently investigating allegations that he evaded taxes and foreign exchange regulations.

In May 2005, the weekly magazine *Veja* uncovered a bribery scandal in the Brazilian Postal Service.[4] Reporters revealed a secretly filmed videotape showing the former chief of the contracts and supplies department, Maurício Marinho, receiving a US $1,250 'cash advance' from private companies seeking contracts. The opposition petitioned for a parliamentary inquiry, which the government consented to after initial resistance. Roberto Jefferson, a member of Congress and president of the Brazilian Labour Party (PTB) – which is allied with the ruling party – was allegedly implicated in the scandal.

Jefferson was also involved in the next scandal to break. In May 2005, the media reported allegations by Lídio Duarte, former president of the state-run Brazilian Reinsurers Institute (IRB), that Jefferson had tried to pressure him to hire a number of his associates.[5] The scandal deepened after Duarte accused Jefferson of also demanding a monthly kickback to the PT of R400,000 (US $170,000) as a 'thank you' for giving him the IRB post.

In response, Jefferson accused the governing PT of using undeclared funds to pay campaign costs and bribe legislators. Lacking a majority in Congress, the PT was accused of paying a monthly allowance of R30,000 (US $12,500) to congressmen from two allied parties in return for their votes. The two parties implicated are the Progressive Party (PP), led by Severino Cavalcanti, the low-profile ultra-conservative chairman of the Chamber of Deputies; and the Liberal Party (PL), whose president, Waldemar Costa Neto, became the first lawmaker to step down in the widening corruption scandal.

Dirceu resigned as the president's chief of staff in June 2005 and returned to his seat in the Chamber of Deputies where he is under investigation by the Chamber of Deputies Ethics Committee.

As the political crisis escalates and election campaign financing irregularities are being revealed, calls for political and campaign financing reforms gain force. There is a consensus that if anything positive can result from Brazil's worst political crisis in a decade, it is the approval of comprehensive political reforms that address problems associated with private financing, inadequate disclosure of campaign accounts and the failure to impose proportionate sanctions when breaches of political finance rules are found to have occurred.

Ana Luiza Fleck Saibro (Transparência Brasil)

Further reading

Rogério Bastos Arantes, *Ministério público e política no Brasil* (Public Prosecutions and Politics in Brazil) (São Paulo: Sumaré, 2002)
David V. Fleischer, *Corruption in Brazil: Defining, Measuring, and Reducing* (Washington DC: Center for Strategic and International Studies, 2002)
Transparência Brasil, 'Vote Buying in the 2004 Elections', www.transparencia.org.br

Transparência Brasil: www.transparencia.org.br

Notes

1. www.brazzil.com/2004/html/articles/jul04/p135jul04.htm
2. www.congressoemfoco.com.br/arquivo_especiais/12fev2004_rochamattos/rocha_respostas. aspx, and www.economist.com/world/la/displayStory.cfm?story_id=2542089
3. UPI (USA), 6 October 2004.
4. *Veja* (Brazil), 14 May 2005.
5. *Estado de São Paulo* (Brazil), 20 May 2005.

Burkina Faso

Conventions:
AU Convention on Preventing and Combating Corruption (ratified March 2005)
UN Convention against Corruption (signed December 2003; not yet ratified)
UN Convention against Transnational Organized Crime (ratified May 2002)

Legal and institutional changes

- In March 2005, the National Ethics Committee submitted its report for 2003 to the prime minister after a delay of one year. It highlighted the lack of professionalism, weak governance and corruption in public service, and recommended the adoption of **public sector codes of conduct** for the departments of public administration, health, education, security and finance. The nine-member committee also conducted ethics training with parties, ministries, parliamentarians and civil society organisations throughout 2004. With the publication of its second report, the committee has now gained a degree of public confidence, but it remains to be seen if its recommendations will be implemented.

- In December 2004, the government issued a decree on the **conduct of the national police force** that sets standards for behaviour and provides disciplinary sanctions for breaches of conduct. It is expected to increase public awareness of police officers' duties and the rights of citizens to file complaints about illegal acts committed by officers, including corruption.

Challenges faced by anti-corruption bodies

Despite government promises to facilitate anti-corruption efforts by creating new institutions and ratifying several international conventions, the continued failure to disclose reports into official corruption and a culture of relative impunity cast doubts on these efforts in 2004–05.

A case in point was the 2004 report by the High Commission for the Coordination of Anti-Corruption Activities (HACLC) in March 2005, which remained as confidential as its predecessor in January 2004 in spite of an agreement that HACLC findings should be publicly available.[1] Also in March, a document setting out the priorities of a national campaign against corruption, initiated by the HACLC and validated during a seminar attended by 200 people in December 2004, was presented to the government. Its two main recommendations were the creation of a national anti-corruption assembly, bringing together delegates from the public and private sectors and civil society, and the creation of a higher authority to refer corruption-related matters to the courts when necessary.[2] At the time of writing, the government had not responded to its recommendations.

The HACLC, which officially began work in 2003, faces a series of challenges to its effective functioning and is viewed by some as weaker than other anti-corruption bodies, such as the National Ethics Committee and the Public Accounts Court (see below). Several ministers and project managers were implicated in the misappropriation of public funds amounting to FCFA3 billion (US $5.5 million) in its first report.[3] The official response has been limited, although three corruption-related cases were referred to the courts on the instructions of the prime minister. Critics saw the gesture as a political move to gain popularity before the presidential elections in November 2005 and to wrong-foot the opposition's campaign against corruption.

On submission of its second report, the HACLC's president, Honoré Tougouri, was quoted as saying that 'the commission has not received any tangible response to the recommendations in the 2003 report, taken as a whole, that would have enabled it to direct, correct, amend, reorganise, energise or even slow down its activities'. Speaking of the HACLC's operational difficulties, Tougouri stressed that the main problem was the government's slow reaction to its requests. With respect to its budget of nearly FCFA1 billion (US $1.8 million), he said: 'Even if the HACLC budget has risen slightly, it does not cover its essential activities, i.e., those that justify its creation.'[4]

The HACLC's problems are not limited to the lack of financial and human resources; it also suffers from a lack of direction. It is not clear, for instance, whether it should coordinate the fight against corruption, as stipulated in its governing provisions, or act in all areas related to anti-corruption, such as raising awareness, investigation, lobbying and interagency cooperation. Its work should be much better coordinated with the activities of the National Ethics Committee, the Public Accounts Court (PAC) and other courts, the General State Inspectorate (GSI) and the committee responsible for monitoring the GSI's recommendations.

Despite these difficulties, the HACLC deserves credit for producing activity reports on a regular basis and for the professionalism of its nine members. Moreover, there has been a significant increase in public awareness of the importance of the fight against corruption, and citizens now expect greater integrity in public affairs.

The PAC, established in 2002, has played a key role in the oversight of public finance management in the past few years. It has tried to compensate for the failings of the former Accounts Chamber by producing three draft laws governing the state budgets for 1999–2001, 2002 and 2003. Although the preparatory reports for these laws are supposed to be public, when the court is asked to produce them officials reply that they are not authorised to do so. Nevertheless,

every MP receives a copy and substantial extracts can be found in the press.

The PAC's investigations have led to the discovery of irregularities that cost the public purse dearly. According to an October 2004 report by the finance and budget committee of the National Assembly, routine checks revealed that 151 retired civil servants in various ministries were still receiving their salaries.[5] Apparently unaware that the staff concerned had retired, the finance ministry continued to pay the salaries, a blunder that cost more than FCFA450 million (US $860,000).

The PAC has planned to submit its first report to President Blaise Compaoré in the first half of 2005. Preparations for its publication have involved the inspection of the budgets of a number of public institutions, local authorities and public companies, including many where the press had already reported poor management, embezzlement and fraud.

The judiciary comes under fire

A string of corruption scandals in 2004–05 raised expectations that prosecutions of senior officials would follow, but the courts handed down only a limited number of verdicts. From January 2004 to April 2005, the Council of Ministers imposed sanctions on officials accused of corruption, dismissing some and moving others to different posts. Judicial proceedings were undertaken in the most serious cases, involving nearly 20 state accountants, financial controllers, collection agents and court registry officials. The steepest penalties were imposed on the mayors of Ouahigouya and Zorgho, both members of the ruling Congress for Democracy and Progress (CDP). They were removed from office and charged with corruption in February 2005. This could be interpreted as a settling of scores within the CDP, given that other mayors suspected of corruption were not charged. In February, several cases of embezzlement of public funds were also heard before the criminal courts. One involved the misappropriation of some FCFA11 million (US $21,000) from a public fund for health and nutrition by state accountant, Jean Paul Balbéogo. He admitted the charges and was sentenced to five years in prison.[6]

Nevertheless, the judiciary was widely criticised for delaying alleged corruption investigations involving senior officials, such as director generals, high commissioners, MPs and ministers, even when there was overwhelming evidence against them. The sacrosanct rule of separation of powers is not sufficiently observed: judges face difficulties in opening such investigations and corruption cases are rarely tried before the courts. This has led to a public perception that high-ranking officials enjoy impunity, and the finger of blame points at the judiciary.

Allegations of corruption have recently been made against the judiciary, whose performance has never been lower in the annual corruption perception rating of REN-LAC, a nationwide anti-corruption network of 30 civil society organisations. In December 2004, the magazine *Evénement* published the findings of an investigation into corruption that accused judges of attempted extortion from litigants; lawyers of robbing their clients; court officials of embezzling funds; and other auxiliaries of tampering with court files and other documents.[7] The exposé led to a massive outcry. Professional lawyers'

associations denounced their colleagues, while others supported the justice ministry, denying that corruption existed in their ranks.

In the face of mounting public pressure, the Higher Council of the Judiciary, chaired by the president, created an ad hoc commission of inquiry into corruption in the judiciary in June 2004. Chaired by Kadiatou Dakoure, who also chairs Council of State meetings, it filed its findings in March 2005 which confirmed that graft was widespread. Corruption was found to be prevalent in the courts of Bobo-Dioulasso and Ouagadougou, which deal with the more serious cases. The commission found more than 30 cases of 'questionable practices' and 'suspicious behaviour' implicating judges, lawyers, police officers, intermediaries or 'touts', and other users of the judicial system, including accounting firms and liquidators. The report concluded that no strategy to combat corruption would be effective without genuine political will.[8]

In the meantime, the bar association imposed sanctions on two of its members in April 2005. One, Maître Djibril Lankoandé, was suspended for extorting FCFA1 million (US $2,000) from a client on the grounds that the sum was needed to 'motivate' the judge in charge of the case.[9] The judiciary was shaken by this and other cases, but no official steps have been taken to address the findings of the commission of inquiry.

Luc Damiba (REN-LAC)

Further reading

REN-LAC, *Rapport 2004 sur l'état de la corruption au Burkina Faso* (2004 Report on the State of Corruption in Burkina Faso) (Ouagadougou: Editions REN-LAC, 2005)
'Médiateur du Faso, Rapport final des conférences du médiateur du Faso sur la gestion du patrimoine public' (Final Report on the Conferences of the Faso Mediator on the Management of Public Assets) (Ouagadougou, 2004)
HACLC, *Document cadre de la politique nationale de la lutte contre la corruption* (Framework Document for the National Policy on Ways to Combat Corruption) (Ouagadougou: HACLC, 2004)
Conseil Supérieur de la Magistrature, 'Rapport de la commission d'étude sur la corruption dans le secteur de la justice, mars 2005' (Report of the Commission Charged with Studying Corruption in the Judiciary, March 2005)

REN-LAC: www.renlac.org

Notes

1. *Global Corruption Report 2005*.
2. 'National Seminar on the Proposed National Policy to Combat Corruption', Summary Report, 13–15 December 2004.
3. HACLC Press Conference, 10 January 2004, published in *L'Observateur Paalga* (Burkina Faso), 11 January 2004.
4. *San Finna* (Burkina Faso), 4 April 2005.
5. National Assembly, Report No. 2004/030/AN/COMFIB, File No. 16; see also *Bendré* (Burkina Faso), 17 October 2004.
6. www.aib.bf/siteaib/revuearch2.htm
7. *Evénement* (Burkina Faso), 10 January 2005, www.cnpress-zongo.net/evenementbf/pages/dossier_1_59.htm
8. Conseil Supérieur de la Magistrature, 'Rapport de la commission d'étude sur la corruption dans le secteur de la justice, mars 2005' (Report of the Commission Charged with Studying Corruption in the Judiciary, March 2005).
9. www.lefaso.net/article.php3?id_article=8270

Cameroon

Conventions:
AU Convention on Preventing and Combating Corruption (not yet signed)
UN Convention against Corruption (signed December 2003; not yet ratified)
UN Convention against Transnational Organized Crime (signed December 2000; not yet ratified)

Legal and institutional changes

- A law passed in September 2004 instituted a **new procurement code** (see below).

- A decree in February 2005 laid down the rules for a **new committee to coordinate the fight against fraud, smuggling and forgery**. Its remit is to review existing regulations and propose changes; initiate administrative investigations; combat the import and sale of products derived from fraud, smuggling or forgery; devise and monitor the implementation of prevention programmes; protect tax and customs receipts; and centralise information about illegal commercial practices. The committee, chaired by the Minister of Trade, includes representatives from other concerned ministries, the unions, the employers' federation, the security services and the department for external research. It will also have inspectors at its disposal to carry out activities in the provinces.

- A presidential decree in February 2005 established a **special supervisory department** (Division spéciale de contrôle des services) in the **national security service** with responsibility for investigating the 'confidentiality, state of mind, morale and loyalty' of members of the national and local police. If the new body were given real powers, it would yield an immediate boost in public confidence since the police force is allegedly one the most pernicious sources of everyday corruption.[1] It is doubtful the new department will prove effective, however. A similar unit was created in the past but dismantled at short notice, without proving its value.

- In March 2005, the government promised to **lift the secrecy** surrounding its **oil revenues** by signing up to the Extractive Industries Transparency Initiative and promising to publish comprehensive, quarterly figures about its production, sales prices and revenues (see below).

Procurement: will independent audits help?

Sixteen months after ratifying the UN Convention against Corruption, the government introduced a Procurement Contracts Code in September 2004 to replace the three decrees from 1995 and 2002 that had regulated public tendering poorly. The new code increases the responsibility of contractors, establishes a mechanism to regulate the system and strengthens supervision before and after contracts are allocated by submitting them to independent observers and an independent auditor. Article 2 enshrines 'equality of access to public orders', 'equality of treatment for bidders' and 'procedural transparency' as the code's guiding principles.

The code is intended to deal with a multitude of procurement-related corrupt practices, including: breaches of rules regarding publication of offers, limiting competition; failure to respect confidentiality when bids are examined; lack of precise criteria by which candidates and offers are chosen; acquisition of interests by the supervisory authorities through the creation of fictitious companies; skewing of the selection procedure; abuse of the purpose of contracts; fictitious deliveries; payment for contracts not performed; and the splitting of orders to circumvent procedures by remaining below the minimum required threshold. Such practices make regular appearances in the courts, most notably in the 'Mounchipou case' in 2003 when a former minister of telecommunications was found to have colluded in the fraudulent award of a public works contract that involved order splitting, fictitious delivery of contracts and overpricing.[2]

To combat these practices, the government proposed two measures to improve the performance of the Procurement Contracts Commission (CPM), which is responsible for providing contractors with technical support and supervision in all departments, including state-owned companies and diplomatic missions. The first is a new sub-commission within the CPM to analyse and classify bids in purely technical and financial terms. It will be supported by four specialist bodies with supervisory responsibility for monitoring procurement procedures in roads and infrastructure, buildings and collective facilities, general supplies, and intellectual services.

The code's other innovation is the recruitment of an independent observer through an international call for bids by the Agency for the Regulation of Procurement Contracts (ARMP), whose role is to ensure that all regulations, transparency rules and principles of fairness are respected in procurement processes. The ARMP will also recruit an independent auditor of 'untarnished reputation' to conduct annual audits of all procurement contracts above FCFA500 million (US $940,000) and a 25 per cent sampling of contracts worth FCFA30–500 million. While the recruitment method provides some assurance that the independent observer will be truly independent, the weight of administrative practice and pressure from senior politicians (such as that exerted on the NGO Global Witness when it was appointed independent observer in the forestry sector) could jeopardise the post's impartiality.

Cameroon should be congratulated on the new procurement code, but it remains to be seen how effective it will prove in the absence of an independent judiciary, the body ultimately responsible for enforcing the law and sanctioning illegalities. Lack of human and financial resources, and the complexity of procedures invariably lead to judicial delays while eroding the integrity of staff. Successful implementation requires that the commissions created by the new law should be staffed by people of integrity, as required by article 8 of the UN Convention against Corruption.

Arguably, the weakest link in the monitoring chain is the ARMP, which oversees its application, recruits external observers and auditors, and appoints chairmen to the four supervisory bodies. As a state agency, it has close ties with the political elite, and thus does not have the independence necessary to carry out the delicate tasks entrusted to it. There is also the danger of 'operational drift' by the regulatory authority. At the time of writing, a first generation of observers appointed in 2001 to oversee procurement had not been paid for nearly two years, a state of affairs that clearly exposes them to temptation.[3]

Finally, with respect to contracts, departmental price lists cannot be used as a reliable basis for assessing suppliers' invoices. State agents are well accustomed to corrupt practices and the official list for office supplies, to take one small example, constitutes prima facie evidence of overpricing, because it contains prices four times higher than normal market rates. External audits and reviews are imperative if the hidden commissions that litter price lists are to be weeded out before the new code becomes operational.

Cameroon signs up to EITI

In a month that saw 500 civil servants referred to a disciplinary council on charges of fraud or misappropriation[4] and news that 3,000 fictitious officials had been stripped from the payroll,[5] the government gave further evidence it was taking corruption seriously by signing up to the Extractive Industries Transparency Initiative (EITI) on 17 March 2005. In a letter to the IMF on 30 March, Prime Minister Ephraïm Inoni reiterated that commitment and promised to post quarterly data on oil production, sales prices and revenue since 2000 on the website of the state-owned Société Nationale des Hydrocarbures by the end of June 2005, and to update it regularly.

In the light of these undertakings, civil society organisations are in the process of setting up a contact group to monitor the publication of oil revenues. It comprises the Centre for the Environment and Development (CED), the Cameroonian Women's Foundation for Rational Environmental Action (FOCARFE), Transparency International Cameroon (TIC), the Catholic Relief Service (CRS) and the Commission for Justice and Peace of the Episcopal Conference of Cameroon (CJPCEC). The EITI initiative provides potential for civil society to play the role of objective observer.

Breaking the secrecy surrounding oil revenues will have a direct impact on the recently completed Chad–Cameroon pipeline, providing communities in the regions that it crosses with vital information against which to measure the government's performance in developing the country. The pipeline is expected to have a major economic effect. By one account, the salaries and income derived from the supply of goods and equipment during the three-year construction phase increased national GDP by 2 per cent, and an annual 1 per cent increase is anticipated during the 25–30 years of its lifespan.[6] In 2004, the Cameroon Oil Transportation Company (COTCO) paid Cameroon some FCFA23 billion (US $43 million) in transit fees, a figure included in the budgetary framework as required by international lenders, particularly the IMF and the World Bank.

For many observers, while sustained efforts are required to reduce the extent of corruption, the EITI initiative forms part of a raft of measures recently introduced to clean up public sector management and promote professional ethics. The test will be in implementing them.

Jean-Bosco Talla and Maurice Nguéfack (TI Cameroon)

Further reading

Cameroon National Governance Programme, *Cameroun: les chantiers de la gouvernance* (Cameroon: The Workshops of Governance) (Yaoundé: PNG, 2004)

Lucien Ayissi, *Corruption et gouvernance* (Corruption and Governance) (Yaoundé: PUA, 2003)

Charles Manga Fombad, 'The Dynamics of Record-Breaking Endemic Corruption and Political Opportunism in Cameroon', in John Mbaku and Joseph Takougang (eds), *The Leadership Challenge in Africa: Cameroon under Paul Biya* (Trenton, NJ: Africa World Press, 2004)

Friedrich Ebert Stiftung, *Lutte contre la corruption: Impossible n'est pas camerounais* (Combating Corruption: Everything is Possible in Cameroon) (Yaoundé: PUA, 2002)

Pierre Titi Nwel (ed.), *De la corruption au Cameroun* (Corruption in Cameroon) (Yaoundé: Gerddes-Cameroun and Friedrich Ebert Stiftung, 2001)

Babikassana and Abissama Onana, *Les débats économiques du Cameroun et d'Afrique* (Economic Debates about Cameroon and Africa) (Yaoundé: Prescriptor, 2003)

Notes

1. See *Global Corruption Report 2005*.
2. Ibid.
3. *Mutations* (Cameroon), 28 April 2005.
4. *Cameroon Tribune* (Cameroon), 1 March 2005.
5. *Le Messager* (Cameroon), 1 April 2005.
6. Roger Tsafack (ed.), *Le pipeline Tchad–Cameroun et l'emploi. Quelles leçons?* (The Chad–Cameroon Pipeline and Employment. What Lessons Can Be Learned?) (Yaoundé: PUA/FES, 2003).

China

Conventions:
UN Convention against Corruption (signed December 2003; not yet ratified)
UN Convention against Transnational Organized Crime (ratified September 2003)

ADB-OECD Action Plan for Asia-Pacific (endorsed April 2005)

Legal and institutional changes

- On 19 September 2004, the Fourth Plenary Session of the 16th Central Committee of the Communist Party of China (CPC) adopted a resolution on **governance capacity building** that called for more accountability of members through broader citizen participation, greater separation of government from the management of businesses and the creation of more democratic evaluation systems. The resolution included a call for **whistleblowers' protection**, a right officially enshrined in an ordinance that came into effect on 24 October (see below).

- In January 2005, the CPC Central Committee released guidelines for a national system of corruption prevention that entails a three-pronged approach of **ethics education, institutional accountability and civil monitoring**. The system is due to be in place by 2010. This is the first time Chinese leaders have laid out a comprehensive blueprint for a national anti-corruption campaign (see below).

- Given that more and more corrupt officials settle their families abroad before joining them with their ill-gotten gains, the Central Commission of Disciplinary Inspection (CCDI) began a scheme in July 2004 under which senior officials must declare in advance any **overseas visits by spouses and children**. A pilot project is currently operational in Xiangfan, Hubei province, Suzhou in Shanxi and in a factory and power station belonging to the Shenhua Group. Officials who do not declare such visits will be denied promotion.

- In April 2005 the standing committee of the 10th National People's Congress (NPC) approved the country's **first civil servant law** to define officials' rights and responsibilities. The law covers such areas as duties, posts and ranks; recruitment, training, salaries and assessments; and punishments and related issues. The law stipulates that all public servants should be recruited through just, open and fair examinations. At present, some people become civil servants by directly engaging or transferring from civilian organisations. In addition, the law provides for a more stable rewards system by ensuring that salaries are raised in line with economic growth.

Planned improvements to the strategic system against corruption

Shenzen, the site of China's first special economic zone, is to be the test-bed for the CPC's blueprint for checking internal corruption before it is rolled out to the rest of the country by 2010. The 'implementation guideline for the establishment of a national system of punishing and preventing corruption', unveiled in January 2005, calls for further development of democracy and legal institutions with the goal of bringing power to closer public account. Among the guideline's targets are more dynamic anti-corruption tactics; broader channels for public oversight and civil society monitoring; protection of whistleblowers and citizens' rights to criticise; and increased transparency of public policy. Five ordinances were introduced in 2004 with the aim of increasing the accountability of high-ranking officials, including two designed to promote greater meritocracy in the selection and promotion of party and government officials, and another that specifies complaints procedures for party members.

The guideline calls for improved responsibility systems for the administrative and judicial sectors, and a three-pronged programme of ethics education, institutional accountability and civil monitoring. Ethics education will be incorporated into general school curricula; the Central Commission of Disciplinary Inspection (CCDI) will be responsible for accountability capacity building; and the Party Congress will encourage whistleblowing by party members, accountability in the public administration and a code of conduct for the judicial sector.

In particular, it prioritises enhanced auditing in targeted sectors and ministries, and introduces efficiency auditing for high-ranking officials. All audits will be published, building on an existing trend towards more active and open auditing processes. Notably, in June 2004, the state audit office publicly released a report on central government spending that disclosed that 41 out of 55 central departments audited were suspected of embezzlement and appropriation of public funds, including funds earmarked for the China Olympic Committee and disaster relief fund. The report led to disciplinary action against 545 people and more than 80 judicial hearings, including cases against the former director of the Beijing Municipal Power Supply bureau and against two vice-presidents of the Agricultural Development Bank. In July 2004, the state audit office announced plans to audit all CPC central committee departments and all central government ministries, commissions and departments that receive funds from central government.

The guideline foresees the creation of a checks-and-balances institution to ensure the accountability of investment decisions by state companies and agencies, and to monitor their projects. Those responsible for investment policies will be held accountable. In a similar vein, it proposes introducing a 'real name' bank accounts system to limit cash transactions, a warning system for high-volume cash movements and improved information sharing to contain money laundering.

Whether the guideline's grand designs will translate into action is debatable. Beijing has tended to advocate mostly administrative measures to combat corruption. Moreover, party investigators will find it difficult to investigate their own bosses.

Corruption amongst party cadres

Ever since the late 1990s, when the party chief in Zhanjiang, Guangdong province and two mayors in the autonomous region of Anyang, Henan province were convicted of corruption, the practice of selling promotions for cash has been on the rise. Despite passing a series of regulations to streamline its system of selection and appointments in 2000 and 2002, the CPC has failed to stamp out 'power trading', as it is known, though the detection rate may have slightly improved. In 2000, Ding Yangning was convicted of trading posts for money during his three-year term as party chief in Zhenghe, Fujian province, a case that incriminated 246 officials on charges of bribery. This 'record' was soon beaten by Wang Hulin of Changzhi City, Shanxi province, who allegedly sold 278 government or party posts in a single month.

In 2004, five more ordinances aimed at closing institutional loopholes in the accountability of officials were issued, among them 'interim regulations on open selection of party and government officials', 'interim provisions on promotion via open competition' and another on 'party or government officials who take occasional jobs in enterprises'. At the same time, the Central Committee sent out five teams on inspection tours to monitor senior leaders at provincial and ministerial level. In a sign that power trading still thrives, Ma De, former party chief in Suihua city, Heilongjiang province, was charged in March 2005 with taking bribes worth US $726,000 from 260 officials over his six-year tenure of office. The conviction of Ma – known as the '10,000 yuan chief' for his daily income from bribes – sent shock waves

through political circles and later ensnared the provincial heads of the high court and prosecutor's office, a deputy governor, the chair of the provincial congress and the head of the local party secretariat. Tian Fengshan, a former minister of land and resources, was also implicated.

The inspection teams exposed the extent of corruption at all levels of administration. *Xinhua* and *China Daily* reported almost daily on officials scamming the system, ranging from the Xintian education officials who owned luxury cars in an impoverished county in Hunan province, or accusations that officials in Fuzhou displaced impoverished land owners without compensation and sold their plots to developers at prices lower than market value. Examples of this are legion. The NPC publicised the arrest of crooked party cadres and officials at banks and other state-owned enterprises, claiming more than 150,000 corrupt members had been disciplined and the misuse of public funds of over US $300 million had been uncovered in 2004.

Further substantiation that lack of accountability is endemic among officials is provided in a survey released in January 2005 by Wang Jianxin, an expert at the Law School of the Jiangxi University of Finance and Economics in eastern China.[1] Wang's survey of village officials demonstrated that there has been an increase in officials' abuse of power and related economic crimes, with cases of corruption by high-ranking and grassroots officials cropping up in quantity. Such cases involved bribes valued at thousands, tens and even hundreds of thousands of yuan (from US $240 to US $1.2 million).

Massive graft plagues some of China's banks

China's banking system suffered a string of graft allegations involving senior executives at major state banks in 2004–05, and was weakened by high levels of bad debt and low rates of capitalisation. In January, investigators found 1 billion yuan (US $120 million), missing from deposits at a local branch in Ha'erbin city after the branch's director fled abroad. In March, a staff member in the Dalian branch of the Bank of China was found to have misappropriated US $6 million and staff at the Baotou branch of China's Industrial and Commercial Bank were accused of a conspiring to loan illegally 300 million yuan (US $37 million). On 16 March, the chairman of China Construction Bank, Zhang Enzhao, resigned amid reports that he had allegedly received a US $1 million kickback and other monetary favours from US companies in return for granting loans. Zhang is under investigation. His predecessor, Wang Xuebing, was jailed for corruption in 2002. China Construction Bank, the country's top property lender, had been the shop window of China's efforts to reform its debt-ridden banking sector, having received US $22.5 billion late in 2003 to recapitalise its balance sheet following aggressive bad-loan write-downs. According to a survey by the Research Bureau of the People's Bank of China, 81.5 per cent of people think corrupt dealing is a common feature of China's banking system.

In April 2004, the media exposed another fraudulent loan scandal. Two years earlier, an internal investigator at the Beijing branch of the Bank of China had found a loan case in which Real Estate Ltd used its employees' names, forged purchase contracts and proof of income declarations to apply for 199 separate loans from the bank worth 645 million yuan (US $78 million). The fraud resulted in the abandonment of 273 unfinished luxury apartments. This scandal highlighted the vulnerability of China's banking system, which is groaning under a mountain of bad loans. In 2004, credit risk was increasing because bank lending continues to tilt towards large real estate and capital construction projects, favouring medium- and long-term loans, and monopolistic industries, such as highways, railways, airports, power and communications. The capital adequacy rate of most banks in China is well below the 8 per cent Basel Standard. These two factors are severe impediments to further reform of the banking sector.

The China Banking Regulatory Commission (CBRC) announced a new crackdown on corruption following the resignation of Zhang Enzhao. The CBRC says it will enact a range of investigative checks, including the monitoring of mortgage, consumer and infrastructure project loans to help address the problems. Meanwhile, it warns banks to tighten their own checks to prevent new cases of corruption emerging. Between 2001 and 2005, courts sentenced 27,000 bank employees for finance-related crimes, over 4,000 of them to more than five years' imprisonment, life imprisonment or death. Attempts to solve the bad debt issue by improving monitoring and internal controls have failed because of political leverage on credit decisions.

Guo Yong (Tsinghua University, China) and Liao Ran (Transparency International)

Further reading

Wang Chaunli, *Feel the Pulse of Corruption – Studies of the Correlation between Frequency of Corruption and Control Intensity* (Beijing: Qunzhong Publishing House, 2004)

Li Junjie, 'The Current Status, Development Perspectives and Monitoring of China's Banking System', *International Economic Review* 3–4, 2004

Chi Lo, 'Bank Reform: How Much Time does China Have?', *China Business Review*, March–April 2004

Xie Ping and Lu Lei, 'The Economics of Corruption in China's Financial Institutions: Behaviour and Mechanism Design' (Beijing: People's Bank of China, 2003)

Yan Sun, *Corruption and Market in Contemporary China* (New York: Cornell University Press, 2004)

Zhong Wei, Ba Shusong, Gao Qinghui and Zhao Xiao, 'Evaluation Report of China's Financial Risks', *China Reform* 3, 2004

Li Yifan, 'Strategic Shift of China's Fight against Corruption', *China Outlook* 2, 2004

Guo Yong, 'Strengthening International Cooperation to Deal Heavy Blows against Trans-Border Corruption', *Studies of International Issues* 5, 2004

Note

1. Unpan1.un.org/intradoc/groups/public/documents/apcity/unpan020124.htm

Costa Rica

Conventions:

OAS Inter-American Convention against Corruption (ratified June 1997)

UN Convention against Corruption (signed December 2003; not yet ratified)

UN Convention against Transnational Organized Crime (ratified July 2003)

Legal and institutional changes

- A **law against corruption and illicit enrichment** in the public services was approved in October 2004. The law defines and provides sanctions for crimes including influence peddling, international bribery and appropriation of gifts to the state, which formerly were not defined and therefore rarely prosecuted. The new law also provides detailed requirements for public officials to declare their assets.

- The **Office of the Special Attorney for Ethics and Public Services**, established by law in 2002, became operational when the post was filled in 2004. The budget for the office was increased following a series of high-profile scandals in 2004 (see below), and its remit expanded to include supervising implementation of the OAS Convention against Corruption, and helping the public prosecutor with ongoing investigations into allegations of corruption against four former heads of state.

Trust in political institutions wanes as the cover is pulled off corruption

Costa Rica, hitherto the most stable democracy in Latin America, had been able to boast low levels of corruption until a recent spate of scandals drew the public's attention to decades of shady financing of politicians and parties. It now faces the challenge of rebuilding public trust in its political institutions.

The first scandal erupted in October 2004 when former president Miguel Angel Rodríguez was forced to resign as Secretary-General of the Organization of American States less than three weeks after he had taken up office. He stepped down after allegations implicated him in a bribery scheme involving the French telecommunications company, Alcatel. In mid-2004, details emerged that Alcatel had been awarded a contract to improve the country's cellular phone system allegedly after its officials successfully bribed José Antonio Lobo, Rodríguez's protégé and a former director of the state electrical company, Instituto Costarricense de Electricidad (ICE), with a US $2.4 million 'prize'. Lobo said he had been 'advised' to accept the sum by Rodríguez, who is reported to have then demanded 60 per cent of it.

Digging deeper into Alcatel's dealings, allegations emerged that it had attempted to influence previous Costa Rican politicians as well. José María Figueres, a former president, was forced to step down from his senior position at the World Economic Forum in Geneva in October 2004 following allegations that he had received a US $900,000 bribe from Alcatel during his years of public service. And current President Abel Pacheco has been asked to explain an undeclared US $100,000 donation to his presidential campaign, also by Alcatel. In total, the authorities believe that Alcatel, which enjoys a near monopoly of telecommunications services in the country, has paid more than US $4.4 million to Costa Rican politicians and officials.

Money flowed to party coffers from foreign governments as well. Rodríguez's Panama-based investment company, Inversiones Denisse, allegedly received two payments of US $500,000 from the Friendship Company, which has strong ties to the Taiwan government. When he was president, he is alleged to have received US $200,000 from Taiwan on two separate occasions and his party, the Social Christian Unity Party, has been questioned over donations worth US $500,000 from companies with connections to Taiwan.

A separate scandal embarrassed another former president, Rafael Angel Calderón, who is accused of receiving nearly US $450,000 from a US $40 million loan from the Finnish government to subsidise the state-run social security system (see 'Grand corruption in Costa Rica', Chapter 2, page 26).

These scandals – along with evidence produced through monitoring campaign spending – suggest that the sums of 'off the record' money flowing to campaign chests dwarf the amounts legally declared and scrutinised by the electoral authorities.

Current legislation requires parties to report donations received and campaign spending, sets limits on both and forbids parties from accepting money from foreign sources. Most of these regulations were violated in the recent elections in April 2002, according to TI Costa Rica, but the authorities failed to sanction the abuses. Civil society groups found it difficult to obtain information about party financing that should be made public.

The legislature responded by setting up special commissions to investigate irregularities in the financing of the recent campaign and to draft reform bills to tighten up the legal framework. This is a start, but more is needed if the public is to regain confidence in the country's political institutions, especially given the gravity of the allegations against former presidents.

Levels of abstention are expected to increase in the next elections. A poll taken in the first quarter of 2005 showed that one in two people does not support any of the potential candidates one year ahead of elections, compared with one in three people in 2001 and one in five in 1997.[1] According to a second poll in January 2005, corruption is the biggest public concern (37 per cent of people polled put it first), while violence and crime were the primary concern of just 5 per cent. In July 2004 the opposite was the case, with 26 per cent placing violence and crime at the top of their worries, and only 5 per cent expressing concern about corruption.[2]

Two positive developments have been increased public involvement – a massive march against corruption took place in October 2004 – and the increased credibility of the judiciary. The public prosecutor has shown a great deal of independence from political pressure in his investigations, and polls by the University of Costa Rica show increased confidence in the judiciary.[3]

Access to information: the citizens' tool against corruption

Access to information has been confirmed as a critical tool in the fight against corruption, thanks to a series of rulings by the Constitutional Court rejecting attempts to limit access to public information. Prior to the rulings, access was limited to what officials permitted.

One major advance was lifting bank secrecy provisions. This was effected through a writ against public and private banks that appealed to bank secrecy rules to prevent access to information. The Constitutional Court ruled that where the funds of political parties or candidates were concerned, banking secrecy did not apply. The ruling made reference to a constitutional reform in 2000 stating that public institutions must be accountable and held up to public scrutiny.

The newspaper *La Nación* requested information about non-contributory pensions to the board of directors of the social service agency, Caja Costarricense de Seguro Social. The reporters wanted an electronic copy of the database, including the names of beneficiaries and details about their pension entitlement. The request was denied in September 2002 on the grounds that it was information about third parties whose confidentiality should be respected.

The reporters filed a writ of habeas data requesting the information, which they argued is public. The court agreed in March 2003, asserting that transparency is a constitutional requirement for public administration, and only limited exceptions apply. The journalists were granted the information as a result.

Not only should information be made publicly available when requested, the court ruled, but the government should actively disseminate information that is in the public interest.

While the court's attitude is important in prising open public records, obstacles continue to be put in the way of accessing information and a law clearly delineating the right to access information is necessary. Several access to information bills exist in draft form but have yet to be adopted.

Roxana Salazar (Transparencia Costa Rica)

Further reading

Casals and Associates, *El financiamiento de los partidos políticos en Argentina, Chile, Costa Rica y México: Lecciones para América Latina* (Financing of Political Parties in Argentina, Chile, Costa Rica and Mexico: Lessons for Latin America), 2004, www.respondanet.com/spanish/boletines/pdf/issue41.pdf

Carlos Eduardo Serrano Rodríguez, *La corrupción como fenómeno social en Costa Rica* (Corruption as a Social Phenomenon in Costa Rica) (San José: Escuela de Administración Pública, 2004)

Roxana Salazar (ed.), *Corrupción: una visión desde la sociedad civil* (Corruption: A View from Civil Society) (San José: Editorial Fundación Ambio, 2004)

Roxana Salazar, *Mapas de riesgo de corrupción en el sector forestal* (Corruption Risk Maps in the Forestry Sector) (San José: Editorial Fundación Ambio, 2004)

Jorge Vargas and Luis Rosero-Bixby, *La cultura política de la democracia en Costa Rica* (The Political Culture of Democracy in Costa Rica) (Nashville: Vanderbilt University, 2004), www.dec.org/pdf_docs/PNADB407.pdf

Transparencia Costa Rica (TI Costa Rica): www.transparenciacr.org

Notes

1. *El Financiero* (Costa Rica), 28 March 2005.
2. *Ojo* (Costa Rica), 12 and 30 January 2005.
3. University of Costa Rica, 'Sondeo sobre corrupción de las élites políticas costarricenses: la ciudadanía valora positivamente las acciones contra la corrupción' (Survey on Corruption by Costa Rican Political Elites: Citizens React Positively to Actions against Corruption), Instituto Investigaciones Sociales, Proyecto Investigación en Opinión Pública, November 2004.

Croatia

Conventions:
Council of Europe Civil Law Convention on Corruption (ratified June 2003)
Council of Europe Criminal Law Convention on Corruption (ratified November 2000; Additional Protocol ratified May 2005)
UN Convention against Corruption (ratified April 2005)
UN Convention against Transnational Organized Crime (ratified January 2003)

Legal and institutional changes

- In September 2004, parliament passed a **law on the financing of the presidential campaign** that prohibits campaign donations from foreign powers, state-owned and public companies, unions, employers' associations, civic organisations, public institutions and companies partly or entirely owned by local governments. A significant innovation is article 6, which requires candidates to declare the amount and sources of their campaign funding. Although the law represents some progress towards a more transparent election process, it sets no upper limit on campaign costs (see below).

- The Prevention of **Conflicts of Interest** in the Exercise of Public Office Act (PCIA), passed in October 2003, underwent two alterations in July 2004 and April 2005. The first reduces the amount of base capital a serving public official may retain in a company from 25 per cent to 0.5 per cent. Fines for violating the law were raised, and the list of liable officials expanded to include the Croatian president, the secretaries of the supreme and constitutional courts, the deputies of secretaries of parliament and the government. The second amendment closed a loophole on the declaration of gifts by including presents of less than 500 kunas (US $80), presents to relatives, and national and international awards. Since April, officials are also obliged to report in their personal declaration forms on how they acquired their assets and the sources of the funds with which they purchased properties (see below).

- In August 2004, the Ministry of Justice and the State Geodetic Administration launched a €62 million (US $74 million) project to **digitalise the country's land register** with the twin aims of resolving hundreds of thousands of disputes over ownership, and drawing up an accurate and more accessible land registry database. Assisted by EU grants and a credit from the World Bank, the Ministry established 107 land registry departments to work with 105 land registry courts with a view to settling the 351,046 cases then in progress. The old system of registering property was cumbersome and offered a platform for corruption by public officials in land offices and the judiciary. By February 2005, the new system had successfully resolved 62,000 property registry claims. The first electronic land register was expected to be published in June 2005.[1]

- An amendment to the law on the Office for Prevention of Corruption and Organised Crime (USKOK) in February 2005 gives the agency complete jurisdiction in all felonies involving **corruption and organised crime**. County attorney offices and police will conduct preliminary investigations into cases bearing the hallmarks of these offences. If they establish reasonable suspicion, they will pass the case up to USKOK. It is hoped that the amendment, which was sponsored by an USKOK working party set up in March 2004, will make the office more efficient by eliminating cases that are not under its jurisdiction.

In 2004, USKOK investigated 117 cases of corruption of which 65 went to court, but only 20 ended in prison sentences.[2]

- Progress in implementing the 2003 **Right of Access to Information Act** was fitful with high numbers of requests on one hand, but slipped deadlines and non-existent reporting on the other. While the Central Office for State Administration (COSA) did issue regulations concerning the organisation of official records, which was a prerequisite for implementation of the law, the government published a list of the bodies to which the act applies six months late. The report on implementation of the law, published by COSA in May 2005, showed that ministries had received a combined 4,302 requests in 2004, of which 16 were refused; other government offices received 1,174; and COSA itself redressed 13 requests it had previously rejected.[3] The opposition criticised the report's brevity, saying it did not provide adequate information on why requests were being refused. One opposition member claimed that 180 municipalities had not handed in their reports on the act and some had not even appointed information officers to deal with requests.

Political financing: a free-for-all

The presidential elections of January 2005 threw a spotlight on Croatia's less than transparent system of financing political parties and their electoral campaigns.

Financing of the election process is based on two laws: the Law on Political Parties, which came into force in 1993; and the Law on Financing of the Presidential Campaign, adopted in September 2004 in preparation for the presidential election of January 2005. Given the lack of will by politicians to disclose details of their own financial arrangements, neither provides very satisfactory regulation, although the more recent of them was undoubtedly an improvement.

The Law on Political Parties disposes of the entire topic in a few curt clauses. Article 19 describes the methods of processing financial transfers that parties receive from the national budget and article 20 obliges parties to declare their sources of funds, and their designated uses, within one year. But the law does not prohibit specific types of financing (foreign governments, corporations, unions, and so on), nor determine a figure above which a party is obliged to make the donor's identity known. Nor are there limits on expenditure during electoral campaigns.

The new Law on Financing of the Presidential Campaign regulates some of these issues. It makes donations from foreign sources, state-owned companies, unions and public institutions illegal, while article 6 requires candidates to publicly declare the amount of funds used in campaigns, and their sources. The law is an undoubted improvement on the 1993 political party law, but it still fails to set a ceiling on electoral expenditure. Another major flaw – and one with which the public is very familiar – is that there is no independent office responsible for verifying whether a party's declaration of funding and sources is true, and no provisions for sanctions in the event it proves false.

Consider the presidential campaign of January 2005 when there was much speculation in the media about the expenditure of Jadranka Kosor, the HDZ (Croatian Democratic Union) candidate.[4] Civil society, led by local NGOs GONG (an election monitoring watchdog) and TI Croatia, applied in January and February 2005 to Croatian National Television (HRT) to publish the cost of promotional videos and electoral advertising purchased by all candidates. HRT refused, claiming the information was protected by rules of commercial confidentiality. This was implausible, given that HRT is a state-owned institution with a duty to make information of public interest available under the Right of Access to Information Act. HRT refused to provide the same information to its own Council, creating the impression that its executives were trying to shield a candidate from public scrutiny. HDZ later claimed that Kosor had spent 6 million kunas (US $979,000) on her campaign, but a market research agency reportedly estimated her expenditures to be twice as high,[5] although this figure in turn has been contested. Due to public pressure, information on the costs of television advertisement of the campaigns of Kosor and other candidates was officially issued by Croatian National Television in May 2005. But there is still no independent regulator with powers to investigate and verify the financial reports of electoral campaign expenditure, and to apply sanctions on those who violate regulations.

Other anomalies exist in the auditing of the state's contributions to party finances. Though required to deliver budget reports to a parliamentary committee (Standing Orders and Political System), the information is not published in the official gazette. A number of specialist observers claim that several parties do not meet even this minimal legal requirement, but were not sanctioned. Parties who file on time do so in the knowledge that their reports will not be subject to an independent audit. There is a clear need for root-and-branch reform of the legal framework of party and election finance. The Law on Political Parties needs revision, with particular focus on the source and size of donations, public accounting of the use of state and private contributions and the creation of an independent oversight body. Only then will transparency be improved in what is currently a murky electoral process.[6]

The 'Imostroj affair'

Since it was passed into law in October 2003, not a single high ranking public official has been brought to book under the Prevention of Conflicts of Interest Act (PCIA), although the public has become increasingly concerned about corruption and abuse of power by those in high office. This is only partly explained by the resignation of the commission responsible

for implementing the PCIA in late 2004 due to internal political disputes, with the result that it did not start work properly until February 2005.

The most controversial conflict of interest allegation in 2004–05 was the 'Imostroj affair', whose chief protagonist was the then minister of foreign affairs, Miomir Žužul. The local media alleged that Žužul took a bribe from a friend and businessman in return for pushing the cabinet to cancel the debts of Imostroj, a company the man planned to buy.[7] Although the State Attorney and Audit Offices did not identify any conflict of interest, the public remained sceptical.

In parliament, the opposition Social Democrat Party (SDP) and Croatian People's Party (HNS) demanded the minister's resignation. The majority Croatian Democratic Union (HDZ) turned the tables by appointing a committee to inquire into conflicts of interest by senior officials during the 2000–03 coalition government, naming Zlatko Tomčić, leader of the Croatian Peasant Party (HSS) and former parliamentary speaker, and Radimir Čačić, a former minister of public works and member of HNS, as ripe for investigation. Miomir Žužul, considered Prime Minister Ivo Sanader's right-hand man and head of the team negotiating Croatia's entry to the EU, resisted calls to step down for two more months, but finally resigned in January 2005, several days before the presidential election. In his letter of resignation, he defended his innocence but recognised that the allegations had inflicted some political damage on the government. His resignation was a demonstration of the power that public pressure can exert when conflicts of interest arise – real or perceived. Nevertheless, he remained in charge of coordinating negotiations with the EU for some time after.

While the allegations against Žužul fell in the fallow period before the commission for investigating conflicts of interest resumed work, the case demonstrated Croatia's bare-knuckle approach to allegations of political impropriety: when accused of corruption, accuse back. In spite of the PCIA and recent amendments to it, the technique appears to work. Though he was forced to resign, the allegations against Žužul have not been investigated and therefore cannot be proved either way.

Ana First (TI Croatia)

Further reading

Davor Derenčinović, *Comments on UN Convention against Corruption* (Zagreb: University of Zagreb Law Faculty, 2005)

Viktor Gotovac and Đorđe Gardašević, *Regulation of Free Access to Information* (Zagreb: TI Croatia, 2004)

Josip Kregar, 'Financing of Political Parties and Election Campaigns', *Collected Papers of Zagreb Law Faculty No. 5/2004* (Zagreb: University of Zagreb Law Faculty, 2004)

Josip Kregar, *Introduction to the National Integrity System Country Study: Croatia* (Zagreb: TI Croatia, 2004)

TI Croatia: www.transparency.hr

Notes

1. www.pravosudje.hr
2. Transparency International Croatia, 'Analysis of National Integrity System: Croatia 2005' (Zagreb: TI Croatia, 2005).
3. www.sabor.hr/Download/2005/03/22/IZVJESCE.pdf
4. www.gong.hr/eng/Downloads/Predsj_05_izborniproces_en.pdf
5. www.index.hr
6. For further discussion of this, see Josip Kregar under 'Further reading'.
7. *International Herald Tribune* (France), 5 January 2005.

Ecuador

Conventions:

OAS Inter-American Convention against Corruption (ratified June 1997)
UN Convention against Corruption (signed December 2003; not yet ratified)
UN Convention against Transnational Organized Crime (ratified September 2002)

Legal and institutional changes

- Secondary legislation implementing the **Law on Transparency and Access to Public Information** has been drafted by a working group comprising the attorney general, auditor general, prosecutor general, defence minister, secretary general for national security, national archive, commission for women, tax and telecommunications offices and civil society representatives. The law, which entered into force in May 2004, requires all public entities, government contractors, trade unions, and public secondary and higher education establishments to make information public. The guiding principle of the law is that all public sector information is the property of the general public, with a few exceptions that are specified in the law. The law was drafted by the Ecuadorean Association of Newspaper Publishers.

The democratic crisis in Ecuador

A constitutional crisis that culminated with the resignation of President Lucio Gutiérrez has forced the country to rethink its institutions, particularly the way in which the politicisation of the judiciary had left the country vulnerable to corruption.

The crisis began a year after Gutiérrez took office in January 2003. A former coup leader, he had run for office on a platform of anti-corruption and social reform pledges. His victory was all the more surprising since his campaign, supported by indigenous groups, had succeeded in dislodging the country's traditional parties of power.

However, with little political experience and in a state with a recent history of presidents failing to reach the end of their terms of office, Gutiérrez soon began to barter with his former electoral opponents to drum up support for his policies.

In December 2004, the government managed to gain the 52 legislative votes needed to dismiss via a 'resolution of unconstitutionality' the 31 Supreme Court judges, and to form a new court. Congress also resolved that the National Judicial Council, which is responsible for the administration of the justice system, would be restructured within 15 days, and a shortlist of three candidates for the post of prosecutor general would be drawn up. Congress also re-established its powers to impeach and censure members of the Supreme Court and National Judicial Council. These powers had been rescinded following a process of popular consultation in 1997.

Gutiérrez's response to these decisions was to affirm that the existing court members would stay in place for three months, during which time the government would try to push through a political reform supporting the changes – making manifest the attempts by the executive branch to exert influence over the judiciary. The Constitutional Court and Supreme Electoral Court were also reconfigured in the government's favour during this period.

These decisions by Congress violated the constitution in a number of ways. Article 202 grants tenure to Supreme Court judges and was not respected; Supreme Court vacancies cannot be filled through negotiations between political parties; and the independence of the judiciary must not be violated by political parties seeking to further their own interests.

The attempts to stack the judiciary along partisan lines unleashed a crisis of democracy. People took to the street in protest. Civil society groups including Corporación Latinoamericana para el Desarrollo (the national chapter of Transparency International) and Participación Ciudadana called on car drivers to toot their horns as they drove past the court. This generated interest and awareness about themes that are not usually a matter of popular interest, such as the rule of law and the separation of powers.

As the number of protesters swelled, the government's popularity ratings plummeted. The UN special reporter for the independence of judges and lawyers visited Ecuador and described the destitution and replacement of Supreme Court, Constitutional Court and Electoral Court magistrates as unconstitutional. The reporter called for respect for the UN standard on the need for the judiciary to be independent of political influence, and for transparency in the selection of magistrates.

By April, the political situation had become unsustainable in Quito where most of the protests occurred. Popular discontent converted into outrage when the de facto court annulled judicial processes for embezzlement that were being launched against former president Abdalá Bucaram, as well as corruption charges against former president Gustavo Noboa and his former vice-president, Alberto Dahik. At this point, the focus of protest changed from promoting respect for the rule of law to demands for Gutiérrez's resignation. By April, demonstrators were demanding not just the resignation of the president, but of the entire political class.

Protesters organised loosely and peace-fully around Quito, setting up platforms for people to express their discontent and suggest ways forward. Though not organised along party lines, these informal gatherings were sufficient to convince Gutiérrez to step down. They also demanded that Congress take stock of the ways it had overstepped the boundary with the judiciary, provoking the crisis in the first place; and that the judiciary seek a constitutional way to review the independence of its members in response to concerns by society.

Street protests disappeared soon after the president stepped down, and political parties have since regained their position at the centre of public life, though it remains to be seen how they will respond to public demands for increased probity and transparency in their functions. The new government, headed by Gutiérrez's former vice-president, Alfredo Palacio, is expected to introduce deep political reforms, including changes to government structures that are particularly vulnerable to corruption. There are high expectations that civil society, which was so active in bringing about the change in government, will be allowed to play a significant role in proposing and debating the badly needed reforms in the fields of corruption and transparency.

Andrés Tobar (Corporación Latinoamericana para el Desarrollo, TI Ecuador)

Further reading

Corporación Latinoamericana para el Desarrollo (TI Ecuador): www.cld.org.ec

Finland

Conventions:
Council of Europe Civil Law Convention on Corruption (ratified October 2001)
Council of Europe Criminal Law Convention on Corruption (ratified October 2002)
OECD Anti-Bribery Convention (ratified December 1998)
UN Convention against Corruption (signed December 2003; not yet ratified)
UN Convention against Transnational Organized Crime (ratified February 2004)

Legal and institutional changes

- In May 2005, parliament passed a law that **criminalises accepting a bribe**. A company found guilty of accepting a bribe can be sanctioned, but only if the bribe has caused damage to another company. The law was expected to come into effect in July 2005.[1]

- An **amendment to the public procurement act** came into effect in February 2005 ruling that a public contract can be signed only 21 days after a decision has been made and the bidders have been informed, allowing the latter time to appeal the decision. It also requires that all public procurement contracts and any decisions made prior to awarding the contracts be put in writing. Both changes open procurement-related decisions to greater scrutiny. The government is preparing further amendments by January 2006 to meet the requirements of the European Court of Justice.

- In March 2005, the police formed a **special unit for pre-trial investigation of economic crimes**, including cases of alleged corruption in Helsinki and its surrounding areas. Prior to its formation, units investigating alleged economic crimes in Helsinki municipality were severely overstretched. In 2004, 582 cases were pending in the municipality alone.[2]

Blowing the whistle on cartels

Finland is routinely ranked among the least corrupt countries in the world in Transparency International's Corruption Perceptions Index, and a public debate began last summer on whether graft was an issue in the country at all. Classic examples of corruption generally entail petty bribery of officials. For example, an employee of the Directorate of Immigration was sentenced in February 2005 for accepting payments of €12,000 (US $15,500) over four years from immigrants seeking to speed up their residency applications.[3] Similarly, an employee of the Defence Staff was prosecuted for accepting free tickets worth more than €1,500 (US $2,000) to the opera, golf tournaments and other events from a supplier of office equipment.[4] The highest-profile corruption case in recent years involved the Finnish Maritime Administration and came to a close in July 2004 when the Supreme Court decided not to examine an appeal. The head of the administration and two other managers were sentenced in August 2003 to conditional discharge for bribery through accepting trips and other gifts, and using credit cards given them by a client.[5]

Although bribery through direct monetary gifts is undoubtedly rare, there is increasing evidence of Finnish companies forming cartels. While cartels are not necessarily a form of corruption, they undermine the goal of open, public tenders. Their possible link to corruption is two-fold. First, the formation of cartels involves collusion, which is a deception of the public. Collusion results in public tenders being manipulated and public funds being wasted. Second, companies may use corrupt means to secure cartel arrangements, for example by bribing insiders of the contracting agency to get confidential information on acceptable prices.

In May 2004, an amendment to the competition law came into force to fulfil EU requirements.[6] Under the new legislation, if a company blows the whistle on a cartel in which it has participated, it can avoid a fine, or see its fine reduced. The law has proved unusually successful in uncovering the use of cartels. The first firm to denounce a cartel was a timber products company, UPM-Kymmene, which admitted in May 2004 to participating in a price-fixing agreement with forest sector giants Stora Enso and Metsäliitto. EU investigators raided the latter's offices looking for evidence of agreements made by company executives on price and production quotas during informal meetings.[7] The investigation is ongoing.

In another case, the Finnish Competition Authority ruled in March 2004 that seven companies controlling 70 per cent of the tarmac market had agreed on prices, participation in public tenders, customers and geographical sectors from 1994 to 2002, at an annual cost to the public purse of €30 million (US $39 million).[8] A number of municipalities have begun legal action to reclaim the wasted funds and the Market Court (a special court hearing market law, competition and public procurement cases) is investigating.

According to Matti Purasjoki, former head of the Finnish Competition Authority, price cartels have been a standard business practice for decades, having originated in the post-war reconstruction period. In the 'mixed economy' era, the state encouraged companies to collaborate, primarily to compete against foreign firms. Price cartels and monopolies became illegal in 1992 when Finland joined the EU, but the culture persists.[9]

In September 2004, the European Commission fined the metals and technology corporation Outokumpu €36 million (US $46 million) for participating in a price cartel for copper pipes with KME, Sanco, Boliden, IMI, Mueller, Halcor SA, HME Nederland BV, KKE and Wieland Werke from 1988 to 2001.[10] According to the Commission, the cartel was a 'traditional' one in which members colluded on production quotas, market segments, target prices and price rises during informal meetings at airports.[11]

In accordance with OECD recommendations,[12] Juhani Jokinen, head of the Finnish Competition Authority, has proposed that executives incriminated in price fixing ought to be personally liable since the current system of fining has not deterred them from forming cartels. Trade and Industry Minister Mauri Pekkarinen confirmed that the amended law had contributed towards rooting out cartels, but more severe penalties were required for those who participated. In March 2005, ministries were considering a proposal to punish executives as individuals. In addition to a lack of appropriate penalties for forming cartels, there is no clear system for individuals to denounce them. Companies brought all the recent revelations to public attention under the amended act; a system for individual whistleblowers would further strengthen the authorities' ability to uncover other cartels.

Finnish companies drop no-bribes policy abroad

Bribery is as rare as corruption within Finland's borders, but there is substantial evidence that Finnish companies use bribes when doing business abroad, particularly in Russia and the Baltic States, as highlighted by the 2002 report on the application of the OECD Anti-Bribery Convention.[13]

A guidebook to doing business in Russia, entitled *Tak ili kak – venäläistä tapakulttuuria suomalaisille* (A Little of This, a Little of That: Russian Customs for Finns), published by the Finnish-Russian Chamber of Commerce in 2003, outlines in detail instances in which bribes may be paid and gives examples of their size and kind. In January 2005, the guidebook was taken off the market following widespread media criticism. The fact that such a book had ever been published by a reputable trade organisation funded by the government scandalised the public, as it openly acknowledged that Finnish companies break the law when operating abroad.

A sales manager of Wärtsilä, a ship power supplier, is currently under investigation for alleged bribery amounting to €1 million (US $1.3 million) in deals with a Swedish shipbuilding company, Rederi AB Gotland, between 1999 and 2001. Wärtsilä maintains that the company was misled and the sum was not intended for a private individual.[14] Another scandal erupted after it was alleged that Instrumentarium Corporation Medko Medical had bribed officials in a €32 million (US $41 million) deal to supply medical equipment to Costa Rica that had been supported by €12 million (US $15 million) in interest subsidies from the Ministry of Foreign Affairs' aid budget (see Chapter 2, page 26). According to Costa Rican media, a €6.5 million (US $8.5 million) commission was paid to a company called Fischel and ended up in the accounts of the heads of the Costa Rican social security office and the family of former president, Rafael Ángel Calderón.[15]

When Finnwatch, an NGO that monitors Finnish company activities overseas, demanded an inquiry, the Ministry of Foreign Affairs opened an investigation. On 4 March, Foreign Trade and Development Minister Paula Lehtomäki declared that the purchasing price had been 'fairly high' and that the quality of the equipment delivered by Instrumentarium was not '100 per cent up to scratch'.[16] The case demonstrated that the activities of independent watchdog agencies like Finnwatch need to be strengthened and that monitoring mechanisms need to be institutionalised in all state-aided schemes involving Finnish companies abroad to ensure public funds are not misused.

Santeri Eriksson (TI Finland)

Further reading

Corruption: A Risk to the Effectiveness of Bilateral Development Cooperation (Helsinki: State Audit Office, Performance Audit Reports 77/2004, 2004). Abstract (in English): www.vtv.fi/chapter_images/2985_772004_Corruption.pdf; document in full (in Finnish): www.vtv.fi/chapter_images/3664_772004.pdf

Olli Mäenpää, *Hallintolaki ja hyvän hallinnon takeet* (Administrative Procedure Act and the Guarantees of Good Administration) (Helsinki: Edita, 2003)

Organisation for Economic Co-operation and Development (OECD), *Economic Survey of Finland 2004* (Paris: OECD, 2005), abstract available at www.oecd.org/document/26/0,2340,en_2649_201185_33750554_1_1_1_1,00.html

Preventing Corruption. A Handbook of Anti-Corruption Techniques for Use in International Development Cooperation (Helsinki: Ministry for Foreign Affairs, 2002), global.finland.fi/english/publications/pdf/preventing_corruption.pdf

Values in the Daily Job – Civil Servant's Ethics. A Handbook for the State Administration (Helsinki: Ministry of Finance, State Employer's Office, 2005), www.vm.fi/tiedostot/pdf/en/91383.pdf

Notes

1. *Helsingin Sanomat* (Finland), 18 May 2005.
2. *Helsingin Sanomat* (Finland), 24 June 2004.
3. *Helsingin Sanomat* (Finland), 19 February 2005.
4. *Helsingin Sanomat* (Finland), 17 December 2004.
5. *Helsingin Sanomat* (Finland), 30 August 2003.
6. The law amended the 1992 legislation on controlling competition (*Laki kilpailunrajoituksista*).
7. *Helsingin Sanomat* (Finland), 26 May 2004.
8. *Tekniikka and Talous* (Finland), 31 March 2004.
9. See the speech by Matti Purasjoki and Juhani Jokinen, available at www.kilpailuvirasto.fi/cgi-bin/suomi.cgi?sivu=kilpailupolitiikan-odotukset.html
10. www.eureporter.co.uk, 3 September 2004.
11. *Helsingin Sanomat* (Finland), 4 September 2004.
12. OECD Economic Survey, Finland 2004.
13. OECD Directorate for Financial, Fiscal and Enterprise Affairs: *Finland, Phase 2, Report on Application of the Convention on Combating Bribery of Foreign Public Officials in International Business Transactions and the 1997 Recommendation on Combating Bribery in International Business Transactions* (Paris: OECD, 2002).
14. *Helsingin Sanomat* (Finland), 17 November 2004.
15. *Helsingin Sanomat* (Finland), 13 October 2004.
16. *STT* (Finland), 4 March 2005.

France

Conventions:

Council of Europe Civil Law Convention on Corruption (signed November 1999; not yet ratified)

Council of Europe Criminal Law Convention on Corruption (signed September 1999; not yet ratified; Additional Protocol signed May 2003; not yet ratified)

OECD Anti-Bribery Convention (ratified July 2000)

UN Convention against Corruption (ratified July 2005)

UN Convention against Transnational Organized Crime (ratified October 2002)

Legal and institutional changes

- In July 2005, a law was passed to **align the judicial system with EU legislation** in the following areas: improving access to cross-border justice; introducing the concept of international repeat offences in the field of counterfeiting; rules on combating corruption in the private sector; and the freezing of assets and the gathering of evidence. These new provisions should reduce the impunity enjoyed by corrupt officials who hide the evidence, or proceeds of their crimes, abroad or in France.

- Two laws passed in March 2005 authorise the approval of the May 2000 Convention on Mutual Assistance in Criminal Matters between the member states of the European Union and its protocol on banking information signed in October 2001.[1] The convention, initiated by France, aims to make **cross-border judicial cooperation** more rapid and flexible, while the protocol gives the judicial authorities improved access to banking information, an important tool for increasing the efficiency of transnational criminal investigations and the detection of money laundering. The laws should facilitate cooperation between judicial, police and customs authorities in other EU states and make the prosecution of cross-border crimes, including corruption, easier. An earlier law (*loi Perben II*), passed in March 2004, introduced a number of changes in the criminal justice process. It will strengthen the investigative powers of the police and public prosecutors, provided that the case is classified as an investigation into organised crime, and introduces a new mechanism for determining penalties. This could have an impact on offences involving corruption, as the penalties imposed are less likely to be reduced after a certain period of time.

- An interdepartmental directive issued in October 2004 outlined plans announced in late 2003 to create and operate a **central anti-corruption squad** within the criminal police. Composed of some 20 officers specially trained in economics and finance, the squad will operate in conjunction with the economic and financial branches of the national police and the gendarmerie.

- A circular from the justice minister to public prosecutors and judges in June 2004 set out the principle that 'the fight against corruption is a fundamental element in the fight against economic and financial crime'. It reaffirmed the direction of France's **criminal policy** in relation to the detection, prosecution and punishment of corruption. Some of the circular's main points reaffirm that: public sector employees and auditors must inform immediately the public prosecutor's office of any evidence of corruption; prosecutors must investigate with care all complaints of corruption and follow through quickly with criminal proceedings; and the state reserves the right to confiscate all proceeds of corruption.

Public procurement and the Ile de France trial

The Ile de France trial, one of the biggest trials involving alleged corruption in public procurement ever held in France, opened in March 2005. Seven years of investigations were required to expose an extensive system of corruption in procurement contracts for the construction or renovation of 300 of the 470 high schools in the Ile de France, the region around Paris. The case involves 47 defendants, who if found guilty face up to 10 years in prison for collusion, conceal- ing corruption and influence peddling. The accusations centre on allegations that companies paid major political parties to win contracts to renovate schools around Paris. The defendants include a former coop- eration minister, an ex-president of the Ile de France regional council and a former labour minister, as well as the former treas- urers of three political parties and business executives.[2]

Following a decision by the Ile de France regional council to upgrade the school facilities, it reportedly signed 114 10-year construction and maintenance contracts valued at close to €1.4 billion

(US $1.68 billion) in total, with only five multinational companies. It was alleged that these companies made an unofficial and secret deal, involving the payment of 2 per cent of the value of the contracts to various political parties: 1.2 per cent to the ruling Rassemblement Pour la République and 0.8 per cent to the Socialist Party, with smaller allocations to the Republican and Communist parties. The payments took the form of apparently legal gifts to finance the parties' campaigns. Between 1991 and 1996, some €30 million (US $36 million) were paid out under the scheme.

The scandal highlights the role played by the media in denouncing corruption. Having assumed a surveillance and detection role in the field, the media constitutes a major power centre in its own right, and its revelations frequently lead to judicial enquiries. The public reaction to the Ile de France trials illustrates how opinion has become more sensitive to corruption than it used to be. Elected representatives now proclaim their willingness to fight corrupt practices.

As a consequence, a number of standards, mechanisms and bodies have been created since the mid-1990s, using EU legislation as a model, to control and monitor the implementation of public works, and sanction corruption. Moreover, financial authorities, such as the Cour des comptes (Court of Auditors) and the Chambres régionales des comptes (Regional Courts of Accounts), are playing an increasing role in corruption prevention by issuing frequent notices on the management of private and state-owned companies and, more generally, on the management of public funds. Regulatory authorities have also played a role. The regulatory authority for telecommunications, for example, has encouraged the sector to open up to competition and adopt regulations to increase transparency.

The new procurement code that came into force in January 2004 restates the principle of freedom of access to public tendering and equal treatment of bidders, and includes stricter publication rules. The threshold beyond which publishing bids is mandatory has been drastically reduced from €90,000 (US $110,000) in the previous code to the ceiling required for very small purchases by a public body – which is usually around €10,000 (US $12,000) and depends on the size of the body. An added transparency measure requires public purchasers, including local governments, to publish details of all contracts signed in the past year, including the name of the contractor.

The courts do not hesitate to cancel contracts or procedures that do not comply with these principles. Bidders who fail to win contracts are able to find out why, and may refer the matter to court if the process appears improper. France's highest administrative court, the Conseil d'état, recorded an increase of 35 per cent in the number of suits filed in the field of public contracting in 2004: 180 cases were recorded in that year as compared to 133 in 2003.

The new procurement code was followed by the development of public–private partnerships in June 2004, making it easier to involve private companies in public sector projects. Though an interesting development, Transparency International France, among other civil society organisations, have criticised such contracts for being vulnerable to financial abuse, inter alia because of their complexity, which increases the risks of corruption. But they, too, are supposed to be subject to the principles of transparent, open and competitive bidding, and the allocation procedure for such contracts is strictly regulated and monitored by a judge.

The public contracting system in place when the Ile de France procurement was negotiated has now effectively been superseded. The introduction in the 1990s of the offence of favouritism also played a preventive role in fighting corrupt practices in contracting.[3] Nevertheless, the continuing importance of negotiated contract procedures – closed public bids allowed under article 35 of the new procurement code – could increase the risk of corruption.

The 2004 procurement code has not had a direct impact on reducing corruption, but it has streamlined and simplified the rules.

Hence the ethical conduct of both public purchasers and contracting parties should receive more prominence. Transparency International France has encouraged elected representatives to ask bidding companies to sign a no-bribes 'transparency pact', through which they pledge not to offer bribes, and to require public purchasing agencies to subscribe to a code of conduct. Although it is true that public outcry against political party financing through public procurement contracts has motivated change, there is still a great deal to be done. The mechanisms for the allocation of public procurement contracts need to be monitored, particularly when contracts are part of major projects. This scrutiny should be extended to subcontractors.

Antoine Genevois (Docteur en droit, Université Paris-Sorbonne, member of the Laboratoire de Droit Economique Francophone)

Further reading

Thierry Beaugé, *Le nouveau code des marchés publics. Commentaires et analyse des réformes de 2001 et 2004* (The New Public Procurement Code. Commentaries and Analysis of the 2001 and 2004 Reforms) (Paris: AFNOR, 2004)

Daniel Dommel, *Face à la corruption. Peut-on l'accepter? Peut-on la prévenir? Peut-on la combattre?* (Can Corruption be Accepted? Can it be Prevented? Can it be Fought?) (Paris: Karthala, 2003)

Bruno Fay and Laurent Olivier, *Le casier judiciaire de la république* (The Republic's Criminal Record) (Paris: Ramsay, 2002)

Antoine Genevois, *L'efficacité internationale des droits anti-corruption* (The International Effectiveness of Anti-corruption Laws), 2004, PhD thesis pending publication by Presses Universitaires de la Sorbonne

GRECO (Group of States against Corruption), Council of Europe, *Evaluation Report on France, Second Evaluation Round,* 2 December 2004, available at www.greco.coe.int

Eva Joly and Laurent Beccaria, *Est-ce dans ce monde-là que nous voulons vivre?* (Is This the World in Which We Want to Live?) (Paris: Les Arênes, July 2003)

TI France: www.transparence-france.org

Notes

1. See http://europa.eu.int/scadplus/leg/en/lvb/l33108.htm
2. BBC News, 21 March 2005.
3. This offence was introduced into French law in 1991 and its application was extended in 1995.

Georgia

Conventions:
Council of Europe Civil Law Convention on Corruption (ratified May 2003)
Council of Europe Criminal Law Convention on Corruption (signed January 1999; not yet ratified)
UN Convention against Corruption (not yet signed)
UN Convention against Transnational Organized Crime (signed December 2000; not yet ratified)

Legal and institutional changes

- Two sets of laws adopted as part of a package on **judicial reform** are intended to augment the independence of the courts and strengthen the government's ability to prosecute corrupt judges. A law passed in February 2005 elaborated the government's disciplinary response to violations by judges. Two other laws adopted in December 2004 raised the salaries of judges in the Supreme Court and the Constitutional Court to the level of state ministers. Higher salaries were one of the new government's most important measures for fighting corruption among civil servants.

- Parliament adopted a **revised tax code** in December 2004. Though too early to assess, the new code should reduce corruption by streamlining the existing system and increasing the capacity and incentives for tax payment. Changes include the introduction of a flat tax rate of 12 per cent, replacing a higher progressive income tax and potentially reducing the tendency of wage earners to hide their income. However, the new code could also contribute to Georgia's smuggling problem. Large increases in tax – up to 180 per cent on cigarettes and 67 per cent on alcohol – were intended to boost state revenues by 95 per cent, but excise returns from January and February 2005 are down, indicating increased smuggling. Smuggling is a critical issue in Georgia and there are indications that senior officials have been involved.[1]

- Also in December, Minister of Education Alexandre Lomaia pushed through parliament a law that standardises the **university admissions system** and is aimed at eliminating the practice of students securing their place in college by paying bribes. State support for universities will now depend on the number of students admitted, reducing the opportunities for rectors to keep as personal income arbitrary sums from the ministry. A number of rectors have been fired or have resigned amid a wave of corruption charges since the law was adopted.

- A presidential decree in January 2005 established an **anti-corruption working group** with the goal of developing an anti-corruption strategy. Though fighting corruption has been one of the government's main aims, it has notably lacked any targeted legislative or policy initiatives. The new working group, composed of members of government and NGOs, falls under the auspices of the recently established Anti-Corruption Policy Coordination Department in the National Security Council and is required to come up with a strategic plan by June 2005 (see below).

Adhering to Georgia's anti-corruption initiatives

President Mikheil Saakashvili, who led the campaign to remove Eduard Shevardnadze in the 'rose revolution' of 2003, has successfully altered perceptions of corruption in Georgia. According to TI's Global Corruption Barometer 2004,[2] Georgia saw the highest increase in optimism of all countries surveyed that corruption would diminish over the next few years. Recent polls, however, suggest that Saakashvili's popularity is waning and critics have accused him of assuming too much power, and weakening both parliament and the judicial system. The unexpected death in February 2005 of Prime Minister Zurab Zhvania, considered the only counterweight in government to the president, further destabilised the country. Zhvania had pushed for a coherent anti-corruption strategy and his demise has lessened the momentum for reform.

One problem is the sheer number of anti-corruption recommendations to which the government has made a commitment without, in the view of domestic NGOs, making much progress. None of its recommendations has been institutionalised, while individual ministries reform themselves at their own pace. The government has not instituted national-level anti-corruption initiatives, such as reform of the civil service, the streamlining of existing anti-corruption laws or the creation of an independent anti-corruption agency. It took steps in this direction by creating a Ministry of Economic Reform and an Anti-Corruption Policy Coordination Department at the National Security Council, and by reviving the formerly disbanded Public Service Bureau. The latter, re-established after the state transferred to a ministerial system of government, envisions resolving the overstaffing and low wages that increase the frequency of bribe-taking and corruption in the public sector.

Georgia enjoyed unprecedented levels of international support in 2005. President George W. Bush's visit in May 2005 was a triumph for bilateral relations, and the US Millennium Challenge Corporation has signed a compact with Tbilisi worth US $295.3 million. Anti-corruption goals, however, are not tied to aid or any other leverage mechanisms, which diminishes the incentive to implement them. Georgia has signed a partnership agreement with the G8 on promoting transparency and combating corruption, implementing the recommendations from the Council of Europe's Group of States against Corruption (GRECO) and the OECD's Anti-Corruption Network for Transition Economies. It also presented a report describing its anti-corruption achievements and outlining its future activities in the field at an EU donor meeting.

Compliance with these documents has not been as brisk as their adoption, however. In the government's defence, anti-corruption targets have been overshadowed by the campaign to restore Georgia's territorial integrity through the reintegration of South Ossetia and Abkhazia. The documents, moreover, are vague, set forth contradictory information and lack specific details on timeframe or implementation, making them wish-lists more than feasible plans.

Whether the new anti-corruption working group will be able to establish a workable anti-corruption plan remains to be seen. Though established in mid-January 2005, it met for the first time in March, and only after its NGO members published an open letter urging it to convene. The working group covers much the same ground as other anti-corruption initiatives, with the significant difference that it must come up with deadlines for activity completion and details about the responsible institutions, expected outcomes and finance required. This attention to specifics may ensure a more constructive plan for developing a national policy to curb corruption, but the group had made little progress by April 2005.

Plea bargains: new possibilities for corruption?

The government's use of 'plea bargains' to confiscate illegally obtained funds from public officials was welcomed as a valuable new tool in the fight against corruption when introduced in February 2004. Georgians are now considering the ethical dimension of plea bargains and asking whether the amendment that made them possible truly upholds the rule of law.

In spring 2004, the Saakashvili administration went after a number of officials known to have taken millions of dollars in some of the country's most famous cases of public sector graft. But the idea behind the campaign – to penalise individuals protected by the so-called 'impunity syndrome' – is viewed by the more cynical as a means of raising additional funds for the budget.

Plea-bargaining, a deliberately vague addition to the Criminal Procedures Code, allows a defendant to 'cooperate with the investigation' rather than plead guilty to a crime. While a guilty plea means automatic jail time, 'cooperation' is an informal arrangement whose outcome is decided by officials in the prosecutor's office.

Increasingly, the issue has developed into a debate about methods and goals. Saakashvili's administration argues that it has held corrupt officials accountable, but others – including the influential NGOs Georgian Young Lawyers Association and Institutional Reform and the Informal Sector (IRIS) – claim that lack of information on plea bargains and the arbitrary manner in which they are being handled creates far greater concern about the protection of civil liberties.

Crucial details in plea-bargaining cases, including the identity of the individuals in question, the number of cases and the sums of money restored, are only partly documented at present. Since cases are settled arbitrarily by prosecuting officials, it is evident that plea-bargaining could lead to other forms of corruption.

The prosecutor's office created a special fund from the monies it recovered from corrupt officials for use by the law enforcement bodies. But the fund's division between these bodies, and the total amount involved, are both unknown. One estimate puts the seized funds at 55.7 million lari (US $31 million) from January to November 2004.[3] Nor are there accurate figures on how many cases have been heard since the amendment came into force: the prosecutor's office puts the number at 100, but lawyers involved say it is closer to 1,000. Even when a case has ended, information is no easier to obtain, leading people to question the administration's secrecy. 'There is no system of monitoring and none of the information is transparent', said David Usupashvili, head of IRIS and chairman of the Republican Party of Georgia. 'The procedural rules are meaningless and, as a result, human rights violations and levels of corruption will only increase.'

The government recently made a further amendment to the criminal procedures code that somewhat improves the existing law. Though informal discussions had taken place with a view to removing the amendment altogether, the current compromise has been to reduce pre-trial detention from a maximum of nine to four months from January 2006. Five months is a significant difference for defendants in Georgia, where prison conditions are notoriously squalid. Indeed, pre-trial detention is used to scare people into paying their way out of jail before being sentenced. Moreover, the authorities use preliminary detention as a sign of guilt; officials make statements accusing detainees of corruption before their case has even been heard.

Corruption is down, but crime is not

The most visible sign of Georgia's progress this past year was the overhaul of the police patrol force, the largest of the interior ministry's many units, in August 2004. Equipped with American-style uniforms, modern cars and special-issue equipment at a total cost of US $4.7 million, the new force is a ubiquitous and oddly juxtaposed presence on Tbilisi's gently decaying streets.

Police reform is no small feat in Georgia where law enforcement ranked as its most corrupt institution in TI's Global Corruption Barometer 2004. Extortion flourished under the previous system in which a bloated force was forced to survive on wages as low as US $20 per month. Prior to reform, the ministry employed 54,000 personnel, or one officer per 89 civilians, a figure more reflective of a police state than a democracy. As MP Giga Bokeria said, 'The state was giving the policemen torn uniforms and a gun, and telling them to shakedown drivers and bring a share to us.'[4]

The ministry drastically cut personnel to one third of its previous size, reducing the officer:civilian ratio to 1:214; fired all employees suspected of corruption; and offered significant salary raises to the remaining staff. Other moves included streamlining the ministry's internal organisation and the transfer of two of the units most notorious for corruption, the financial police and civil registration, to the ministries of finance and justice respectively. In July 2004, it abolished four units with overlapping responsibilities – the transport police, traffic police, public order police and ecological police – and replaced them with police patrol units.

The civil registration unit was a source of insidious corruption in the regions. Many Georgians simply refused to register rather than pay the bribes that were demanded, with the result that the country's demographic records remain incomplete, increasing the potential for tax evasion and for misrepresentation of the number of ethnic minorities living in the country.

The government has coasted along on these reforms, holding them up as a tangible benefit of its reform-friendly environment, but the new force is not without problems. Crime rates have doubled since the 2003 revolution and, while the ministry claims this is the result of improved crime registration, others claim that the new force simply lacks the expertise of officers they have replaced.

Daria Vaisman (TI Georgia)

Further reading

Georgian Opinion Research Business International (GORBI), *Corruption Survey* (Tbilisi: GORBI, 2003), www.gorbi.com

Alexandre Kukhianidze, Aleko Kupatadze and Roman Gotsiridze, 'Research Report on Georgia' (Tbilisi: Georgia Office of the American University's Transnational Crime and Corruption Center, 2003)

TI Georgia: www.transparency.ge

Notes

1. In March 2005, President Mikheil Saakashvili dismissed more than 20 police officials in Shida Kartli after accusations they had engaged in smuggling with traders in the breakaway region of South Ossetia (RFE/RL Newsline 9 (49), part I, 15 March 2005). The media also reported allegations of smuggling of timber by senior officials in the Ministry of Interior (RFE/RL Newsline 9 (52), part I, 18 March 2005).
2. See www.transparency.org/surveys/index.html#barometer
3 RFE/RL Newsline 9 (2), 5 January 2005.
4. *AmCham* (Georgia) 3, 2004.

Greece

Conventions:
Council of Europe Civil Law Convention on Corruption (ratified February 2002)
Council of Europe Criminal Law Convention on Corruption (signed January 1999; not yet ratified; Additional Protocol signed May 2003; not yet ratified)
OECD Anti-Bribery Convention (ratified February 1999)
UN Convention against Corruption (signed December 2003; not yet ratified)
UN Convention against Transnational Organized Crime (signed December 2000; not yet ratified)

Legal and institutional changes

• In response to a wave of corruption scandals involving the judiciary, parliament adopted a new law in March 2005 that introduces increased monitoring and transparency within the branch.[1] Under the new legislation, the **bribing of judges** will no longer be treated as a 'delinquency' but a felony, raising the maximum prison sentence from five years to life. The law also includes stipulations for safeguarding transparency in the selection of judges who preside over criminal courts and rule on cases involving injunction measures (see below).

- Under an amendment to the constitution passed in 2001, any allegation of wrongdoing by a government minister, even if unfounded, must be directly forwarded to parliament, rather than being investigated by the prosecuting authorities. In October 2004, the first parliamentary inquiry was set up to investigate **allegations of corruption in arms contracts** signed in the late 1990s. The inquiry examined allegations that a former defence minister and other officials had accepted bribes from Russian arms dealers to sign contracts for the procurement of anti-aircraft missiles. According to a parliamentary committee, the deals allegedly cost taxpayers €300 million (US $373 million). The inquiry concluded its work in January 2005 after deciding that the evidence uncovered did not suffice to initiate a prosecution.

- A new code of conduct for police officers was adopted by presidential decree in December 2004.[2] Under the code, officers are obliged to **refuse offers of bribes** or to use their positions to obtain advantages for themselves, or their friends and relatives. The code stipulates that police officers should report acts of corruption immediately to the competent authorities.

Corruption scandals rock the judiciary and the church

A series of corruption scandals in the judiciary and the Greek Orthodox church has tarnished their reputation and led to widespread public outcry. In March 2005, the reported discovery that a priest, Archimandrite Jacobos Josakis, had bribed three judges to obtain rulings in his favour in cases involving the misappropriation of antiquities and illegal excavation appeared to be an isolated case.[3] But journalists investigating related cases uncovered evidence suggesting that this might only be the tip of the iceberg.[4]

At the time of writing, 32 cases involving Josakis were under investigation. In addition to accusations of partiality by the judges ruling in these cases, the court proceedings against him, all in Piraeus, took longer than expected. The priest has been remanded in jail while awaiting trial.

Judicial proceedings in Greece are usually very slow, but the authorities have been remarkably quick in probing this scandal, given the unprecedented level of corruption.

In February 2005, four judges came under investigation. One of them, Antonia Ilia, was fired in June 2005 and charged on seven counts, including money laundering and accepting a bribe.[5]

The Josakis investigation led to the discovery of a series of other scandals involving alleged bribery of the judiciary. The media reported that a judge from Chania in Crete apparently accepted bribes on a regular basis to issue biased rulings. The authorities claim to have evidence that a local businessman had deposited €60,000 (US $73,380) into his account to obtain a favourable ruling. The same judge had taken a vacation aboard a yacht belonging to another individual whose case he had presided over, and other suspect, albeit smaller, amounts of money were deposited in a similar manner.[6]

A common feature of these cases was the overwhelming amount of evidence uncovered. Previous exposure of corruption in the Greek judiciary has been extremely rare, but, although the number of judges named in the current scandal is small (15 of the country's 2,700 to date),[7] the stories rocked society and prompted massive media coverage. Greece's judiciary once enjoyed a reputation as a corrupt-free institution with strict moral values and a keen sense of duty, despite occasional reports to the contrary,[8] and this reputation remains to a great extent merited. But the Josakis case highlighted systemic flaws in the judiciary that could facilitate corruption.

At the time of writing, four judges had been fired for alleged corruption (mainly bribery) and three other cases were pending before the Supreme Court. Constantina Bourboulia faces charges of receiving 40 million drachmas (US $143,000) for a favourable ruling in a stock market case in June 2001.[9] In June 2005, a case was filed against appeals court judge Kyriakos Karosas for bribery and breach of duty in cases involving 15 defendants, including Josakis. In the same month, allegations were made against a Supreme Court judge and president of the judges' union, who is under investigation for allegedly having his summer house built by a contractor to whom he gave a favourable ruling.[10]

Both the Supreme Court and justice ministry responded to the crisis in confidence with remarkable speed, implementing measures to address systemic defects, as well as taking preventive action to reduce further scandals. The justice ministry has proposed a draft law which was adopted by parliament in March 2005. Its aim is to introduce measures to strengthen internal monitoring and transparency in the judiciary. It stiffens penalties for bribing judges, elevating it from a misdemeanour to a felony, and raises the maximum sentence from five years in prison to life. The law also includes stipulations for safeguarding transparency in the selection of judges to preside over criminal court cases and injunction measures. The Supreme Court, which is responsible for evaluating the selection of judges, also proposed a preventive measure for the relocation of 70 judges and 15 prosecutors who had served in the same location for over eight years.[11] Since it was based on the hypothesis that working in the same place for many years could lead to partiality and corruption of the judiciary, this decision sparked a fierce outcry in the legal community. Judges and their union objected, saying any judge relocated would automatically fall under suspicion of involvement in corrupt activities.

Public scrutiny of the activities of the Greek Orthodox church is another development to have come out of the corruption scandals. Indeed, questions of corruption or lack of transparency in the church were taboo until the recent events. In addition to the arrest of Archimandrite Josakis, there were allegations that the Bishop of Attica had suspicious deposits of 1 billion drachmas (US $3.6 million) in his bank account, of which 100 million drachmas were allegedly misappropriated from a monastery.[12] He was dismissed in February 2005. At the same time, four bishops were asked to give explanations regarding allegations of possessing fortunes that cannot be justified. The scandals apparently led to the resignation of the Bishop of Thessaliotidos in February 2005; though not directly involved, he had introduced accused persons to the archbishop and proposed that the church should employ them.

Another scandal involved the Chrysopigi organisation, founded in the 1970s by the current archbishop and some of his bishops, who are still members of the organisation. According to media reports, members of the Chrysopigi organisation are alleged to have unduly influenced elections in the church, including the Patriarchate selection process in Jerusalem.[13] Though the allegations have not been proven, the organisation is to be audited for financial irregularities by both the church and state authorities.

The string of scandals highlighted the institution's complex and unique set of regulations. Under the constitution, the Orthodox church is an autonomous and self-regulating legal entity with its own auditing and monitoring mechanisms, and sanctions. But the church is also a public institution. Priests are public employees, subject to criminal law, although criminal offences by priests are adjudicated by state high courts.[14] The exposure of corruption in this important institution has led to a series of chain reactions.

In March 2005 the government announced that church finances would henceforth be audited and that the legislation requiring MPs, ministers, judges and senior public employees to declare their income and assets would in future apply to bishops.[15] The issue of financial auditing came up in parliament and is to be regulated by a joint decision of the education and finance ministers. The main problem is that the body charged with the task, the Synodos, includes among its members the very bishops that have been accused of abusing their positions.

Meanwhile, the church announced on several occasions in March 2005 that it would take measures to fight corruption within its ranks. The fact that many priests and other bishops have actively demanded that disciplinary action be taken bodes well for the church's future transparency.

Markella Samara (TI Greece)

Further reading

Levteris Drakopoulos, *State and Organised Crime* (Athens: Ekati Publications, 2002)
Nestor Kourakis, 'Corruption as a Problem of Greek Criminal Policy', *Poinikos Logos* Issue 1/02 (Athens: Ant. N. Sakkoulas Publishers, 2005)
Vassiliki Prigkouri, 'Corruption in the Greek Public Administration', unpublished master's thesis, University of Athens, 2004

TI Greece: www.transparency.gr

Notes

1. Law no. 3327/2005.
2. Presidential decree no. 274/2–3.12.2004/A243.
3. It should be noted that the media presented tapes containing evidence, but the prosecuting authorities will not admit their contents, which were acquired illegally. Instead, the charges will be based on legitimate means of evidence, such as witnesses, bank accounts, and so on.
4. The following information is based on newspaper articles and public statements. As the cases are very new, no court decisions or formal documents on the issue have been published yet.
5. www.lawnet.gr, 23 June 2005.
6. *Kathimerini* (Greece), 10 March 2005.
7. Author's interview with justice ministry officials.
8. In February 2005, *Kathimerini* newspaper published a document from 1993 written by a Supreme Court judge and addressed to the current president of the parliament, warning of the high level of corruption in the judiciary.
9. *Kathimerini* (Greece), 17 June 2005.
10. www.lawnet.gr, 17 June 2005.
11. *Ta Nea*, 15 March 2005.
12. *Kathimerini* (Greece), 1 April 2005.
13. *Kathimerini* (Greece), 27 February 2005.
14. For previous bribery cases, see Thessaloniki Court of Appeals 55/61, published in *Poinika Chronika IA' 282* (in Greek).
15. *Kathimerini* (Greece), 11 and 12 March 2005.

Guatemala

Conventions:

OAS Inter-American Convention against Corruption (ratified July 2001)
UN Convention against Corruption (signed December 2003; not yet ratified)
UN Convention against Transnational Organized Crime (ratified September 2003)

Legislative and institutional changes

- A proposal to **reform the penal code**, drafted by the Presidential Commission for Transparency and against Corruption, the public prosecutor's office and the NGO Acción Ciudadana, was made public in February 2005. It has yet to be submitted to the legislature. The reforms would bring the legal framework into line with the Inter-American Convention against Corruption by defining existing corruption crimes, adding new crimes such as transnational bribery and illicit enrichment, and increasing penalties for corruption by public officials. However, the reforms are unlikely to dent corruption unless accompanied by additional measures, such as the approval of an access to information law; increased powers for the auditor general to analyse asset declarations and make them public; mechanisms to identify and resolve conflicts of interest; and more transparent public contracting mechanisms.

- In February 2005 Congress passed a law guaranteeing the **impartiality of appointment commissions**. Public officials are forbidden from hiring, nominating or authorising the appointment to a position within their institution of any of the members of the appointment commission involved in hiring them. Members of appointment commissions are allowed to apply for positions through the ordinary competitive processes provided they fulfil advertised requirements for the job. The law is especially significant for protecting the independence and impartiality of the heads of the Supreme Court, the auditor general, the public prosecutor and the supreme electoral court.

- The **Commission for Transparency and against Corruption**, established as a temporary presidential body in 2004, had its mandate extended for another year from March 2005. The commission is responsible for advising the president, drafting anti-corruption policies and legislative reform proposals and promoting the creation of the Multidisciplinary Council for Transparency, made up of members of government and civil society. The prolongation of the commission reflects positively on the government's commitment to anti-corruption, though changes to the commission's structure and operation are needed. Of concern, is the absence of norms outlining the competencies of the commission and its independence from the president.

- In February 2005, Congress created an **Extraordinary National Legislative Commission for Transparency**, at a time when the auditor general (Contraloría General de Cuentas, CGC) was in crisis, following the dismissal and prosecution of its two former heads and the failure to appoint a successor. The commission is empowered to conduct studies, including monitoring the CGC, issue recommendations and draft legislative proposals. Concerns have been raised about the overlap between the commission's work and the work of the Commission on Probity, which was set up in 1994 and could also have looked into problems at the CGC. Indeed, a memorandum of understanding was signed in September 2004 between the civil society organisation Coalition for Transparency, the Commission on Probity and the CGC on their commitment to work jointly with the aim of strengthening the two signatory public bodies.

Electronic system helps fight corruption in public contracting

Guatemala's Internet-based public contracting system, GUATECOMPRAS, was launched in September 2003 amid expectations that it would help clean up an area of government that has long been the subject of numerous corruption scandals. Its inception was complicated; it was created two months before general elections by a government that had been repeatedly accused of corruption by the media.[1] Fears that the new party in power would scrap the project proved unfounded, however. Instead, GUATECOMPRAS has been extended and strengthened.

When initially launched, government bodies could opt voluntarily to put their contracting processes online. In February 2004, President Oscar Berger issued a government agreement within his council of ministers that reformed implementing regulations for the Law on State Contracting, making use of the GUATECOMPRAS system mandatory. Since then, all information related to the purchase, sale and hire of goods, services and public works must be put online.[2]

The use of GUATECOMPRAS has increased notably over the past year. It was used by 305 government agencies in April 2005, compared with just 75 in July 2004. Around 60 per cent of municipalities currently use the system, as well as 89 per cent of central government bodies.[3]

But the success story of its usage is qualified by GUATECOMPRAS' structural weaknesses. It operates within the framework of the Law on State Contracting, which includes significant exemptions to transparency requirements. Chief among them is an exemption for the Ministry of Defence, which is not required to participate in GUATECOMPRAS, and did so on only six occasions from October 2004 to May 2005. In only two of these cases were contracting processes finalised.[4]

Another weakness is that GUATECOMPRAS' legal status is weak because it was regulated by a ministerial agreement and not a legislative vote. This has caused problems. For example,

in October 2004, the national association of municipalities (ANAM) requested that the system be suspended on the grounds that they lacked the necessary computers and Internet facilities to use it. They also argued that making GUATECOMPRAS mandatory violated municipal autonomy since it was based only on an executive agreement.[5] After a month's debate, the president's office stated that the municipalities would continue to use the system, given that 147 had managed to by October 2004, and 47 per cent of contracting processes had been completed without problems.[6] The communiqué has not encouraged some municipalities with large budgets to use the system, however, including the capital city and the municipality of Mixco.

Another weakness with the current legal framework is that the contracting process is split into four processes depending on the sums involved, with larger contracts subject to greater scrutiny. This has led to contracts being sub-divided in order to avoid the highest degree of scrutiny. Also of concern is that the Law on State Contracting exempts from transparency requirements the social investment funds created from international loans or donations from private, international or national bodies, and institutions. These funds are considerable, but may be spent on public goods and services in processes that fall outside of the reach of the Law on State Contracting and the GUATECOMPRAS system.

The Law on State Contracting needs to be reformed to strengthen GUATECOMPRAS. Various reform bills exist: one of the best was drafted by the Presidential Commission for Reform, Modernisation and Fortification of the State (COPRE) which, if adopted, would go a long way to correcting shortcomings in the system.[7] Civil society organisations consider the system to be an effective tool to fight corruption and promote transparency in state contracting and purchases. But it remains to be seen whether Congress will give it the necessary support to enable it to perform its task to the full.

Access to information: a right still to be enshrined in law

The right of citizens to access public information has been enshrined in the constitution, which states that all administrative acts should be public and that every citizen has the right to request any public document or file at any time.[8] But the right is eroded by the fact that despite constitutional recognition, there is no law regulating provision or facilitating access to information held by public institutions. Access to information is crucial to fighting corruption, since monitoring by civil society depends on information about how money and power are used by public or political bodies.

In the absence of an access to information law, requests for information are dealt with haphazardly and inefficiently. While it is possible to file a complaint before the Constitutional Court if public information is denied, this rarely happens since few know about the process.

The constitutional right is continuously violated, according to studies by the NGOs Acción Ciudadana (Citizen Action) and Observatorio Ciudadano para el Libre Acceso a la Información (Citizens' Observatory for the Free Access to Information). They found that between October 2002 and June 2004, 6 of every 10 requests for public information were denied. The rate of denial of requests for information increased during the electoral period, when 78 per cent of requests were rejected, while in the post-electoral period the rate went down markedly to 32 per cent.[9] In April 2005, Acción Ciudadana monitored access to information about social investment funds. They found that half of all requests for information were denied or not answered, while only one in four was answered appropriately.[10]

In November 2004 another report on implementation of the Inter-American Convention against Corruption found that the institutional and legal framework did not help citizens to seek information that was their constitutional right and, worse, acted as an incentive for officials to violate the constitutional requirement that they make information available. The fact that there is no express obligation to organise, publish and provide official information; the absence of procedures for accessing information; ambiguous definitions of information exempt from the right to access; the lack of public bodies to enforce the right; and the lack of sanctions when the right is violated, all lead to a situation where the right to access to information is continuously violated, the authors asserted.[11]

The legislature has shown a lack of political will to tackle the problem. There is still no access to information law, though seven drafts have been submitted to Congress since 2000.[12] One of the bills to get further in the legislative process was Bill Number 2594, called 'Law of Free Access to Information'. It was submitted to the legislature in 2001 and went through all of the appropriate legislative processes until the last phase in March 2003, when the process stagnated and the bill was shelved.

There was hope that the new parliament would take a different approach to the issue after the December 2003 elections. A broad group of civil society organisations worked expectantly on a new proposal, which as well as including access to public information and a writ of habeas data provision, included stipulations concerning the classification and declassification of reserved information. This proposal was presented in November 2004 by Congressmen Eduardo Zachrisson and Nineth Montenegro, and debated by the plenary in February 2005.[13] Despite being given an official bill number and title, the 60-day period given to the congressional commission to analyse the bill expired without it ever being properly debated. The bill was still awaiting discussion at the time of writing.

Alejandro Urizar (Acción Ciudadana, Guatemala)

Further reading

Acción Ciudadana, *Manual anticlientelar para la fiscalización y control parlamentario de los fondos sociales* (Anti-clientilistic Manual for Parliamentary Auditing and Control of Social Funds) (Guatemala City: Editorial Magna Terra, April 2005)

Acción Ciudadana, *Manual para la fiscalización parlamentaria de las contrataciones públicas a través del sistema GUATECOMPRAS* (Manual for Parliamentary Oversight of Public Contracting through the GUATECOMPRAS System) (Guatemala City: Editorial Magna Terra, April 2005)

Acción Ciudadana, 'El régimen disciplinario en el Sistema de Justicia y la lucha contra la corrupción' (The Disciplinary Regime of the Judicial System and the Fight against Corruption), February 2005, www.accionciudadana.org.gt

Acción Ciudadana and partner NGOs, *Informe independiente de seguimiento a la implementación de la Convención Interamericana contra la Corrupción* (Independent Report on the Follow-up of the Inter-American Convention against Corruption) (Guatemala City: Editorial Magna Terra, 2005)

Asociación de Investigación y Estudios Sociales (ASIES), 'La cultura política de la democracia en Guatemala' (The Political Culture of Democracy in Guatemala), March 2003, www.asies.org.gt/informes.htm

Coalición por la Transparencia, *Los conflictos de interés en el sector público* (Conflicts of Interest in the Public Sector) (Guatemala City: Editorial Magna Terra, August 2004)

Acción Ciudadana (Guatemala): www.accionciudadana.org.gt

Notes

1. Agreement no. 386–2003 of the finance ministry, published in the official gazette on 25 September 2003.
2. Agreement no. 80–2004 of the executive body, published in the official gazette on 23 February 2004.
3. www.guatecompras.gt
4. Ibid.
5. 'Boletín Municipal', *Inforpress Centroamericana* 85, Guatemala, November 2004.
6. *Diario de Centroamérica* (Guatemala) 36, 302, 3 November 2005.
7. Presidential Commission for Reform, Modernisation and Strengthening of the State and its Decentralised Entities (COPRE), 'Formal Proposal of Reforms to the Law of State Contracting', April 2005.
8. Article 30 of the constitution. The constitution, however, grants important exceptions to the right to information: military or diplomatic matters that are considered national security, or information involving individuals who have been given a guarantee of confidentiality do not need to be disclosed.
9. Acción Ciudadana and Observatorio Ciudadano para el libre acceso a la información, *El acceso a la información pública en Guatemala, informe de tres experiencias piloto* (Access to Public Information in Guatemala: Report on Three Pilot Experiences) (Guatemala City: Editorial Magna Terra, 2004). A total of 268 requests were issued to central government or municipal authorities. Just under half of the requests were made in the name of individuals and the rest in the name of the institutions involved in the study.
10. Acción Ciudadana, *Manual anticlientelar para la fiscalización y control parlamentario de los fondos sociales* (Anti-clientilistic Manual for Parliamentary Auditing and Control of Social Funds) (Guatemala City: Editorial Magna Terra, 2005).
11. Coordinated by Acción Ciudadana, *Informe independiente de seguimiento a la implementación de la Convención Interamericana contra la Corrupción* (Independent Report on the Follow-up of the Inter-American Convention against Corruption) (Guatemala City: Editorial Magna Terra, 2005).
12. www.congreso.gob.gt
13. It has been given bill number 3165 and is called 'Law on Access to Information and Classification and Declassification of Reserved State Information'.

Ireland

Conventions:
Council of Europe Civil Law Convention on Corruption (signed November 1999; not yet ratified)
Council of Europe Criminal Law Convention on Corruption (ratified October 2003; Additional Protocol ratified July 2005)
OECD Anti-Bribery Convention (ratified September 2003)
UN Convention against Corruption (signed December 2003; not yet ratified)
UN Convention against Transnational Organized Crime (signed December 2000; not yet ratified)

Legal and institutional changes

• The Proceeds of Crime Act was ratified in January 2005 to amend the 2001 Prevention of Corruption (Amendment) Act and **increases the powers of investigation** of the Criminal Assets Bureau (see below).

• The Commissions of Investigation Act, passed in July 2004, provides for the creation of **Commissions of Investigation** that will investigate 'matters of significant public concern', including corruption. One of the main reasons for the legislation was to provide an alternative mechanism to the Tribunal of Inquiry (see below).

• The Central Bank and Financial Services Authority of Ireland Act, passed in July 2004, complements the Central Bank and Financial Services Authority of Ireland Act, approved in 2003. It provides for the establishment of an **independent Financial Services Ombudsman** to deal with consumer complaints against financial institutions, and provides for greater transparency and accountability in the financial sector.

• The Public Service Management (Recruitment and Appointments) Act of October 2004 **reforms the recruitment process in the civil service** and other public bodies under its remit for the first time since 1926. It replaces the Civil Service and Local Appointments Commission with two new bodies: the Commission for Public Service Appointments (CPSA) and the Public Appointments Service. The CPSA publishes codes of practice for recruitment to a number of public service bodies and grants licences to some of them to recruit on their own behalf, allowing for more flexible and locally focused hiring arrangements. Concerns have been raised that the relocation of recruitment might 'facilitate a culture of local favouritism in appointments to departments located outside Dublin' and politicise appointments in the civil service.[1]

• A Civil Service Code of Standards and Behaviour for Ireland's 30,000 civil servants was published in December 2004. It places in a single document matters related to the principles of integrity, impartiality, effectiveness, equity and accountability. The Civil Service code establishes a 12-month moratorium and an outside appointments board to **address possible conflicts of interest** when civil servants take positions in the private sector. It also advises civil servants how to deal with gifts received, and prohibits civil servants from engaging in outside business or activities that would conflict with the interests of their departments, or abuse their official positions to benefit themselves or others.

- The Garda Síochána (Police Service) Bill 2004 has passed the upper house of parliament and is likely to come into effect before the summer 2005 legislative recess.[2] It provides for the establishment of the three-person **independent** Garda Síochána **Ombudsman Commission** for the purposes of ensuring openness, transparency and accountability in the way complaints against the police are investigated (see below).

- An Irish chapter of Transparency International was launched in December 2004, reflecting increased concern about corruption following a series of legislative changes and a string of parliamentary, tribunal, civil society and international reports on corruption.

- An independent organisation, the **Centre for Public Inquiry**, was established in February 2005 with a brief to investigate matters of importance within Irish political, public and corporate life, and to heighten public awareness of the need for whistleblower protective legislation. The centre has high-profile directors, including former high court judge Feargus Flood, and generous funding from the Irish-American charitable foundation, Atlantic Philanthropies. Political figures, including the leader of the Seanad Eireann (upper house of parliament), have expressed reservations about the Centre's broad terms of reference, particularly its lack of accountability for the focus and direction of potential investigations.

Reform of the tribunals

The Houses of the Oireachtas (parliament) established the Mahon Tribunal (formerly the Flood Tribunal) in 1997 to investigate allegations of corruption involving political and business interests in the planning process.[3] Its work has been frustrated and constrained by the archaic structures it must operate within and by the persistent non-cooperation of key witnesses.

Justice Mahon acknowledged this non-cooperation by his use of discretion in granting costs to witnesses who, though involved in corruption, had chosen to cooperate with the tribunal. In the absence of whistleblower legislation, this was interpreted as a 'whistleblower's charter'.[4] As further evidence of the constraints of the tribunal of inquiry method, eight legal challenges have been filed against the process. These have proved time-consuming and disruptive.

In a climate of mounting criticism, the difficulties of the tribunal acts have finally been addressed and their investigative powers strengthened. The commissions of investigation, established under a 2004 act, will have powers to compel witnesses to give evidence, search premises and remove documents. This new body will operate alongside the tribunals. A commission of investigation will primarily be a private investigative process designed to encourage cooperation by moving away from the adversarial approach that applies within the courts and tribunals. There is less likelihood of a need for legal representation. A commission established under this act must submit a report on its findings and be timely and cost-effective. In April 2005, the first commission of investigation was established to investigate alleged collusion in the Dublin and Monaghan bombings of 1974.

The Tribunal of Inquiry into Certain Planning Matters and Payments Act 2004 removes the obligation of the tribunal to inquire into every matter before it. The tribunal now has power of discretion over what it investigates. Its final report has been given a deadline of 31 March 2007. If it is not met, the tribunal will continue to work but barristers' fees will drop from €2,500 (US $3,058) a day to €900 (US $1,100).

The far-reaching Proceeds of Crime (Amendment) Act 2005 eliminates existing legislative difficulties that require that a specific instance of corruption must be linked to a specific payment and a specific favour. The act increases the powers of the Criminal Assets Bureau (CAB), which now requires a lower burden of proof to confiscate the assets of corrupt individuals and seize a gift suspected of being a bribe.

The two acts not only challenge the lengthy, costly and complex nature of the tribunals, they eliminate the need for the tribunal inquiry method altogether. These departures are overdue, but represent a closing of the stable door after the horses have bolted.

Even the sternest critics of the tribunals acknowledge their catalytic role in focusing cultural change in Irish society toward corruption since they began in 1997. No individual has successfully been convicted on corruption charges arising from the tribunals, but George Redmond, the former assistant city and county manager for Dublin, will face new corruption charges in December 2005.[5] Former minister Ray Burke was convicted for making false tax returns identified by the tribunal and began a six-month jail sentence in January 2005.

Morris report points to need for further police reforms

The Morris Tribunal issued a damning report into corruption in the Donegal County An Garda Síochána (police) in July 2004. The government dismissed one superintendent and a chief superintendent resigned after the tribunal found they had been motivated by career ambition to plant ammunition and hoax explosives. The report cited 17 members of the Donegal force for varying degrees of culpability ranging from gross negligence to being uncooperative. The report highlighted failures in management, accountability and standards.

As the Mahon Tribunal also reportedly experienced, the principal obstacle to the Morris Tribunal was the culture of non-cooperation in the Garda Síochána, which the justice minister described as a 'hedgehog culture'.[6] The report suggested that Gardaí

primarily feel loyalty to their colleagues, rather than the law, and cooperation is withheld from disciplinary investigations and tribunals.

The Garda bill was initiated in February 2004 and is anticipated to pass before the summer 2005 legislative recess. It will replace all laws pertaining to the police since 1924 and is the first serious effort in the history of the state to reform policing structures. Though long overdue, many regard the bill as a missed opportunity to engage in a broader and deeper reform programme.

The bill proposes the creation of an independent Police Ombudsman Commission to replace the inadequate Police Complaints Board. The commission will investigate public complaints against members of the Garda, initiate investigations in matters in the public interest and examine Garda practices, policies and procedures. Legal experts branded a proposal to establish a hybrid between an ombudsman and a commission as 'misconceived'.[7] This departure from the ombudsman model, as adopted in Northern Ireland, to a multi-member model, 'will detract from its capacity to take a robust and decisive approach to the investigation of complaints against Gardaí and public concerns about policing'.[8] This is evident from structural weaknesses of the ombudsman commission, in particular, the absence of specificity in qualifications for appointment and the fact that appointments will be made by the government, rather than through open competition.

The Garda bill was subsequently amended to provide for the establishment of an independent civilian inspectorate that will give advice and support to the ministry, audit management systems and introduce international standards, practice and performance benchmarks. The fact that the inspectorate answers directly to the justice minister drew particular criticism from the Garda Representative Association and the opposition that it was 'using the excuse of the report of the Morris Tribunal' to obtain 'a hands-on approach'.[9] The proposals do not allow inspectorate reports to be publicly available as is the case in the United Kingdom. Nor do they provide for the Garda commissioner to be directly accountable to the Dáil (lower house of parliament) on operational policing matters.

The Morris Tribunal hopes to deliver a second report on its findings before June 2005. In an attempt to speed up proceedings, it introduced a five-point ruling that banned oral objections and applications, and limited cross-examination. However, a number of obstacles could potentially prevent the work of the tribunal. In March 2005, it cancelled planned public sittings in Donegal when a key witness, Frank McBrearty, refused to cooperate after he was denied free legal representation.[10] The issue of costs is now before the European Parliament.

In January 2005, a key witness for the tribunal had tapes stolen during a robbery at her home. No other items were taken. Reflecting the general loss of faith in Donegal's police, the witness has taken High Court proceedings to have Garda from outside the county investigate the case. This had not been resolved at the time of writing. It remains to be seen whether the tribunal will report as expediently or as comprehensively as it hopes.

Whistleblower protection still elusive

The reported systemic nature of corruption within the police force and planning process, as the Morris and Mahon Tribunals have identified, warrants the introduction of whistleblower legislation more than ever.

Despite momentous change in the Irish statute books since 1995 and various tribunals of inquiry and parliamentary investigations, whistleblower legislation remains elusive. It has been on the legislative books since March 1999. Six years later the initiator of the bill concluded: 'This bill probably holds some form of parliamentary record as the longest-standing bill on the Dáil's order paper.'[11]

Following a lengthy investigation, three reports were published in 2004 regarding alleged financial malpractice at the National Irish Bank Limited and National Irish Bank Financial Services Limited (NIB) and Allied Irish Bank (AIB).[12] These incidents involved complicity in widespread tax evasion at the NIB and the AIB's failure to comply with regulatory obligations over a period of eight years. Although these episodes were not directly corrupt, they served to illustrate the systematic culture of non-compliance that dominated sectors of Irish life in the 1980s and 1990s. As with the Mahon and Morris Tribunals, the NIB report cited frustration regarding a lack of full cooperation.[13]

Acknowledging this, the Irish Financial Services Regulatory Authority has advocated a change in cultural practice regarding hostile attitudes to whistleblowing. 'Staff members of financial institutions should not feel that they have to go to outside agencies in order to raise issues of importance to that institution', said chief executive Liam O'Reilly in January 2005. 'They should feel comfortable raising issues up the line. Those who wish to raise such issues should not be held responsible for the issue they are highlighting, simply because they have raised the matter.'[14] Whistleblower legislation is vital to combat an engrained cultural acceptance of corruption in Ireland.

Elaine Byrne (University of Limerick, Ireland)

Further Reading

Neil Collins and Mary O'Shea, 'Political Corruption in Ireland', in M. J. Bull and J. L. Newell (eds), *Corruption in Contemporary Politics* (Basingstoke: Palgrave Macmillan, 2003)

Council of Europe, 'GRECO, First Evaluation Round, Compliance Report on Ireland' (2003), www.greco.coe.int/evaluations/cycle1/GrecoRC-I(2003)14E-Ireland.pdf

Paul Cullen, *With a Little Help from my Friends: Planning Corruption in Ireland* (Dublin: Gill and Macmillan, 2003)

Justice Feargus M. Flood, *The Second Interim Report of the Tribunal of Inquiry into Certain Planning Matters and Payments* (Dublin: Government Stationery Office, 2002), www.flood-tribunal.ie

Colm McCarthy, 'Corruption in Public Office in Ireland: Policy Design as a Countermeasure', in Economic and Social Research Institute, *Quarterly Economic Commentary* (2003), www.esri.ie/pdf/QEC1003SA_McCarthy.pdf

Justice Frederick R. Morris, *Report of the Tribunal of Inquiry set up pursuant to the Tribunal of Inquiry (Evidence) Acts 1921–2002 into certain Gardaí in the Donegal division* (Dublin: Government Stationery Office, 2004), www.morristribunal.ie

Gary Murphy, 'Payments for No Political Response? Political Corruption and Tribunals of Inquiry in Ireland, 1991–2003', in John Garrard and James Newell (eds), *Scandals in Past and Contemporary Politics* (Manchester: Manchester University Press, 2005)

TI Ireland: www.transparency.ie

Notes

1. Dáil Debate 578, (2) 21 January 2004, Joan Burton, TD, debates.oireachtas.ie/Xml/29/DAL20040121.PDF
2. Minister for Justice, Equality and Law Reform, Michael McDowell, address at the Garda College Graduation Ceremony, Templemore, 28 April 2005, www.justice.ie/80256E01003A02CF/vWeb/pcJUSQ6BVKH8-ga
3. See *Global Corruption Report 2005*.
4. *Irish Times* (Ireland), 1 July 2004.
5. See *Global Corruption Report 2005* for details of the charges against him.
6. *Irish Times* (Ireland), 16 July 2004.
7. Professor Dermot Walsh, 'The Proposed Garda Síochána Ombudsman Commission: a Critique', *Irish Criminal Law Journal* 14(1), 2004.
8. Ibid.
9. *Irish Times* (Ireland), 6 August 2004.
10. *Irish Times* (Ireland), 22 March 2005.
11. *Irish Times* (Ireland), 25 April 2005.
12. The Irish Financial Services Regulatory Authority Interim Report (July 2004) and Final Report (December 2004) into the affairs of Allied Irish Bank (AIB); High Court Inspectors Report into the affairs of National Irish Bank Limited and National Irish Bank Financial Services Limited (July 2004).
13. *Irish Times* (Ireland), 31 July 2004.
14. www.ifsra.ie

Israel

Conventions:

UN Convention against Corruption (not yet signed)

UN Convention against Transnational Organized Crime (signed December 2000; not yet ratified)

Legal and institutional changes

- A Supreme Court ruling in November 2004 set a precedent for the interpretation of the offence of **breach of trust**.[1] In a special appeal, Shimon Sheves, a former director general in the Prime Minister's Office, was found guilty in two cases of using his position to promote the financial interests of friends. The case established norms for the behaviour of civil servants by prohibiting senior officials from involvement in serious conflicts of interest. It also placed breach of trust at the centre of efforts to combat corruption.

- In October 2004, the attorney general directed ministers and deputies in the Knesset not to promote the private interests of members of their party's central body or any other institution that helps choose their lists of candidates. This follows the regular appearance of instances of **conflicts of interest** where ministers have juggled their obligations as public servants with their vested interests of gaining party members' support. The directive also provides guidance for the conduct of ministers where conflicts of interest may arise.

- In March 2005, the ministerial committee on legislation approved a private bill that, if passed, would increase the range of '**trustee positions**' to extend to positions including the treasury accountant general, the director of capital markets, the anti-trust commissioner and the head of the National Security Council. This definition is currently limited to posts such as secretaries and director generals, and is taken by political practice in Israel as a licence to appoint non-professional and partisan members. If the bill is approved, some of the highest-ranking jobs in the civil service will be turned into political appointments (see below).

Money, elections and corruption

In February 2005, Attorney General Menachem Mazuz indicted Omri Sharon, son of Prime Minister Ariel Sharon and a member of the Knesset, for campaign finance violations during his father's campaign for the leadership of the Likud party in 1999 and, allegedly, the 2001 national elections.[2] The attorney general, however, stopped short of indicting the prime minister. According to the state comptroller, Ariel Sharon took illegal donations of NIS5.9 million (US $1.3 million) to enhance his chances of winning the 2001 national elections. The money was funnelled through a number of 'straw' companies, including a US corporation, Annex Research Ltd, founded by Sharon's lawyer, Dov Weisglass, and run by Omri Sharon.[3]

Sharon said the money was used to finance a campaign against Benjamin Netanyahu, a fellow Likud member, and not the former prime minister, Ehud Barak, whom he defeated in the 2001 election.[4] His lawyers argued that the Parties Law, which governs internal party campaigns, should be applied to the case, rather than the Party Financing Law, which relates to election campaigns between parties.[5] The importance of this is that a violation of Party Financing Law can

result in a prison sentence, while violating the Parties Law invokes only a monetary fine. The comptroller accepted Sharon's defence regarding the lion's share of the donation, but insisted that 20 per cent of it, or NIS1.4 million (US $310,000), be charged against Likud.[6]

Sharon took steps to return the illegal contribution in October 2001 by borrowing NIS4.2 million (US $920,000) from the bank.[7] This led the attorney general to open an investigation in October 2001 that resulted in charges being brought against Omri Sharon for violating both the Parties Law and the penal code. However, in January 2002, when long-term family friend, South African businessman Cyril Kern, paid US $1.5 million into the account of his other son, Gilad Sharon, a second scandal erupted. While running the first investigation, the attorney general launched an investigation in January 2003 into the more serious suspicions that Kern did not have sufficient resources to raise such an amount, and may have only been a cover for another wealthy businessman with investments in Israel.[8] The investigation into the 'Cyril Kern affair' is still ongoing. The matter is complicated by the fact that the funds were transferred from Austria and South Africa, neither of which has a cooperative framework of investigation with Israel, while Gilad Sharon retains the right to silence.[9]

Although Israel's political and legal systems have relatively tight supervision over parliamentary election campaigns, intraparty contests are mired in inefficiency and influence peddling. Politicians can resort to illicit means – including at times violating the law – to win a favourable place on their party list in order to get into parliament at all.[10]

Politicisation of the civil service?

The private bill to confer 'trustee' status on a number of influential government posts, proposed by Likud deputies in March 2005, is part of a wider concern that the civil service is at risk of becoming more politicised. Public service in Israel has always been exploited for patronage to some extent.[11] The past three years, however, have seen the Likud central committee, a body of 2,500 delegates elected by party members, attain even greater influence over decision-making. The committee's power emanates from its responsibility to select party candidates for the Knesset, which arguably creates a dangerous influence on members once they are elected. The problem is made more acute by the size of Likud, by far the country's largest political group with more posts in government than any other. Although there have been minor cases of politicised appointments not connected to Likud,[12] this party is the most closely associated with the practice.

The growth in power of Likud's central committee provided the basis for a damning report by State Comptroller Eliezer Goldberg in August 2004 that examined Tzachi Hanegbi's use of public resources to appoint Likud central committee members and their relatives while serving as minister of environment in 2002.[13] Political appointments, some by Hanegbi and others at the order of the then director general of the environment ministry, Shmuel Hershkovitz, were found highly suspicious. Although Hanegbi defended himself by

arguing that his actions were in line with the ministry's 'norms', Goldberg rejected this saying that it was the minister's duty to stamp out unacceptable norms. According to the comptroller's report, methods used to appoint his cronies included appointing acting officials to positions that should have been filled through tenders; presenting single candidates for positions exempt from tenders; giving associates preference in external tenders; and increasing the number of jobs at the minister's and director general's bureaus. Falsification of information also occurred in order to tailor jobs for associates.

By the time the report was published, Hanegbi had moved to become Minister for Internal Security, thus becoming head of the police as well. Following Goldberg's report, Attorney General Menachem Mazuz ordered a criminal investigation against Hanegbi for breach of trust and electoral bribery. This investigation was under way at the time of writing. Hanegbi resigned in September 2004 following advice from Mazuz. He was replaced by Gideon Ezra, who received a warning from the attorney general for interfering with police investigations (see below).

String of defeats for law enforcement bodies

Although the law enforcement agencies have tried to tackle conflicts of interest within the civil service, they have been less active in confronting more complicated cases such as those involving allegations of grand corruption. A series of events in the past year suggest a clear reluctance to challenge potential abuses.

In June 2004, the newly appointed attorney general, Menachem Mazuz, decided to close a case involving bribery allegations in which Prime Minister Ariel Sharon was considered a major suspect. The 'Greek island affair' centred on allegations that Sharon and his son, Gilad, had accepted bribes from businessman David Appel between 1997 and 2003 in return for 'favours' from Sharon in his capacities as prime minister, foreign minister and minister of infrastructure.[14] The charges revolved around the alleged support of two of Appel's real estate ventures in return for political support for the Likud primary for the Knesset slate in February 1999 and the Likud leadership contest in December 1999.[15] Furthermore, Appel allegedly hired Gilad to help implement the island project, paying him hundreds of thousands of dollars as a means of getting to Sharon. Ariel Sharon was twice seen having dinner with officials supposedly for the purpose of supporting Appel's projects. Having written a draft indictment against Ariel Sharon before leaving office, ex-attorney general Edna Arbel held that the dinners were rewards for the payment of Gilad and the political support that Appel had given Sharon.[16] In other words, those meetings were part of quid pro quo relations between Sharon and Appel.

The new attorney general concluded that Appel had hired Gilad because he genuinely believed he was a good worker, adding that the fee was not disproportionate to those paid to others in the project. Concerning the allegation that Appel had bribed Ariel Sharon by helping him in the two election campaigns, Mazuz concluded that asking for support and promising support are all a part of politics that no one takes 'too seriously'. Mazuz rejected allegations that Sharon had intervened to save Appel's real estate ventures.

While reading out his decision, Mazuz reproached former state prosecutor Edna Arbel, who had recommended indicting the prime minister.[17] Mazuz's decision to close the case led to strong criticism by one of Israel's most respected legal experts, Professor Mordechai Kremnitzer, who added his name to a group manifesto that expressed 'shock and anxiety' at Mazuz's attack on the legal system.[18]

Another significant blow for the law enforcement system was the dismissal in November 2004 of the head of the Criminal Investigations Department, Moshe Mizrahi, a leading figure in the fight against corruption.[19] On the recommendations of Mazuz and a former attorney general, acting Minister of Internal Security Gideon Ezra reportedly discharged Mizrahi over his handling of an investigation in the late 1990s. Mizrahi had placed court-approved wiretaps on Knesset member Avigdor Lieberman when the police were investigating suspicions of Russian mafia activities.[20] Mizrahi was allegedly 'overly enthusiastic' about transcribing conversations that lacked substantive relevance to the investigation.[21] Although the then chief of police and the former state prosecutor recommended that Mizrahi receive only a departmental warning for his actions, he was dismissed. In direct contrast a few months later, Ezra asked the police to give special treatment to one of the Likud central committee's most powerful members, Uzi Cohen. In March 2005, the attorney general warned Ezra against interfering any further in police investigations, adding that this was all the more essential when a fellow Likud member was involved.[22]

Another case of the legal system being overshadowed by political figures was the prosecution of former public prosecutor Liora Glatt-Berkowitz for leaking information about the Cyril Kern inquiry (see above) to the *Ha'aretz* daily before the 2003 elections. Glatt-Berkowitz only received an eight-month suspended sentence and a NIS10,000 (US $2,200) fine in March 2005.[23]

The Greek island affair, Mizrahi's dismissal and the sentence on Glatt-Berkowitz seem to indicate that the law enforcement system is backing away from challenging the immunity of leading political figures.

Doron Navot (TI Israel)

Further reading

Daphne Barak-Erez, 'Judicial Review of Politics: the Israeli Case', *Journal of Law and Society* 29(4), Tel Aviv, 2002.

Menachem Hofnung, 'Fat Parties-Lean Candidates: Funding Israeli Internal Party Contests', in Asher Arian and Michal Shamir (eds), *The Elections in Israel* (New Brunswick, NJ, and London: Transactions Publications, 2005)

TI Israel: www.ti-israel.org

Notes

1. The offence of 'breach of trust', set out by legislation from 1977, establishes prohibitions on civil servants aimed at limiting conflicts of interest. But in its current form, it is too wide and poorly worded.
2. Attorney general's decision, in 'The primaries in the Likud (Annex Researches)', 17 February 2005. See www.justice.gov.il. The indictment was submitted to court on 28 August 2005, see: *Ha'aretz* (Israel), 29 August 2005.
3. State comptroller's report, 30 September 2001.
4. Ibid.
5. *Ha'aretz* (Israel), 21 November 2004.
6. According to the state comptroller's report on the 2001 elections: 'The prime minister, while head of the opposition, employed a team of advisors who were paid by overseas donors to advance his position and his public image ... His personal political activity is the activity of the party. The chairman of the party is also allowed to prepare for primaries, as long as they make the distinction clear between their activity and the activities of the party's own mechanisms. That distinction was not made in Sharon's case.'
7. *Ha'aretz* (Israel), 7 January 2003; BBC News (UK), 13 January 2003.
8. Attorney general, 'The Primaries in the Likud', article 1.
9. *Ha'aretz* (Israel), 11 December 2003.
10. See Menachem Hofnung, 'Fat Parties-Lean Candidates: Funding Israeli Internal Party Contests', in Asher Arian and Michal Shamir (eds), *The Elections in Israel 2003* (New Brunswick, NJ, and London: Transactions Publications, 2005).
11. For a description and analysis of the relations between partisan members and politicians and the civil service, see David Nachmias, 'Israel's Bureaucratic Elite: Social Structure and Patronage', *Public Administration Review* 51(5), 1991.
12. *Ha'aretz* (Israel), 18 April 2004, reported on Avigdor Lieberman's efforts to appoint a close associate as a director of the civil aviation service.
13. State comptroller, 'Auditing Report on Political Appointments and Inappropriate Appointments in the Environment Ministry', August 2004. In May 2005, the publication of yet another report by the State Comptroller led Attorney General Menachem Mazuz to order an investigation into suspicions that illegal appointments were made in the agriculture ministry.
14. Attorney general's report on the 'Greek island affair', published 15 June 2004.
15. Ibid.
16. Attorney general, 'Opinion on Prime Minister Ariel Sharon Issue', 28 March 2004.
17. *Ha'aretz* (Israel), 16 June 2004; BBC News (UK), 15 June 2004.
18. *Ha'aretz* (Israel), 1 August 2004.
19. *Ha'aretz* (Israel), 7 November 2003.
20. Attorney general, 'The Tapping Affair in National Unit to Investigate International Relations: Superintendent Moshe Mizrahi', 23 October 2003.
21. Ibid.
22. *Ha'aretz* (Israel), 15 March 2005.
23. *Ha'aretz* (Israel), 17 March 2005.

Japan

Conventions:
OECD Anti-Bribery Convention (ratified October 1998)
UN Convention against Corruption (signed December 2003; not yet ratified)
UN Convention against Transnational Organized Crime (signed December 2000; not yet ratified)

ADB-OECD Action Plan for Asia-Pacific (endorsed November 2001)

Legal and institutional changes

- Amendments to the **unfair competition prevention law**, the legislation that enforces the OECD Anti-Bribery Convention, came into effect in January 2005 and introduce a jurisdiction based on nationality to the offence of bribing foreign public officials. Two months later, the OECD published a review of the implementation of domestic legislation that found Japan has not demonstrated sufficient efforts to enforce the offence of bribing a foreign public official. It said it would carry out a further review in 2005.

- Although the Diet (parliament) approved the ratification of the UN Convention against Organized Crime in 2003, an implementing **bill to amend the penal code** and laws related to the prevention of transnational and IT crimes are still pending. The amendment would make it a criminal offence to conspire in organised crime and to bribe court witnesses; strengthen powers allowing the seizure of the proceeds of crime; and apply jurisdiction based on nationality under the penal code to some other offences, including bribing public officials. The bill is expected to clear the Diet in 2005.

- In March 2005, the government announced that the public interest discloser protection law, the **whistleblower protection legislation** enacted in 2004, will be enforced from April 2006. Besides the seven laws in the penal code already designated, 407 laws have been identified to which the whistleblower protection law is also to be applied. Those include the commercial code, the labour standard law, the anti-monopoly law, the unfair competition prevention law, and laws stipulating codes and ethics for professionals such as doctors and lawyers.

- The cabinet approved revisions in March 2005 to the **public service officials ethics code**, enacted in 1999. They include provisions prohibiting a public official from: accepting any fees for compilation or supervision of the publications funded or subsidised by the government; from accepting fees from publications of which more than half the issues are procured by the ministry or agency to which the official belongs; from knowingly receiving or enjoying the proprietary benefit that another official gained in violation of the ethics code; and from not reporting to the authorities when there is reasonable suspicion that a violation of the ethics code has taken place.

Social Insurance Agency in the eye of the corruption storm

With its rapidly greying population, reform to the national pension system is an increasingly sensitive issue in Japan as a diminishing number of younger workers struggles to carry the pensions load. Growing public concerns over a possible collapse in the existing system were compounded last year by a series of corruption and mismanagement scandals.

The Social Insurance Agency, which is affiliated with the Ministry of Health, Labour and Welfare, has been roundly criticised for wasting pension insurance contributions on the construction of staff accommodation, the payment of membership dues for a prefecture association and even the payment of golf course fees. Employees of the agency were also in the habit of receiving fees from private companies for compiling books and videos produced with government subsidies. An in-house investigation in October 2004 found that 1,475 officials of both the ministry and the agency had been paid ¥750 million (US $6.8 million) over five years for supervising the work. The vice-minister and other senior officials who received sums surrendered part of their salaries because they admitted their actions had undermined public trust, though they had not actually broken the law. The investigation further revealed that 1,500 agency employees, or 8 per cent of its total staff, had accessed other people's pension records – including the prime minister's – out of sheer curiosity.

In September 2004, a manager of the ministry responsible for pensions management and a company president were indicted for bribery in procuring cash registers, while two other senior ministry officials were disciplined for receiving dubious money from lawmakers amid a scandal involving the Japan Dental Association.

Public anger at this series of mini-scandals persuaded the government to consider overhauling the Social Insurance Agency as part of a broader programme for pensions reform. The problem is how to do this. In a recent blueprint, the government outlined a privatisation in the near future, but the ministry balked at anything so drastic. The most recent information suggests the government is likely to keep the agency as an independent public body, and not privatise it. Whatever is decided, pensions reform is an issue that will not go away.

¥100 million donation scandal of an LDP faction

In July 2004, a newspaper report revealed that a political faction led by former prime minister Ryutaro Hashimoto of the ruling LDP falsified its 2001 political accounts report, by failing to report a ¥100 million (US $900,000) donation from the Japan Dental Association (JDA). Allegedly, Hashimoto received the cheque from the JDA president at a meeting in a Tokyo restaurant in 2001 when other faction members, including LDP heavyweights Mikio Aoki and Hiromu Nonaka, were present.

After the disclosure was made, the faction admitted receiving the money and Hashimoto resigned as its head. The opposition DPJ filed a complaint against Hashimoto, Aoki and Nonaka with the Tokyo Prosecuting Office. The prosecuting authorities instead indicted the faction's treasurer and Kanezo Muraoka, a former LDP secretary general and MP, for violation of the political funds control law, but dropped all charges against the other three politicians for lack of evidence. Muraoka, who was the faction's deputy chairman at the time of the donation, said that he had been made a scapegoat by the other three who initially received immunity from the authorities. He pleaded innocent in court.

The Tokyo District Court sentenced the treasurer to a suspended 10-month prison term in December 2004. The opposition parties tried to bring the issue up in parliament by summoning Hashimoto and five others to answer questions about the 'cover up' in sworn testimony before the Diet, but the ruling coalition refused to do so.

This was not the end of the story, however. An independent watchdog panel, charged with reviewing prosecutors' decisions, concluded in January 2005 that they had indeed erred when they decided not to indict Hashimoto and his associates. They resumed their questioning of Hashimoto, Aoki and Nonaka in February 2005.

Traditional 'money politics' has always played an important role in the Japanese model of corrupt practices, and corporate control of politicians has been a recurring factor for years. In this case, the JDA had allegedly donated the money to Hashimoto's faction, because its membership had become increasingly worried about Koizumi's structural reform policies. More importantly, the government sets the level of fees for health services in Japan and the dentists were trying to have their fees raised by buying political influence.

The issue of political funding is sensitive. No party or politician follows the requirements of the political funds control laws attentively. Funds are given and taken in secret and the presence of 'black money' in political life means donors and recipients alike further their interests to the detriment of voters. There have been moves by political parties to reform political finance regulations in response to the scandal, by introducing limits on individual contributions, for example, but commentators suggest that this will do little if external accounting is not introduced and money is not required to be routed through accounts rather than in cash.

Changes have been promised in the political donation sphere, but few people expect much from a system where such problems are endemic, not only in the ruling Liberal Democratic Party but also in many ways in the major opposition party, the Democratic Party of Japan. The ruling Liberal Democratic Party together with its partner, the Komeito Party, has announced plans to introduce new reforms in response to the scandal, primarily limiting the maximum of such contributions to ¥50 million (US $423,000).

Even when political funding scandals erupt, 'small fry' are usually sacrificed for the 'big fish'. In 1991, when Hashimoto was finance minister, his privately funded secretary was involved in transacting an unsecured loan worth more than ¥1 billion (over US $9 million). When questioned, Hashimoto denied all knowledge and escaped without sanction. In the JDA scandal (referred to above), LDP treasurer and faction accountant, Toshiyuki Takigawa, and a former LDP cabinet secretary, Kanezo Muraoka, were accused, while Hashimoto, Aoki and Nonaka denied responsibility.

Osaka's secret allowances

In late 2004, Osaka city government announced it had paid secret retirement allowances and pensions to 20,000 retired employees at a cost of ¥30 billion (US $273 million) over the previous 11 years.[1] The city government also shouldered the life insurance premiums that each employee should have paid at a further cost of some ¥10 billion (US $87 million) over 22 years, and paid ¥130 million (US $1 million) in unjustified overtime for 20,000 other employees between April and October alone.[2]

Analysts said that the fact that the past five mayors of Osaka had won elections with the support of employee unions had helped such collusion take root. After a public and media furore, the city government set up a committee to review the payroll that led to an announcement in March that the city would abolish the special labour allowances and slash ¥16.2 billion (US $141 million) from the fiscal budget for 2005.

Osaka is not the only municipality that hung on to special allowances like these. A survey in 2005 revealed that 37 of the 47 prefectures and 13 city governments had similar practices, but nearly half had decided to abolish them by the end of fiscal 2004.

In a related development, a Kyodo News survey revealed that 23 prefecture administrations had used tax revenues to help employees and their family members pay medical expenses. The finding sparked criticism that local government employees have enjoyed subsidised health benefits while private sector employees have been compelled to pay more.

The central government is proceeding with a programme of decentralisation that will pass the financial burden and its management to local governments, and enforce better governance in the municipalities. It is also pressing ahead with a merger policy that reduced the number of municipalities from 3,200 in 1999 to 2,500 in March 2005, and is expected to further cut their number to 1,800 by 2007. Decentralisation will hopefully lead to trimmer central government and reduced opportunities of corruption.

Alongside the entrenched collusion between unions and city governments, another strand of local corruption exists, known as *dango*, that involves collusion between construction companies in a process of bid-rigging. *Dango* sometimes involves government collusion, whereby government officials leak inside information to bidders who set both the price and the name of the winner. *Dango* has become so endemic that it is close to standard operating procedure and completely defeats the purpose of competitive bidding. To demonstrate how endemic it has become, the Fair Trade Commission (FTC) investigated 5,000 contracts between 1999 and 2003 and found 370 rigged bids in sewage and construction, and implicated 113 companies in bid-rigging scandals. Authorities are taking important steps to reduce such practices.

In October 2004, a senior official in the Niigata municipal government was arrested for leaking the planned spending amounts for a sewage facility to a company to help it win the contract. Takayuki Yuki, a councillor in the urban development bureau who previously headed the sewage construction division, was accused of obstruction of a public tender under the anti-monopoly law. Tadashi Uchida, president of the Niigata-based MSG Uchida Construction, was arrested on the same charges. Information had been leaked through municipal officials. Yuki subsequently committed suicide.

Transparency International Japan

Further reading

Yuu Anekoji, *Corruption Investigation* (Tokyo: Kodansha, June 2003) [Japanese]
Masao Kato, *Confessions of Bid-rigging* (Tokyo: Saito-sha, 2005) [Japanese]
Kazuo Kawkami, *Corruption and Bribery* (Tokyo: Kodansha, September 2003) [Japanese]
Japan Fair Trade Commission, 'A Report on Bidding and Public Contracts in Local Governments', September 2004 [Japanese]
Shin'ichi Yoshida, *Documentary Evidence of Corruption in Local Authorities* (Tokyo: Asahi Shinbun-sha, 2004) [Japanese]

TI Japan: www.ti-j.org

Notes

1. *Asahi Shinbun* (Japan), 31 December 2004.
2. *Asahi Shinbun* (Japan), 31 December 2004.

Kazakhstan

Conventions:
UN Convention against Corruption (not yet signed)
UN Convention against Transnational Organized Crime (signed December 2000; not yet ratified)

ADB-OECD Action Plan for Asia-Pacific (endorsed May 2002)

Legal and institutional changes

- In April 2005, the president signed a **decree on measures to step up the fight against corruption** and to strengthen discipline in the activities of state bodies and officials. Disciplinary councils in all provinces will be restructured, and their work will be more accessible to the public. The finance police are due to present a national anti-corruption strategy for 2006–10 by the end of the third quarter of 2005. The decree also contains provisions aimed at achieving greater transparency in procurement and reducing government interference in business (see below).

- Since January 2005, responsibility for investigating 44 offences has been transferred to the **Agency for Fighting Economic Crime and Corruption**, an innovation intended to avoid duplication between law enforcement agencies. Among the crimes for which it is responsible are bribe-taking and other benefits connected to commercial activity, abuse of authority and smuggling. Thirty other crimes in the 'economic' category remain under the jurisdiction of the internal affairs ministry or the finance police. The transfer places the agency's activities under the president's office, leaving some concern over how it will fulfil its obligations of accountability to parliament. Civil society groups have made repeated recommendations on how to improve the agency's efficiency, including laws that guarantee it an independent budget and define more clearly its powers and goals.

- In November 2004, a presidential decree created a permanent **National Commission on Democracy and Civil Society**, a consultative body aimed at developing national dialogue, increasing the transparency of public bodies and engaging civil society in the decision-making process. The commission's membership includes the heads of all political parties, two deputies from both chambers of parliament and two representatives each from the office of the president and the government. It has held five sessions since November on reforming the judicial system, forming a national programme on the political system and strengthening the role of parliament. The commission involves representatives of civil society, such as TI Kazakhstan, in discussions with politicians and international organisations.

The Baikonur scandal

Local and international media uncovered several scandals involving senior officials in 2004–05, increasing pressure on government to address corruption within its ranks. Although the president signed an anti-corruption decree in April 2005, the new law will have little impact unless it is properly enforced.

One area of concern is public procurement. Despite a reasonably progressive law on procurement passed in May 2002, Kazakhstan has had serious problems in implementing it. This is due in part to the absence of oversight and monitoring of irregularities in contracting processes. In the words of Kairbek Suleimenov, a former internal affairs minister, 'after each tender,

it is confidently possible to lead everyone [involved] to court'.[1]

The alleged embezzlement of funds in an agreement between Russia and Kazakhstan over the use of the Baikonur space facility was a case in point. The case was particularly salient since it appeared to involve the head of the presidential administration, Imangali Tasmagambetov. In August 2004, two deputies from the Russian Federation Duma (parliament), Petr Rubezhanskii and Aleksei Guzanov, wrote to the Kazakh parliament enquiring about Russia's payments for rental of the Baikonur complex in the Kazakh steppes.[2] They described how Russia had provided the state railway concern, Kazakhstan Temir Zholy (KTZh), with a credit of US $65 million in 2003 to purchase equipment, instead of paying cash to rent Baikonur. KTZh awarded the tender to two companies based in Omsk, Russia, to supply it with equipment.[3] According to the deputies, these enterprises had inflated the US $19 million cost of the equipment by an extra US $46 million, and pocketed the difference. As a result, Kazakhstan lost US $46 million, while Russia lost US $13 million in taxes.[4]

In September 2004, Sergey Stepashin, chairman of Russia's audit chamber, announced a joint investigation of the deal in collaboration with the Kazakh audit chamber.[5] In the meantime, the Kazakh newspaper *Respublika* was conducting its own enquiry. In August, it revealed that the one person who could shed most light on the missing funds was Imangali Tasmagambetov, head of the presidential administration, who had been prime minister when the deal was struck, and had both signed the agreement and nominated KTZh as the preferred operator.[6] Moreover, Amangeldy Ermegiyaev, son of the vice-president of the ruling OTAN party, had supervised the tender commission, and Alexander Pavlov, the deputy prime minister, had monitored the execution of the deal. The officials who were allegedly linked to the Baikonur scandal denied any wrongdoing.[7]

In late September, the finance minister, Arman Dunaev, insisted that all the rental money had been paid into the national budget in January and February 2004. However, in February 2005, Omarkhan Oksikbayev, chairman of the Kazakh audit chamber, announced that the findings of the Russian audit chamber had been forwarded to the prosecutor general's office and the finance police. Oksikbayev confirmed that KTZh had used the credit to buy equipment in Russia at prices three times higher than the amount normally demanded by the manufacturers.[8]

Investigations were still continuing at the time of writing, but the situation has been complicated by the lack of coordination between law enforcement bodies and the fact that they often interfere with one another's work in high-profile cases. So far,

the public prosecutor's office has prevented the Agency for Fighting Economic Crime and Corruption from bringing charges against KTZh's executive director, Talgat Ermegiyaev.[9] Whatever the outcome, it is clear that public procurement has a long way to go in Kazakhstan before it can claim to be transparent. Contracting should be monitored by independent bodies, including civil society organisations.

Lack of transparency in the banking sector

Another trend over the past year has been a government tendency to manipulate the courts, regulatory agencies and the media to bring about the collapse of private banks that have 'stepped out of line'. These incidences became more frequent in the run-up to the parliamentary elections of September 2004.

Apart from the state-owned national bank, most banks in Kazakhstan are privately owned and include a range of merchant, investment and retail activities. Under current legislation, banks are allowed to finance political parties and many are controlled by enterprises with political affiliations. However, these loyalties are not always transparent. The names of the real owners are hidden behind figureheads or corporations and, although the Kazakh national bank itself is required by law to disclose the names of its proprietors, it is not required to make this information accessible to the public. One bank recently targeted by the government was Kazkommertsbank, founded in 1990 and the country's largest private bank. In an official press report in May 2004, presidential adviser Ermukhamet Ertysbayev accused Kazkommertsbank of becoming too closely affiliated with the opposition Ak Zhol party and denounced its chairman, Nurzhan Subkhanberdin, as a dangerous person, a rival of the president and a 'power broker'.[10] The latter denied he had provided either financial or political support to Ak Zhol, or any other party. Nonetheless, the tax committee in the finance ministry launched an exhaustive investigation into the bank's tax records, levying fines of US $30 million in June 2004.[11] The pro-presidential coalition of the Agrarian and Civic parties, in collaboration with the newspaper *Express-K*, argued that the politicisation of the bank's top managers and the subsequent persecution of the bank by the tax authorities had pushed it to the edge of bankruptcy, and called for the creation of a commission to protect private investors. However, the managers of Kazkommertsbank interpreted this media publicity as a coalition ruse to damage the bank's reputation and steal their business. The bank promptly took *Express-K* to court and won their case.[12]

At the same time, allegations that senior members of government misuse their positions to influence the management of banks are rife. One notable case concerned the head of the presidential administration, Imangali Tasmagambetov, and the Nauryz Bank Kazakhstan (NBK). According to NBK's chairman, Orazaly Yerzhanov, when Tasmagambetov was prime minister in 2002 he offered to participate in NBK's authorised capital with the sum of US $25 million, together with Yerlan Atamkulov, president of the state railway concern, KTZh. Yerzhanov agreed and US $10 million in cash was immediately transferred, with the expectation that the balance would be paid within 18 months. This did not happen because Tasmagambetov was unable to raise the remaining US $15 million. In March 2004, Tasmagambetov and his partner terminated the agreement and demanded their money back. When Yerzhanov refused, arguing such a large withdrawal would damage the bank, Tasmagambetov allegedly used his influence to set the public prosecutor's office and other state agencies on the bank chairman. Between March and June 2004, the public prosecutor's office investigated the NBK three times for financial irregularities.[13] In June 2004, an opposition MP publicised a letter that Yerzhanov had written to the president, begging protection from Tasmagambetov's arbitrariness.[14] Yerzhanov subsequently left the country.

The investigation of the bank by the Agency for Fighting Economic Crime and Corruption continued, while the compulsory liquidation of its assets was threatened. When the agency submitted NBK's tax records to the public prosecutor's office and the Internal Affairs Ministry, the ministry stayed the prosecution and the agency was told that the investigation was the responsibility of other law enforcement bodies, in contradiction to existing legislation on economic crimes. Then suddenly in January 2005, the Internal Affairs Ministry dropped the case against NBK.[15]

These cases show that the lack of transparency in the Kazakh banking system makes it difficult to monitor the links between commercial banks and political parties, or to rule out the possibility of abuse of such connections for private gain. What is clear, however, is that commercial banks must be seen to be close to the ruling party if they are to have any chance of operating successfully.

Sergey Zlotnikov (TI Kazakhstan)

Further reading

G. S. Maulenov, *Organised Crimes and Corruption* (Almaty: Interlegal Publishing House, 2001)

Transparency Kazakhstan, *Assessment of Corruption in the Field of Private Business of the Republic of Kazakhstan* (Almaty: Interlegal Publishing House, 2002)

Transparency Kazakhstan, *Problems and Prospects of the National Fund of the Republic of Kazakhstan* (Almaty: Interlegal Publishing House, 2004)

TI Kazakhstan: www.transparencykazakhstan.org

Notes

1. www.navi.kz/articles/?artid=4168
2. *Respublika* (Kazakhstan), 18 February 2005, www.kubhost.com/~kubkz/respublika.php?sid=8366
3. Report of Russia's audit chamber on the rental of Baikonur space complex, 20 January 2005, Ref. 01–66/05–1. See also www.rferl.org/reports/centralasia/2004/09/34-140904.asp
4. *Respublika* (Kazakhstan), 20 August 2005, www.kubhost.com/~kubkz/respublika.php?sid=6593
5. www.ach.gov.ru/bulletins/1999/8-10.php; www.rferl.org/reports/centralasia/2004/09/34-140904.asp
6. *Respublika* (Kazakhstan), 7 August 2004.
7. *Vremya* (Kazakhstan), 26 August 2004.
8. www.gazeta.kz/art.asp?aid=56271
9. *Express-K* (Kazakhstan), 29 March 2005, www.procuror.kz/rus/jscrpt/_center/_news_gprk/2005/14-04-05_11.htm
10. *Vremya* (Kazakhstan), 13 May 2004.
11. *Nezavisimaya gazeta* (Russia), 21 July 2004. See www.ng.ru/cis/2004-07-21/5_kazakhstan.html
12. *Express-K* (Kazakhstan), 14 September 2004, and news.kkb.kz/news/show.asp?no=152438
13. Kazkommertsbank press release, available at news.kkb.kz/news/show.asp?no=79746
14. www.eurasia.org.ru, 10 June 2004.
15. *Vremya* (Kazakhstan), 24 February 2005.

Kenya

Conventions:

AU Convention on Preventing and Combating Corruption (signed December 2003; not yet ratified)
UN Convention against Corruption (ratified December 2003)
UN Convention against Transnational Organized Crime (acceded June 2004)

Legal and institutional changes

- John Githongo, President Mwai Kibaki's **special adviser on governance and ethics, resigned** in February 2005. The Minister for Justice and Constitutional Affairs subsequently announced in April that the office would be scaled down because some of its functions were already being performed by the Kenya Anti-Corruption Commission (KACC), which became operational in February 2005.[1] Githongo's resignation and the diminution of his office could weaken the fight against corruption and may signal that corruption is no longer on the president's list of priorities (see below).

- In August 2004, parliament passed a law on **public procurement and disposal**. The law is aimed at establishing transparent and accountable procedures for procurement and the disposal of unserviceable, obsolete or surplus stores and equipment by public entities. It also proposes the establishment of a public procurement oversight authority.

- In June 2004, the Commission of Inquiry into Illegal and Irregular Allotment of Public Lands published a report on **illegal allocation of land under previous governments**. It recommended the need for a redress policy to ameliorate the crisis resulting from the illegal allocation of public land and, in particular, public utility land. The report further proposes the enactment of legislation to ensure that the revocation process is conducted effectively and to modify any existing obstructive provisions in Kenya's land laws. It also proposes the establishment of a land titles tribunal to review suspect cases. At the time of writing, however, very few of these recommendations had been implemented (see below).

Further setbacks to the fight against corruption

There is growing pessimism about the government's fight against corruption. Part of the problem lies in the government's lack of a coherent anti-corruption strategy and its inability to investigate and prosecute new cases of graft. As President Mwai Kibaki, who came to power in December 2002, has been unable to stamp his authority on the fragile National Rainbow Coalition (NARC), he has built new alliances, including some with members of the previous government who are suspected of corruption. This makes it risky for him to take drastic measures against corrupt political and administrative heavyweights, as it could take only a few arrests to make the entire coalition crumble. Indeed, the president's chief adviser on governance and ethics, John Githongo, resigned in February 2005, frustrated by new corruption networks and what was perceived as ineffectual support from the president. In February 2005, the US and German governments suspended millions of dollars of grants they had promised in support of anti-corruption programmes in the wake of Githongo's resignation and the government's failure to deal with known cases of corruption.[2] Other donors stated that they were reviewing their stance, but requested to see steps taken to combat new cases of corruption.[3] Also in February, the British High Commissioner, Edward Clay, announced he had presented a dossier to the authorities detailing alleged graft in 20 procurement contracts, and demanded a full and transparent investigation of them.[4]

This is only the latest in a series of setbacks. The president's main strategy in 2003 was to create new anti-corruption institutions and set up inquiries into past scandals. The new institutions have proved to be ineffectual, however, and inquiries inconclusive. For instance, a report by the Commission of Inquiry into Illegal and Irregular Allocation of Public Lands, presented to the president in June 2004, made sweeping recommendations, proposing changes to the law and demanding that illegally obtained land titles be revoked.[5] Grants of government land were widely abused under the former government. The Ministry of Lands has promised action, but little has been taken since the report's publication, except for the eviction of squatters, which critics see as a political move.[6]

The fate of the Public Officer Ethics Act is also indicative of the weakening fight against corruption. The 2003 law requires public officers to disclose their assets and eschew conflicts between private interests and public duty. But asset disclosures are confidential and inaccessible to the public. In the meantime, the fate of prominent political figures allegedly involved in the Goldenberg scandal, which is estimated to have cost Kenya more than US $600 million, has yet to be decided. These include former president Daniel arap Moi, the former vice-president and current education minister, George Saitoti, and the former finance minister and vice-president, Musalia Mudavadi.[7] In another high-profile case, known as the Anglo-Leasing scandal, six people were charged in February 2005,[8] including senior government officials, but no cabinet members resigned in the wake of the scandal.

Even where reforms have been attempted, as in the judiciary, they are incomplete. For example, tribunals set up in 2003 to investigate High Court and Court of Appeals judges suspended for corruption were halted in late 2004 by a spate of litigation by the judges concerned. This could make it harder to appoint such tribunals in future. In April 2005, the Kenyan branch of the International Commission of Jurists released a report on judicial independence and accountability. It pointed out that measures aimed at fighting corruption in the judiciary were not in accordance with international standards, noting in particular that publicising allegations of corruption against judges and magistrates before they had been notified themselves was deeply irregular. Concerns were also raised about the lack of transparency in disbanding the tribunals set up to investigate judges, and the subsequent creation of new tribunals.[9]

In September 2004, the commissioners of the Kenya Anti-Corruption Commission were appointed with Aaron Ringera, a prominent judge, as its director. While this could restore some public confidence, the KACC lacks the power to prosecute and its investigations depend on the diligence of Attorney General Amos Wako, who is embroiled in a scandal of his own. In July 2005 the High Court of Kenya asked President Kibaki to appoint a judicial tribunal to suspend Wako over alleged misconduct,[10] after the Law Society of Kenya filed a private case against him over allegations of abuse of office and failure to prosecute corruption cases. Wako used his powers to terminate the case, but the legality of this move – when he himself was the subject of the indictment – is before the Constitutional Court.

In the meantime, the alliance between civil society and the government is crumbling and key civic groups have pulled out of joint anti-corruption initiatives. In February 2005, the Child Rights Advocacy, the Documentation and Legal Centre, the Coalition on Violence Against Women, the International Commission of Jurists Kenya, the Kenya Human Rights Commission, the Centre for Minority Rights and Development, TI Kenya, the Federation of Women Lawyers, the National Council of NGOs and the Law Society of Kenya all suspended their participation in the Governance, Justice, Law and Order Sector reform programme, citing loss of faith in the government's commitment to anti-corruption reform. Earlier, representatives of the Federation of Women Lawyers, TI Kenya, *The Standard* newspaper and the Institute for Education in Democracy resigned from the National Anti-Corruption Steering Committee, the government–civil society body launched in May 2004 to lead a national anti-corruption campaign. Its executive director, Jane Kiragu, also resigned, saying the committee needed more logistical support than was available. In August 2005, while opening a meeting for anti-corruption officials in Nairobi,[11] Minister for Justice and Constitutional Affairs Kiraitu Murungi admitted that the NARC government's fight against corruption had lost momentum.

The prognosis for the future fight against corruption is not good. In December 2004, Transparency International published the Global Corruption Barometer 2004, which showed the persistence of corruption in Kenya and low levels of public confidence in the government's ability to deal with it. Some 36 per cent of Kenyans reported that they or their family members had paid a bribe in the past 12 months.[12] The police topped the list of the most corrupt institutions by scoring a figure of 4.3 on an index of 1 to 5. This appeared to correlate to rising levels of insecurity. Political parties, parliament and customs ranked next. Though 41 per cent of Kenyans thought that corruption would decrease, 55 per cent thought that it would stay the same (20 per cent) or increase (35 per cent). TI Kenya's 2005 Kenya Bribery Index paints a similarly gloomy picture. Incidences of corruption have fallen somewhat, but the average size has increased, particularly in dealings with the judiciary and police. More than 57 per cent of those surveyed believed that corruption in Kenya has remained the same.

Wachira Maina and Noelina Nabwire (TI Kenya)

Further Reading

Kivutha Kibwana et al., *Initiatives against Corruption in Kenya: Legal and Policy Interventions 1995–2001* (Nairobi: Claripress, 2001)
Report of the Task Force on Public Collections or 'Harambees' (Nairobi: Government Printer, 2003)

TI Kenya: www.tikenya.org

Notes

1. The directors of the KACC were appointed in September 2004 and its staff in February 2005; see *Global Corruption Report 2005*.
2. *The Standard* (Kenya), 8 February 2005.
3. *The Standard* (Kenya), 19 February 2005.
4. BBC News (UK), 3 February 2005.
5. *Report of the Commission of Inquiry into Illegal and Irregular Allocation of Public Land* (Nairobi: Government Printer, 2004).
6. *The Standard* (Kenya), 16 July 2005.
7. For more details, see *Global Corruption Report 2005*, and http://news.bbc.co.uk/2/hi/africa/4025375.stm
8. *Daily Nation* (Kenya), 17 February 2005.
9. International Commission of Jurists, *Kenya: Judicial Independence, Corruption and Reform*, April 2005, available at www.icj.org/IMG/pdf/kenyareport.pdf
10. *The People* (Kenya), 8 July 2005.
11. *Daily Nation* (Kenya), 10 August 2005.
12. The fieldwork for the Global Corruption Barometer 2004 was conducted between July and September 2004.

Kuwait

Conventions:
UN Convention against Corruption (signed December 2003; not yet ratified)
UN Convention against Transnational Organized Crime (signed December 2000; not yet ratified)

Legal and institutional changes

- In October 2004, the Council of Ministers merged its economic and legal standing sub-committees to address the **issue of corruption within the public sector**. These sub-committees had not previously been delegated with the task of dealing with corruption. However, since corruption had become an important government issue, it was deemed prudent to merge the two committees in order to draw from a wider pool of expertise on corruption-related issues.

- In January 2005, the Council of Ministers set up four working groups in accordance with the joint economic and legal committee's recommendations. The groups will submit a report to the Council by the end of 2005 and will be responsible for: examining measures to standardise **internal government procedures**; putting in place guidelines for procedures for the provision of government services; outlining specific standards for the appointment of senior government officials; and monitoring the progress of e-government efforts. Once this has been done, the Council will focus its attention on creating an independent administrative overview body and/or enhancing the role of the Citizens Services and Governmental Bodies Assessment Agency.[1]

- The government brought in the Infocomm Development Authority of Singapore (IDA) in September 2004 to integrate its different information systems and create a **blueprint for e-government** by June 2005. Current e-government schemes include an On-line Directory of Services that specifies the documents and timeframe required for the delivery of certain government services. The municipality has also established a website detailing its services, as well as publishing building regulations and other information.[2]

- The Council of Ministers set up a committee within the Finance Ministry in December 2004 with responsibility for drawing up a **code of conduct for dealing with unsolicited offers**. Public land is scarce and expensive in Kuwait, leading to a situation in which private sector representatives approach officials with proposals for projects in return for access to public land (referred to as 'unsolicited offers').

- Serving judges will no longer be allowed to act as government advisers due to potential **conflicts of interest**, following a Council of Ministers resolution in February 2005.[3]

- In March 2005, the National Assembly passed the **municipality reform law**, which separates the elected municipal council from the administrative institutions, thereby reducing the influence of individuals in one branch over those in the other. An added check includes the appointment of a new minister to oversee the municipal sector. The law also states that the central plan has to be approved by Emiri decree, rather than the municipality, making it harder for corrupt officials to manipulate.

Corruption no longer taboo

The dichotomy between a critical private space in Kuwaiti society and a stagnant public one is still in the process of being reconciled. One indication of this is the government's long overdue recognition of the problem of corruption, which previously was only discussed openly by individuals and in the private media.

In October 2004, Prime Minister Sheikh Sabah al-Ahmad al-Jabir al-Sabah highlighted that corruption had become a key issue on his government's political agenda.[4] Speaking to the press one month earlier, he criticised the municipal sector, saying incidents of corruption there seemed to outnumber those in all the other sectors combined. These comments should not be viewed as isolated blips on the political radar, but as part of a trend in increasing transparency that became particularly evident last year.

For example, the respected daily *Al-Qabas* published a 'secret' report by the Citizens Services and Governmental Bodies Assess-

ment Agency (C2G) in December 2004.[5] The Council of Ministers, in consultation with the World Bank, had tasked the C2G with reporting on administrative corruption in the public sector and formulating a strategy to combat the phenomenon. The report listed the most common types of corruption, such as bribery and favouritism, and highlighted the government sectors most vulnerable, notably public contracts and procurement. It also identified the following deficiencies in the administrative framework: lack of accountability by leaders and politicians; absence of a code of conduct and a work ethic; absence of deterrents for violators; lack of meritocracy in appointments and hiring; and poor scrutiny of managers and officials. It concluded that 'Political corruption lies at the heart of corruption.'[6]

One peculiarity of Kuwait is that, although there are bodies for monitoring financial and criminal accountability, no real watchdog agency exists to ensure administrative accountability. The C2G was established with this mandate in mind, but its capabilities are inadequate. Not only does it lack institutionalised mechanisms, it has no authority to seize documents or question witnesses without prior consent. The only weapon in the agency's arsenal is its proximity to the office of the prime minister, and its ability to report (and blacklist) uncooperative officials or departments directly. The government is currently weighing the benefits of either a new investigative body for the administrative sector, or giving the C2G greater powers to deter corruption.

After a fact-finding trip to South East Asia in July 2004, the authorities have taken other initiatives to improve transparency, in addition to the blueprint for e-government outlined above. In December 2004, the Council of Ministers set up a committee within the finance ministry to formulate a code of conduct, to deal with BOTs (build, operate and transfer) and unsolicited offers. From January 2005, the C2G began working with the Criminal Investigation Department to establish an anti-corruption police unit.

One illustration of the government's changed response to administrative corruption involved an embezzlement conspiracy at the Ministry of Public Works that came to light in the summer of 2004, when the press published allegations that six employees had been drawing illicit amounts of KD30,000 (around US $100,000) a month from the budget since 1995. The Public Prosecutor's Office subsequently discovered that the network was far more widespread and targeted 35 staff, including senior managers, for investigation. The scam involved the transfer of salaries to other staff above their actual level and requests for the return of the difference, which was then pocketed by the fraudsters. Two of the defendants were sentenced to 10-year prison terms in April 2005. As a result of the case, the government has introduced an electronic system whereby salaries are transferred directly to employees' accounts.

It is essential to understand that it is the Kuwaiti state itself which generates the incentives determining the supply and demand for corruption. The public sector employs an astonishing 94 per cent of the labour force, spans 54 institutions and provides around 3,000 services. An all-inclusive 'cradle-to-grave' welfare system has created unparalleled dependence, while sprawling bureaucracies and excessive regulations give officials a monopoly over a wide range of activities. Streamlining the administration would limit officials' discretionary powers and their ability to seek favours in return for speeding up bureaucratic procedures.

At the crux of the government's dilemma is its concern that reducing corruption would also shrink the functions of state. If it is to fight corruption in earnest, the authorities must be willing to accept this transformation.

Blame without accountability?

Kuwait has a long tradition of civic participation due to the formula of 'joint governing' established at an early stage of development when the al-Sabah family was 'chosen to rule' by other leading families, rather than taking power by force. The *diwaniyas*, or salons, where men gather to talk politics in the evenings, are a vivid illustration of the public's interest in politics. The press is private and does not shy away from contention. Indeed, at first glance, sufficient constitutional guarantees and mechanisms seem to exist to ensure accountability. The Audit Bureau is an independent agency with responsibility for monitoring spending in all ministries and government agencies. A permanent parliamentary committee is charged with the protection of public funds and MPs can question ministers over improprieties, and have them removed when necessary.

However, the critical observer is more likely to see these customs and committees as window dressing, rather than genuine tools of accountability. A recent study of parliamentary investigative committees by Khaldun al-Naqeeb and Ali al-Zuabi of Kuwait University indicated that, despite the sharp rise in the number of committees set up in the 1990s, MPs failed to achieve any decisive achievements with regard to official corruption.[7] Several parliamentary investigations led to dissolution of the legislature to prevent further government scandals being revealed.[8]

Failure to achieve real accountability reflects the fundamental flaws in the political system. Opposition parties are banned, leaving a series of semi-nebulous, shifting factions confined to opposing the government on specific issues, but lacking the continuity or ability to formulate policy alternatives, let alone form a government. This weakness is compounded by the executive's right to dissolve parliament, which makes MPs wary of overstepping the boundaries. Many citizens are dissatisfied with parliamentary interpellations, which they perceive as a tool to bludgeon ministers into acquiescing to questionable patronage, to enhance MPs' popularity or to bully members of opposition factions.

There is also the matter of MPs' accountability, which is achieved at the ballot box in most democracies. The Kuwaiti democratic process is unrepresentative due to the narrowness of its electoral base, and is marred by pervasive vote buying. According to Ghanim al-Najjar, 'the narrow electoral base has created a situation where only 14 per cent participate'. This is due to the law excluding members of the security services, the under-21s and, until 16 May 2005, women.[9] Following that momentous parliamentary session, which granted women the right to vote and run for elections, the voter base will expand to 35 per cent of the population.[10]

The other contentious electoral reform issue that has received significant attention this year involves replacing the current 25 voting districts with 10, as was the case prior to the 1981 Election Law, when the government redrew electoral boundaries according to demographic characteristics that would be in its favour. Proponents of the reform say it would reduce the propensity for corruption and vote-buying, as well as diminishing the scope for reliance on ethnic and personal connections, since candidates would need to appeal to broader coalitions and formulate more ideological platforms across larger districts. The enfranchisement of women could compound this effect by increasing the number of potential voters, as well as further institutionalising the process of political campaigning, since candidates would need to address more formal and open associations to get their message across, rather than resort to the more closed system of addressing male-dominated *diwaniyas*. Increasing constituency sizes could come against resistance from the government, if it believes that such a move would dilute its influence over the Assembly. Others postulate that changing constituencies in such a way would make the government the only credible buyer of votes. Thus rather than reducing the level of corruption, it would merely change its distribution. These issues are still being debated.

The issue of MPs' legitimacy is not helped by lack of transparency in the financing of their electoral campaigns, nor are there laws or restrictions on MPs receiving 'gifts'.[11] Parliamentarians also benefit from immunity, perpetuating the myth that they are above the law. A mechanism exists to strip MPs of their immunity in cases of criminal wrong-doing, but it requires a request from the attorney general to parliament, followed by a majority vote in the chamber.

Nor are there any clear means for ordinary citizens to monitor the state's provision of public services. This is due partly to the absence of laws ensuring access to information by which to measure performance. Another deterrent to more effective auditing is the difficulty in registering new NGOs and civil society organisations, since the Law of Public Benefit Societies gives the government complete discretion to grant, license, ban and regulate any such associations.

Kuwait Economic Society

Further reading

Michael Herb, 'Princes and Parliaments in the Arab World', *Middle East Journal* 58(3), Summer 2004 (Washington, DC: Middle East Institute, 2004)

Mary Ann Tetreault, *Stories of Democracy. Politics and Society in Contemporary Kuwait* (New York: Columbia University Press, 2000)

Kuwait Economic Society: www.economic-society.org

Notes

1. The Citizens Services and Governmental Bodies Assessment Agency was established in October 2002. Its mandate is to evaluate the performance of government bodies in providing public services and in complying with 'the general policy of the state according to the government work programme'.
2. See baladia.gov.kw, c2g.gov.kw, csc.net.kw and www.moi.gov.kw
3. *Al-Watan* (Kuwait), 1 March 2005.
4. Prime minister's speech on 23 October 2004.
5. *Al-Qabas* (Kuwait), 29 November–4 December 2004. The report was secret since the study had been requested by the Council of Ministers and all documents and proceedings within the council are confidential under the constitution.
6. Ibid.
7. Khaldun al-Naqeeb and Ali al-Zuabi, 'The Role of National Assembly in Combating Corruption', *Hewar al-Arab Journal*, 10 September 2005. This analysis of parliamentary investigative committees has rendered disappointing results: of the 38 committees established since 1963, only three cases have been sent to the attorney general, with the rest being ignored or failing to produce any tangible results. There has been a consistent lack of parliamentary follow-up of these cases, and the government has missed opportunities to correct alleged deficiencies or use these instances as momentum for reform.
8. Some of the cases investigated involved the embezzlement of public funds, arms procurement and military contracts, and the misuse of public authority and power.
9. Ghanim al-Najjar, 'The Challenges Facing Kuwaiti Democracy', *Middle East Journal* 54(2), Spring 2000.
10. *Al-Shall Report* (Kuwait) 15(20–1), May 2005.
11. C2G Report, *Al-Qabas* (Kuwait), 29 November–4 December 2004.

Kyrgyzstan

Conventions:
UN Convention against Corruption (signed December 2003; not yet ratified)
UN Convention against Transnational Organized Crime (ratified October 2003)

ADB-OECD Action Plan for Asia-Pacific (endorsed November 2001)

Legal and institutional changes

- Following the overthrow of President Askar Akayev in March 2005, the new government was quick to commit itself to a renewed fight against corruption, having witnessed the role it had played in fuelling the revolution that unseated the former president. In May, the government announced the creation of an **anti-corruption centre** in the mayoralty of Bishkek. Provisionally, it provides for the creation of a monitoring agency, composed of civil society organisations, with oversight for the institutions of local government, including public works and services delivery.

- In August 2004, parliament adopted Law 108 concerning the **income and property declarations of politicians**, their close relatives and the sources of their earnings. Under the law, politicians and senior administrators, including ministers, must publish information on their incomes annually in the media. Though intended to create greater openness about wealth at the highest levels of power, the law establishes no complementary agency to verify whether the income and property declarations are factually accurate. In the event, President Akayev declared his income as US $300 per month and other officials followed with equally dubious claims (see below).

- In August 2004, parliament adopted a law to **regulate and modernise the civil service**. More progressive than the law it replaces, Law 114 contains a number of anti-corruption measures. For the first time, civil servants can be temporarily suspended from duties that present a conflict of interest and managers can exercise increased control in such cases. Regulations concerning the declaration of income by public officials have also been amended. Under Law 114, the civil service affairs agency must ensure access to the income and property declarations of officials, and in some cases their close relatives, by publishing the information in the official gazette and on the Internet. Legal procedures exist to ensure that civil society and media can appeal against anyone who refuses to comply with this regulation. Law 114 also includes provisions for a new state service agency to develop a unified policy on the civil service. The tasks of the agency, established by presidential decrees in September and October 2004, are to secure the stable succession and independence of the civil service; attract qualified staff; increase management effectiveness; participate in the process of improving legislation on government service; create a system of transparency of incomes of government officials and other officers of state bodies; and to protect the rights and legal interests of government officials.

Tulip revolution gains second wind

The year of 2005 will be remembered as the year of the 'tulip revolution' in Kyrgyzstan, when a wave of protests swept away the authoritarian regime of President Askar Akayev after 14 years in power. Government manipulation of the parliamentary elections in February and March was the final straw that sparked the 2005 uprising that was already brewing, due to a combination of the pervasive poverty, corruption and concentration of wealth in the hands of few that had characterised Akayev's time in office. Four weeks after the first show of resistance in the southern city of Jalalabad, on 24 March, thousands of demonstrators stormed the White House, the seat of the presidential administration in Bishkek. Akayev fled the city to Moscow where members of his family later joined him. He

formally resigned on 4 April, apparently assured that he would enjoy the immunity granted under the constitution, but the acting chief prosecutor, Azimbek Beknazarov, denied this was the case since Akayev had fled the country. A formal resignation was needed to pave the way for new presidential elections in July 2005.

One of the Bishkek protesters' first objectives was to free Felix Kulov, who used to head the Ministry of Interior and was the leader of the opposition Ar-Namys (Dignity) Party. Kulov, a northerner, was imprisoned in 2000 before the presidential election campaign of that year on charges of alleged corruption and abuse of power. Although subsequently released for a few months, he was given a 10-year prison sentence in 2001. In the aftermath of the initial protests, Kulov was asked to take charge in Bishkek where there was widespread looting, but he held the post only for a week, telling a Western NGO he 'would not work with the new authorities'.[1] In the meantime, a second potential crisis emerged as both the incumbent and newly elected legislatures vied for legitimacy. On 26 March, the incoming assembly appointed Kurmanbek Bakiev acting president and prime minister. President Bakiev, an economist from the south, was prime minister from 2000 to May 2002, when he resigned after the police shot and killed six demonstrators in the district of Aksy. In April, a special working group of the Supreme Court exonerated Felix Kulov of all charges of corruption, effectively clearing the way for his own bid for the presidency.[2]

In spite of the colourful way they came back into the limelight, President Bakiev and Kulov held positions in Akayev's previous administrations and are veterans at manipulating the north–south divide that plays such an important role in political life. Considerably weaker in the south, the cradle of the revolution, Akayev had also lost popularity in the north since the crackdown in 2002. With Kulov sidelined, however, the opportunity to form a north–south coalition of all opposition forces was lost. President Bakiev and other new leaders began to appoint friends, family and clan members, many from the south, and former or incumbent ministers to high office, essentially repeating the pattern followed by Akayev.[3] 'The chaos in the appointments process has undermined the image of Bakiev', said one NGO leader in Bishkek. 'Who has come to power? The old Communist Party *nomenklatura*, the Akayev *nomenklatura*, and those who participated in the storming of the White House.'[4]

While President Bakiev clearly needed to fill the void left by Akayev's sudden departure, the euphoria generated by the 'tulip revolution' evaporated and ministries became paralysed by what one analyst called 'a wild scramble for power'.[5] The appointment of Tashtemir Aitbaev, a former KGB officer and Akayev stalwart, as head of the National Security Service, disconcerted the International Crisis Group among other civil society actors, who had hoped for a sign of a softer position on human rights. But it was the case of the finance minister Akylbek Japarov that drew most protest. A letter to a local newspaper from a 'group of businessmen' alleged rampant corruption in the ministry as Japarov appointed relatives to key posts in the tax and customs services, and employed members of the financial police as his personal bodyguard.[6]

Similar incidents have occurred in state companies and local governments in different parts of the country, dispelling any hope that the legal and institutional apparatus created to combat Akayev-era corruption would be deployed in the Bakiev presidency very soon. Another trend in the post-revolutionary period has been a series of land seizures in Bishkek by some 30,000 people who began building homes or selling the property despite lacking title deeds.[7]

These political and social tensions appeared set to erupt at a replay of the spring presidential elections, which had been so tainted by the exclusion of candidates, vote-buying, infringements on press freedom and the falsification of results that they sparked a revolution. However, in May 2005, President Bakiev and Felix Kulov unexpectedly announced a coalition agreement that effectively removed the prospect of a more critical north–south rift in the near future. Bakiev would stand for president under the deal and, if he won, appoint Kulov prime minister, but with greatly expanded powers. Indeed, with Akayev stripped of his political rights, the Bakiev–Kulov team won a relatively clean sweep in July 2005.

The first priorities of the post-election presidency will be to regain control of the country; adapt the constitution to accommodate the prime minister's enhanced role; and reshuffle the cabinet and other senior appointments in accordance with the coalition's requirements. With Kulov's support, President Bakiev has an opportunity to begin the process of change required to dismantle the Akayev system and to implement the backlog of anti-corruption legislation that has been sitting largely unused on the statute book. It remains to be seen, however, how long the Bakiev–Kulov alliance will remain intact.

The Akayev investigation

Former president Askar Akayev's last declaration of assets before he was overthrown included a four-room apartment in Bishkek, an old Mercedes and a modest *dacha* in Moscow. A commission set up in April 2005 to investigate the business interests of the ex-president and members of his family is examining an extensive list of properties. These range from newspapers, radio stations and supermarkets, to hotels, banks, an airport and the country's largest mobile telephone company, BiTel, worth an estimated US $250 million.[8] Unravelling the complex web of ownership surrounding these companies has been difficult, the deputy prime minister and commission chairman Daniyar Usenov admitted. The founders of BiTel were three offshore companies registered in the Isle of Man. The founders of those were two companies registered in the Seychelles, and the founders of those are two Liberian companies. 'According to our information,' he said, 'the founders of those companies are, in turn, the Akayev family on the one hand, and [BiTel's] management … on the other.' Other companies have been tracked back to shell companies in Cyprus, the Cayman Islands, Liechtenstein, Panama, Turkey and Germany. Establishing the link between the Akayev family and these alleged business interests, however, may be impossible.[9] Though stripped of his privileges by an act of parliament, Akayev has yet to face prosecution.

Less than 10 days after it was created, the commission announced a 'tentative' list of 42 companies to be investigated for links to the Akayev family. A further 31 companies were added to the original list within days and, by late May 2005, 136 other companies had been added to the original list. The commission is also investigating 'money transfer schemes through offshore zones, schemes for skimming from the budget, and from such enterprises as the Kumtor [gold mine]'. A further 48 companies are under investigation for making arrangements with the tax inspectorate to avoid paying taxes. Usenov suggested that Manas International Service, an aircraft fuel supplier allegedly owned by Aydar Askayev, the president's son, had posted sales of US $30 million a year, but profits of 'only a few thousand dollars'.[10] 'If one calculates the damage done to the country from illegal privatisation, tax avoidance, non-payment of duties, illegal seizure of business from businessmen, in all areas,' Usenov – himself a businessman – said, 'I would assess this at billions of soms.'[11]

The acting general prosecutor Azimbek Beknazarov announced in June that the government had agreed to pay a Vienna-based legal firm US $500,000 and 5 per cent of any monies returned to pursue an out-of-country investigation, because Kyrgyz investigators were not licensed to operate abroad.[12] Earlier in the investigation, the commission sent formal requests to Interpol and the fiscal authorities in the United States and the UK for information about the ex-president's bank accounts.

Although the authorities have launched nearly 120 criminal cases against companies connected with the Akayevs and their circle, not a single one has directly named the former president. In response, he has accused Usenov of exacting vengeance on a former political adversary and launched a defamation case through a Russian lawyer.[13] During a press interview in April 2005 about the tax evasion schemes businessmen used while Akayev was in power, Usenov stressed future compliance rather than past wrongdoing. 'We're not asking about what happened yesterday', he said. 'Otherwise we'll have to put half the country in jail.'[14]

Aigul Akmatjanova (TI Kyrgyzstan)

Notes

1. International Crisis Group, www.crisisgroup.org/home/index.cfm?id=3411&CFID=6511543 &CFTOKEN=86901627
2. http://eurasianet.org/departments/business/articles/pp050505_pr.shtml
3. http://eurasianet.org/departments/insight/articles/eav040805a.shtml
4. International Crisis Group, 'Kyrgyzstan: After the Revolution', 4 May 2005, available at www. crisisgroup.org/library/documents/asia/central_asia/097_kyrgyzstan_after_the_revolution. pdf
5. http://eurasianet.org/departments/insight/articles/eav040805a.shtml
6. *MSN* (Kyrgyzstan), 5 April 2005.
7. http://eurasianet.org/departments/insight/articles/eav040805a_shtml
8. http://eurasianet.org/departments/business/articles/pp050505.shtml
9. http://eurasianet.org/departments/business/articles/pp050505_pr.shtml
10. Ibid.
11. www.iwpr.net/index.pl?archive/rca2/rca2_383_1_eng.txt
12. Ibid.
13. Ibid.
14. http://eurasianet.org/departments/business/articles/pp050505_pr.shtml

Malaysia

Conventions:

UN Convention against Corruption (signed December 2003; not yet ratified)
UN Convention against Transnational Organized Crime (ratified September 2004)

ADB-OECD Action Plan for Asia-Pacific (endorsed November 2001)

Legal and institutional changes

- The Central Bank introduced **two public complaints and redress forums** in 2005. The Financial Mediation Bureau (FMB), launched in January, is an integrated dispute resolution centre for financial institutions. The FMB's predecessors, the Banking Mediation Bureau and the Insurance Mediation Bureau, handled a total of 1,515 cases in 2004. The FMB provides an avenue of redress for a wider spectrum of the public since it covers the consumer areas of Islamic insurance, development finance institutions, as well as non-bank issuers of credit and charge cards. In February, the Central Bank set up a website, LINK, to facilitate a rapid response to the public, as well as small and medium enterprises, on matters related to the financial sector. LINK also has the potential to encourage internal and external whistleblowers to disclose corruption in the financial sector.

- In December 2004, the Treasury issued **new guidelines for public procurement** on infrastructure maintenance projects that outline the selection process for contractors, the use of open tenders and the participation of a broader group of public officials to ensure transparency. Though the guidelines cover one area of public procurement only, they apply to all departments of government (see below).

- The **Anti-Corruption Academy**, first announced in December 2003, is expected to become operational in September 2005. Its main role is to train officials of the domestic Anti-Corruption Agency, but it will function as a regional centre for anti-corruption capacity building, promoting best practice in investigation, monitoring and enforcement, as well as forensic accounting and engineering (see below).

- A number of civil society organisations, including TI Malaysia, formed a lobbying group in October 2004, Infokl, to press for **greater freedom of information**. Housed at the Centre for Independent Journalism, Infokl will draft a freedom of information bill, including provisions for whistleblowers, for submission to government. It will also call for a review of the Official Secrets Act, which inhibits comment on many public sector activities.

The government's anti-corruption campaign

The fight against corruption has been the centre piece of Prime Minister Abdullah Badawi's government since it came to power in October 2003. The campaign has focused on prevention, including the formation of the National Integrity Plan (NIP), the Integrity Institute of Malaysia (IIM) and the Anti-Corruption Academy, but it has punitive aspects as well. It is too early to assess the real impact of the campaign but the signs are encouraging.

In April 2005, the government announced that the IIM would develop a National Integrity Index (NII), to assess progress in areas including corporate governance. The IIM was established in April 2004 to implement an NIP for 2004–08, aimed at reducing corruption and abuse of power, mainly through education and training. Since its inception, the IIM has conducted numerous courses on integrity for the private and public sectors, and in universities and schools.

The Anti-Corruption Academy, which is expected to open its doors in September 2005, is the first of its kind in the Asia-Pacific region. Established by the Anti-Corruption Agency (ACA) to train anti-corruption officials in Malaysia and from across the region, the academy will function as a centre for anti-corruption capacity building, promoting best practices in investigation, monitoring and enforcement, and in newer areas such as forensic accounting and engineering. Although it has yet to begin operations, it has been welcomed by the Asian Development Bank and the Organisation for Economic Co-operation and Development.

Meanwhile, the ACA stepped up enforcement of the Anti-Corruption Act with a 47 per cent increase in corruption-related arrests in 2004, compared to 2003, and 179 new cases registered for trial.[1] Among those charged in 2004 were the former land and cooperative development minister, Kasitah Gadam, and Eric Chia Eng Hock, a businessman closely associated with former prime minister, Mahathir Mohamad, who retired in October 2003 after 22 years in office. The charges were remarkable since the agency had been criticised for targeting only 'small fish', with some observers blaming this on the lack of independence of the attorney general, who held the final decision to prosecute.[2] Other anti-corruption laws have not been enforced so effectively. The first prosecution under the Anti-Money Laundering Act of 2001 was only initiated in 2004, but a spate of prosecutions is expected in the near future.[3]

Despite this, there is continuing concern about the ACA's independence. It forms part of the prime minister's office and, though the king appoints the director general, he does so on the prime minister's advice. This does not necessarily translate into executive interference with its investigations, but the former prime minister did remove ACA director general Datuk Ahmad Zaki in March 2001, in spite of his diligence and record of effectiveness.

Another aspect of the government's strategy has been to limit the opportunities for corruption by improving public service delivery. To this end, an internal circular in November 2004 repealed the 1979 auditing system, setting out new objectives, functions and responsibilities. The new auditing regime will be responsible for all monetary and financial transactions, including verifying all the expenditure, profits, assets and stock managed.

In January 2004, the Public Complaints Bureau (PCB), which many had criticised for the complexity of its procedures, launched the MESRA Rakyat programme whereby it tours the country to listen to local complaints. Heads of government departments are also present at these meet-the-people sessions. At a session in Melaka state in July 2004, 278 citizens met 49 heads of department and raised over 40 issues. The officer in charge reported that of the 40 cases brought up, 37 had been settled, while three were pending. All cases relating to corruption are referred to the ACA for further investigation. The PCB plans to monitor these investigations to ensure that action has been taken.

Procurement policies on the mend

In November 2004, a local newspaper published a front-page story on defective buildings and roads that had cost the taxpayer an estimated MYR2 billion (US $500 million).[4] The response of the public works minister was that the fiasco was not the fault of his department, but of a group of contractors known as Project Management Consultants (PMC), set up in the 1990s and registered with the finance ministry.

PMC comprises several contractors who were awarded projects through direct negotiation, circumventing procurement regulations. A treasury circular in September 2000 sanctioned privileged consortia to cover five regions and exempted government departments from normal procurement procedures.[5] This allowed agencies to implement their own projects through limited tenders or direct negotiations. The usual procedure had been to go through the public works department and, only if the latter were unable to take on the contract, could other contractors be selected. The justification for the new procedure was speedier completion of projects,[6] but the cost doubled in some cases and the construction was seriously flawed. With a consultancy fee fixed at 1.5 per cent of a project's cost,

the PMC concept contributed to massive overruns and individual project failures.[7]

For example, the health ministry was forced to close the MYR500 million (US $133 million) Sultan Ismail Hospital on 27 September 2004 due to structural and design flaws. Repairs to bring it up to safety standards were estimated at MYR8 million (US $2 million).[8] Work on the MYR167 million (US $44 million) Malaysian External Trade Development Corporation tower, due to have been completed in 1997, was not finished until mid-2005 and the costs rocketed to MYR400 million (US $106 million). Defects in the building were estimated to cost MYR28.4 million (US $7.5 million).[9] Even on modest projects, PMCs came in substantially over costs. According to Public Works Minister Samy Vellu, the ministry could construct a classroom for MYR55,000 (US $15,000), but when taken over by a PMC, the bill would soar to MYR120,000 (US $32,000).[10]

The public welcomed the new government's move to abolish the PMC in March 2004. Departments have been directed to comply with current procurement policies that use the tender system to ensure transparency and accountability. New guidelines may be issued to deal with specific contracts. For example, a treasury circular in December 2004 provides guidelines for the selection of contractors for public infrastructure maintenance, applicable to all government departments.[11] The terms detail the use of open tenders and the participation of a more balanced group of public officials, including a representative from the public works department.

These conditions comply with the 'Model Law on Procurement of Goods, Construction and Services', issued by the UN Commission on International Trade Law in 1995, but they do not divide the roles of selection and supervision, as outlined in TI's 'Minimum Standards for Public Contracting'.[12] Even more significant is Malaysia's failure to require companies to adopt a code of ethics against corruption, or to blacklist companies with a track record of corrupt practices.

Police corruption under fire

The Royal Commission on Enhancing the Operations and Management of the Police (RCP), set up in February 2004 to reform the police force, submitted a report of its findings to the king on 19 April 2005. Of the 926 complaints the commission received from the public between March 2004 and March 2005, 98 concerned police corruption.

The RCP's enquiries revealed widespread corruption within the police force, including: monthly kickbacks from illegal factory owners and employers of illegal immigrants; demands for payments in exchange for providing detainees with food, or allowing them to make telephone calls; and accepting bribes to detain innocent people, or to decline from taking action against guilty parties. The report also accuses police personnel of bribing senior officers to obtain promotions or transfers.

The report cited public complaints of the lavish lifestyle some officers enjoy. One is alleged to have declared assets of MYR34 million (US $9 million), but no investigation was conducted to determine how he had acquired such a fortune. Influenced by the finding that corruption awareness is low among police personnel at all levels, the commission recommended that eliminating it must rank high on the reform agenda. It made 125 recommendations, of which 10 relate to corruption.

There were some indications that the government may be 'sitting on' the RCP's report, as it does with reports from the Human Rights Commission. The deputy prime minister announced that it would have to be scrutinised by all central agencies, the finance ministry and the department for public works, before any of its recommendations could be implemented.[13] However, in May 2005, Prime Minister Badawi announced that a task force would meet to determine an order of priority for implementation and, a few weeks later, police were reportedly investigating the corruption cases cited in the report. In late June, five sub-committees were set up to study the recommendations in greater detail. Civil society has welcomed the RCP's findings and is monitoring its implementation.

Mehrun Siraj and Sunita Chima (TI Malaysia)

Further reading

Tunku Abdul Aziz, 'Fighting Corruption: My Mission' (Kuala Lumpur: Konrad Adenauer Foundation, 2005)

Zarinah Anwar and Kar Mei Tang, 'Building a Framework for Corporate Transparency: Challenges for Global Capital Markets and the Malaysian Experience', *International Accountant* 18, 2003

Khaliq Ahmad Mohd Israil and Abul Hassan M. Sadeq, *Ethics in Business and Management: Islamic and Mainstream Approaches* (Kuala Lumpur: Asian Academic Press, 2001)

Mazilan Musa, Izal Arif Zahrudin and Suzanna Che Moin (eds), 'Ethics and Integrity in Malaysia: Issues and Challenges' (Kuala Lumpur: Integrity Institute of Malaysia, 2005)

TI Malaysia: www.transparency.org.my

Notes

1. Keynote address by Prime Minister Abdullah Ahmad Badawi, World Ethics and Integrity Forum, Kuala Lumpur, 28–29 April 2005.
2. Transparency International, *National Integrity Systems Country Study: Malaysia* (Berlin: Transparency International, 2003).
3. Information provided by the deputy public prosecutor in the office of the attorney-general.

4. *New Straits Times* (Malaysia), 21 November 2004.
5. Treasury Circular, no. 4, 2000, at www.treasury.gov.my/design/web/b_pekeliling.htm
6. *Utusan Online* (Malaysia), 14 November 2004.
7. *New Straits Times* (Malaysia), 21 November 2004.
8. *The Star* (Malaysia), 15 November 2004.
9. *Bernama* (Malaysia), 22 October 2004.
10. *Utusan Online* (Malaysia), 14 November 2004.
11. Treasury Circular, no. 7, 2004, at www.treasury.gov.my/design/web/b_pekeliling.htm
12. See *Global Corruption Report 2005*, p. 4.
13. *Bernama* (Malaysia), 17 May 2005.

Morocco

Conventions:

UN Convention against Corruption (signed December 2003; not yet ratified)
UN Convention against Transnational Organized Crime (ratified September 2002)

Legal and institutional changes

- In April 2005, the government announced a new six-point **plan to fight corruption**. One measure will require all senior office holders to make a formal disclosure of their assets and net worth before and after holding public office. Other measures include a proposed new law on money laundering; the creation of an office responsible for keeping track of known corruption cases; and the consolidation of transparency in the process of awarding government contracts to private businesses.

- A law passed in September 2004 replaced the **Special Court of Justice** (CSJ) with five Courts of Appeal.[1] Offences involving corruption, extortion, the dishonest receipt of money by officials, influence peddling and the embezzlement of public funds will be handled by courts of first instance in the case of lesser offences, and the criminal divisions of the Courts of Appeal when offences are deemed more serious. The CSJ had dealt with official corruption since 1965. Under the pretext of greater efficiency, its procedures were faster but had less regard for individual liberties. The penalties were also more severe than those laid down in the Criminal Code. The CSJ was closely dependent on the justice minister, who had sole authority to initiate proceedings. This meant that the decision of whether or not to bring a case to trial was at the discretion of the executive. Non-governmental organisations, including Transparency Maroc, had called for the CSJ's abolition.

- The same law also introduced **changes to the Criminal Code** by stiffening penalties for the offences of corruption, extortion, the dishonest receipt of money by officials, influence peddling and embezzlement. It also provides for the mandatory confiscation by the state of all or part of the assets or income obtained through the offence and, in the case of bribery, the confiscation of the items supplied by the bribe payer. The law exonerates bribers that report an offence before a corrupt official has taken any action, or who are able to show that they were forced to make an illegal payment to achieve a certain outcome.

- In November 2004, a law was passed that is expected to **end the state's broadcasting monopoly** in 2005 and convert the radio and TV stations, RTM and 2M, into companies open to private capital. However, NGOs have criticised some limitations to freedom of expression such as the requirement that media organisations granted licences must promise to 'scrupulously respect the values of the monarchy and the kingdom's achievements in Islamic matters and territorial unity'.[2]

'Rabat Spring?'

When King Mohammed VI was crowned in July 1999, there were high hopes for an all-out assault on alleged corruption by the privileged class during the 38-year reign of his father, King Hassan II. Although delayed, the new king did try to meet some of these expectations, using the partially liberalised press and an emboldened state auditor, Inspection Générale de Finances (see below), as the agents of change. The most remarkable development in 2004–05, therefore, was the media's new freedom to discuss the issue of corruption.

The press has helped to transform domestic perceptions by unravelling complex accounts of reported corruption in parastatal agencies and banks, going as far as examining the business activities of senior officers in the Royal Armed Forces (FAR), hitherto considered unmentionable.

Much of the attention focused on the Hassan II Mosque, the king's giant mausoleum in Casablanca, which was built over a period of 13 years, at a cost variously estimated at US $500–800 million, and finally opened in 1993. That financial irregularities should only come to light more than a decade later is indicative of the restrictive measures imposed on the press during that time. Construction was financed partly by 'voluntary contributions' and partly by the compulsory deduction of employees' salaries, providing ample opportunities for racketeering and the embezzlement of funds.[3] Reporters also investigated irregularities involving suppliers of materials to the mosque, including the Grandes Marbreries du Sud (GMS) in Agadir, which operated a marble treatment plant and whose board was chaired by the deputy to King Hassan's former influential interior minister, Driss Basri.[4] Though no arrests have been made, this example points to a lack of accountability for large sums of public money during the late king's reign.

Nor has the army been immune to revelations of alleged abuse of position, particularly with regard to the fishing industry. The army has unprecedented control over the industry, due to the security role it plays on the coast, in addition to policing the catches of Moroccan and EU trawlers. Suspicions that the fishing industry had fallen into the hands of military officers surfaced in 2001, when the press reported that a number of senior officials in the military and security agencies, and members of their families, owned companies or shares of companies that exported fish to Spain.[5] These allegations resurfaced in a more authoritative article in January 2005 that further detailed these connections, and which alleged the existence of conflicts of interest between the professional duties and private interests of members of the military. How could these officers, it asked, effectively oversee compliance with fishery conservation policies when their trawlers stood to lose millions of dirhams?[6]

The situation in the military is not helped by the fact that the defence budget is approved by the executive without debate in parliament, and that military procurement contracts are – at least in practice – not subject to the law on public contracting, limiting oversight to internal checks only. This does not allow for the transparent management of an important part of the state budget.

Despite the rare publicity afforded to all these cases, not one has come before the new Courts of Appeal, leading to the conclusion that corruption will continue to flourish in the absence of an independent judiciary and impunity of high-ranking officials. A number of NGOs and journalists have called for an independent inquiry to find out the extent of the wealth that was amassed illegally during Hassan's long reign,[7] while others say this is impossible because of the sheer number of business transactions that occurred in the past 40 years. One thing appears certain. Greater freedom of speech has not been accompanied by any significant improvement in accountability. 'Greater freedom of speech is not enough', said journalist Farida Mouha. 'What is needed are effective policies against corruption.'[8]

IGF publishes bold reports, but there is little follow-up

The second weapon in the government's arsenal is the Inspection Générale de Finances (IGF), a once moribund government auditing office of 160 accountants with oversight responsibility for the activities of public sector institutions and funding from donors.

While the auditing activity of the IGF was limited in the past, the IGF's work picked up steam in 2003. Its inspections have revealed evidence of gross financial fraud or embezzlement in banking, social security, agricultural credit, public housing, state contracts, public companies, municipal councils and international aid projects.

Some of the biggest names in the banking firmament – including Credit Immobilier et Hôtelier (CIH), Banque Populaire, Caisse Nationale de Sécurité Sociale and Banque Nationale pour le Développement Economique (BNDE) – have been investigated for alleged mismanagement and corruption. According to the IGF, the BNDE management dipped into its DH19 billion (US $2.1 billion) reserves in the CDG, a fund that can only be used with the agreement of the finance ministry, the Al Maghrib Bank, the Credit Commission and the board of directors.[9] Procedures normally required for withdrawals of this kind were not followed. This case is still ongoing.

A similar theme surrounds the CIH, the prestigious tourism and housing development credit fund that, according to a parliamentary inquiry in 2000, lost DH14 billion (US $1.3 billion) over several years. Fifteen former senior CIH officials were investigated for embezzlement, including the former director general, who blamed the bank's failure on demands for unguaranteed loans from well placed businessmen close to the seat of power. Fictional businessmen using fictional companies obtained credit from the bank and were later declared bankrupt. With so many senior politicians allegedly involved, it is doubtful that full and thorough disclosures will be possible in either case.

In early 2005, the IGF's attention switched to the Office de la Formation Professionale et de la Promotion du Travail (OFPPT), the body responsible for providing 70 per cent of the country's professional training and construction of the infrastructure required, often with the support of donors such as Canada and the European Union. In 2004, an IGF investigation uncovered an extensive web of fictitious training schemes, with misappropriated funds estimated at DH60 million (US $6.7 million).[10] This signalled a complete breakdown of the monitoring systems in place at the OFPPT, but also in other public bodies responsible for oversight. According to the IGF inquiry, between 1996 and 2001, only 45 cases out of a total of 6,247 that received subsidies for training had been monitored at all.

For all of its newfound bravado, the IGF is still critically underfunded and its reports receive little follow-up.[11] When cases involving senior officials are uncovered, the judicial system freezes. Only until the IGF's audits are made fully available for public scrutiny will the warnings become impossible to ignore.

Azeddine Akesbi, Siham Benchekroun, Kamal El Mesbahi,
Rachid Filali Meknassi and Michèle Zirari (Transparency Maroc)

Further reading

Transparency Maroc, *Université de la transparence* (University of Transparency) (Rabat: Transparency Maroc, 2003) (Also available in Arabic)
Transparency Maroc, *La corruption au Maroc: synthèse des résultats des enquêtes d'intégrités* (Corruption in Morocco: A Summary of the National Integrity System Survey) (Rabat: Transparency Maroc, 2002)

TI Morocco: www.transparencymaroc.org

Notes

1. Law no.79–03, published in the *Bulletin Officiel*, 17 September 2004.
2. Reporters Without Borders, *Morocco – 2005 Annual Report*, available at www.rsf.org/article.php3?id_article=13310
3. *TelQuel* (Morocco), 4–10 December 2004.
4. *Al Ayyam* (Morocco), 19–25 January 2005. The article gives precise information about unpaid invoices and people close to the minister receiving large amounts of marble without paying.
5. http://sahara_opinions.site.voila.fr/kbeirouk2001.htm
6. *Al Ayyam* (Morocco), 19–25 January 2005.
7. *Vue Economique* (Morocco), 10 December 2004.
8. *Libération* (Morocco), 14 December 2004.
9. *Ahdat Almaghribia* (Morocco), 7 January 2005.
10. *Assahifa* (Morocco), 30 June–6 July 2004.
11. Interview with IGF director Abdelali Benbrik in *Aujourd'hui le Maroc* (Morocco), 24 January 2005.

Nepal

Conventions:
UN Convention against Corruption (signed December 2003; not yet ratified)
UN Convention against Transnational Organized Crime (signed December 2002; not yet ratified)

ADB-OECD Action Plan for Asia-Pacific (endorsed November 2001)

Legal and institutional developments

- King Gyanendra issued a decree in February 2005 that created a **Royal Commission for Corruption Control** (RCCC). Although the commission was initially formed through a clause in the constitution on the issuing of a state of emergency, the king extended its mandate after the state of emergency was lifted. Though the measure addresses popular grievances about corruption in the country, it has been widely criticised by politicians and civil society. There is general agreement that a measure that gives a single agency both investigative and judicial powers violates the basic principle of separation of powers. The commission has also been criticised as redundant, given the existence of the Commission for Investigation of Abuse of Authority (CIAA), an anti-graft body set up in 1991, which has been seen as increasingly effective (see below).

- In accordance with a directive on public service, 71 district committees were formed in March 2005 to **monitor public service delivery** for, among other things, abuse of authority and bribery. The local administration act was also amended by royal decree to include the appointment of five regional and 14 zonal administrators. The additional provisions were made to ensure that officials are more conscious of their duties and to put a check on bribe-taking. However, the new administrative tiers could clash with previously existing ones, due to overlap of jurisdiction and authority.

- A **draft act against money laundering** was prepared by the finance ministry in July 2004; a draft bill on **public procurement** and regulation was prepared in January 2005 by the general office of the financial comptroller; and draft regulations on the National Vigilance Centre (NVC) were prepared in March 2005 by the NVC. All were in the process of public consultation before being finalised, but have now been put in jeopardy in the absence of a functioning parliament.

The Royal Commission's questionable role in corruption control

On 1 February 2005, King Gyanendra dissolved the four-party coalition government headed by Sher Bahadur Deuba, assumed executive control and introduced a state of emergency under article 115 of the 1990 constitution. The reasons given for this 'royal takeover' were the deterioration in security, the failure of past governments to improve law and order, and rampant corruption. The dissolution of the government was widely criticised for being undemocratic and unconstitutional.

The new government quickly announced a plan to launch a vigorous campaign against corruption and in February 2005 the Royal Commission for Corruption Control (RCCC) was established. Past measures to control corruption have not succeeded due to political instability and weak checks and balances in Nepalese institutions. This most recent initiative is similarly questionable, given the absence of parliament and local government, the non-conducive atmosphere for elections, delayed justice from the courts, continuing conflict and security problems, and the deepening economic crisis.

Many political party leaders, human rights activists and journalists have been detained while political gatherings are strongly discouraged. The promulgation of restrictive measures concerning the press, in particular, has deprived anti-corruption bodies, the media and members of civil society of their right to freedom of speech. Anti-corruption activists have been told that 'their enquiries or watchdog activities should not lower the morale of those in civil service'.[1] Nonetheless, segments of the population are convinced that the king's takeover of government was in the best interests of the nation.

The six-member RCCC is headed by Bhakta Bahadur Koirala, a former government secretary, and enjoys the powers of both the Commission for the Investigation of Abuse of Authority (CIAA) and the Special Court. This goes against the basic principles of justice and the separation of powers. The CIAA was established in 1991 and its powers of investigation were extended to the prime minister and to MPs in 2002. As a prosecuting body, the CIAA investigates charges and refers its cases to the Special Court for trial. The Special Court, formed in 2002, deals specifically with corruption cases.

Since its creation, the RCCC has pursued a number of cases involving high-ranking officials and politicians. Former prime minister Sher Bahadur Deuba was convicted in July 2005 for irregularities committed in the award of a contract related to the US $464 million Melamchi Water Supply Project, whose main financier is the Asian Development Bank. The former public works minister, Prakash Man Singh, and four others were also convicted.[2] Deuba and

Singh were jailed for two years and fined US $1.3 million each. Civil society groups, lawyers and foreign governments criticised the verdicts for their extra-judicial nature.

In another case, in March 2005, the RCCC began the prosecution of six former ministers for misusing the prime minister's relief fund to distribute some NPR4 million (US $57,000) to political supporters in the guise of relief aid to Maoist insurgency victims. The media dubbed the alleged scam the 'Dashain allowance', Dashain being an important Hindu festival. According to the RCCC, the six former ministers misused monies from the relief fund to cover 'Dashain expenses' for 21 party supporters.[3] Then in June 2005, the RCCC made an abrupt U-turn and cleared the former prime minister of these charges, as well as the six members of his cabinet and the 21 beneficiaries of the expenses. According to the RCCC chairman: 'The decision to distribute cash could not be established as a case of corruption under Clause 17 of the Anti-Corruption Act 2002.' Critics saw the move as evidence of the commission's excessive discretionary powers.

The RCCC's investigations invited condemnation from political parties and sectors of civil society, including the Nepal Bar Association, for what was termed an 'arbitrary, political vendetta'. In April 2005, the RCCC issued fresh orders to Nepal's banks to provide the financial records of more than 100 selected politicians and bureaucrats; according to media sources, none of the names belonged to 'loyal royals'.[4]

In the view of its detractors, the RCCC is in danger of becoming an instrument for political manipulation. The RCCC has been further criticised because it sidelines the CIAA, the constitutionally designated anti-corruption agency. The RCCC's life was extended under a clause in the same article in the constitution that lifted the state of emergency in April 2005. It would have been logical to discontinue the RCCC as soon as the state of emergency was lifted. Why this has not happened is a point that continues to baffle politicians, lawyers and civil society.

CIAA gains strength but corrupt officials can still escape justice

The CIAA was established in 1991 and has withstood pressure and political attack in its drive to investigate improper conduct by politicians and officials. The professionalism of the CIAA has resulted in a remarkable 84 per cent conviction rate in the 250 or so cases it has filed at the Special Court since the latter was conceived in 2002. The CIAA has saved substantial revenues, both through the prosecution of individuals and the discovery of financial irregularities.

One recent instance when the CIAA proved its worth was in checking irregularities concerning money owed to the Civil Aviation Authority of Nepal (CAAN). In March 2005, the CIAA issued a directive to Royal Nepal Airlines (RNA) – as well as other airlines – to pay charges owed to the aviation authority following a study that found it was in arrears by NPR540 million (US $8.1 million). The CIAA demanded that the CAAN fulfil its legal obligation to prepare monthly bills for RNA jets landing, parking and using other airport facilities for payment within 21 days. By the end of April, the authority informed the CIAA that it had started to collect arrears.

Anti-corruption activists cite this as a positive example of good practice on the part of regulatory bodies in checking financial irregularities and recovering public monies. The non-payment of dues was apparently a temporary measure undertaken by mutual consent by officials at RNA and the CAAN, but this had been neglected for five years until the CIAA alerted them.

Public confidence in the CIAA also received a boost with action against senior government officials, including the filing of corruption cases in August 2004 against three former chiefs of police. Moti Lal Bohara, Achyut Krishna Kharel and Pradip Shumsher Rana were accused of abusing their office to illegally amass several hundred thousand dollars each.[5] This was the first time that the CIAA had laid charges against the police's top brass, a move that exposed institutionalised corruption in the law enforcement agencies.

For its part, the Special Court was widely acclaimed in 2004–05 for verdicts penalising three senior officials in different corruption cases filed by the CIAA. In July 2004, former public works minister and leader of the Nepali Democratic Congress Party Chiranjibi Wagle was sentenced to two and a half years in prison and a fine of NPR27.2 million (US $411,000) for corruption.[6] This was considered historic in Nepal since no corruption case has ended with such a huge penalty. The CIAA claimed that Wagle had made a fortune of nearly NPR30 million (US $450,000) by misusing his authority. In January 2005, the Special Court convicted Ramagya Chaturvedi, head of the state-owned Nepal Oil Corporation, for corruption, imprisoned him for two years and ordered the confiscation of illegal earnings of over NPR19 million (US $287,000). The CIAA said he had misused his authority to accumulate more than NPR70 million (US $1.1 million).[7] In March, the former chief of Mechi Customs Office, Keshar Jung Khadka, was given a one-year sentence and a fine of over NPR2.5 million (US $35,000) for corruption, and property to the value of US $144,000 was confiscated.[8]

However, all three escaped the court's premises moments before the verdicts were delivered. The fact that these high-ranking officials were permitted to go free was the result of a loophole in the judicial system whereby the Special Court does not have the authority to order the arrest of corruption offenders. Instead, its verdicts must be executed through the relevant district court, which can take some days to effect due to administrative procedures. Hence judgments by the Special Court are not always implemented. Another problem is that the accused are often released on bail, enabling them to strengthen their cases by mobilising their resources. Anti-corruption activists believe that anyone held on serious corruption charges should pursue the defence from prison.

The three cases raised questions about more effective means of implementing Special Court orders. At present, the court is considering more than 150 corruption cases involving senior politicians, administrators and police officials prosecuted by the CIAA. Many are likely to escape justice unless the current shortcomings in the judicial system are fully addressed.

Rama Krishna Regmee (Kantipur City College, Kathmandu)

Further reading

Baburam Dhakal, *Empire of Corruption* (Kathmandu: Baburam Dhakal, 2005)
CIAA and TI Nepal, *Compilations of Anti-corruption Laws*, 2nd edition (Kathmandu: CIAA and TI Nepal, 2005)
Hari Bahadur Thapa, *Bideshi Sahayataka Bisangati* (The Distortion of Foreign Aid) (Kathmandu: National Book Centre, 2004)
Rama Krishna Regmee, *Nepal National Integrity System Study 2004* (Kathmandu: TI Nepal, 2004)

TI Nepal: www.tinepal.org

Notes

1. Author's interview with a district administrator of Pokhara, February 2005.
2. BBC News (UK), 28 July 2005; *Dawn* (Pakistan), 28 April 2005.
3. www.gorkhapatra.org.np/pageloader.php?file=2005/03/24/topstories/main6
4. *Dawn* (Pakistan), 28 April 2005.

5. *Nepal News* (Nepal), 14 August 2004.
6. *Nepal News* (Nepal), 22 July 2004.
7. *The Himalayan Times* (Nepal), 21 January 2005.
8. www.gorkhapatra.org.np/pageloader.php?file=2005/04/05//topstories/main3

New Zealand

Conventions:
OECD Anti-Bribery Convention (ratified June 2001)
UN Convention against Corruption (signed December 2003; not yet ratified)
UN Convention against Transnational Organized Crime (ratified July 2002)

Legal and institutional changes

- In December 2004, four existing laws aimed at promoting **integrity in the public sector** were amended. As a result, the State Services Commission, the agency responsible for overseeing all core government departments, now has explicit responsibility over a far broader range of state agencies than before (see below). Under the new legislation, the commission's annual reports on the agencies' progress in promoting ethical standards must be made available to the public. In early 2005, the commission began drawing up a set of pilot guidelines for the affected agencies.

- In January 2004, New Zealand ceased to use Britain's Privy Council as its final court of appeal. A **new Supreme Court** began hearing cases in 1 July 2004 following the passage of the Supreme Court Act of October 2003. During the transitional period, there was an unprecedented degree of tension between the government and the judiciary over funding for the new court. In May 2004, the Chief Justice made a speech in London criticising the New Zealand government for the funding process, as well as the amount available to the new Supreme Court. The independence of the judiciary is well established in New Zealand, and the controversy over the Supreme Court was seen as a litmus test of the country's standing on good governance.

Corruption gains profile in New Zealand

Transparency International's Corruption Perceptions Index consistently finds New Zealand to be one of the least corrupt countries in the world. In the past year, however, the issue has received unprecedented attention due to a number of allegations concerning the misuse of public funds for community services.

Since reforms were launched in 1984 to reduce state intervention in the economy, successive governments have increasingly contracted out service provision. In some cases, this process of devolution occurred too quickly and community service organisations lacked the capacity to manage funds effectively. This broadened the scope for financial misappropriation and other corrupt activities within such organisations.

One recent and highly publicised case of mismanagement of public funds involved an opposition MP, Donna Awatere Huata, who established a charitable trust in 1999 to promote reading programmes in homes that targeted Maori children. She successfully lobbied government departments to raise funds for the trust, but was then alleged to have used a large part of them for her private benefit. Huata was charged with fraud in November 2003,[1] but at this writing, she had not yet been tried and has continued to deny the allegations. The protracted scandal eventually led to her dismissal from parliament in November 2004, although this was also due to a conflict within her own political party.[2] Allegations of financial impropriety involving MPs are virtually unknown in New Zealand and no one in living memory has hitherto been expelled.

This scandal was followed by allegations of financial mismanagement in the country's largest tertiary education institution, Te Wananga o Aotearoa. Evidence was tabled in parliament that pointed to nepotism in the award of contracts to companies owned by the organisation's senior executives or their relatives.[3] Several inquiries were initiated in the wake of the allegations and are still ongoing. Although media reports suggested that this could be a case of mismanagement rather than actual misappropriation, the case highlighted that such problems could have been avoided if more time and money had been invested in capacity building in the first place.

Periodic instances of misuse of funds by small, government-funded service providers, including Maori organisations, have started to attract more attention, sparking a debate about corruption at the community services level. For example, there have been reports of Maori organisations mismanaging substantial assets, many of which were acquired as compensation for breaches of the Treaty of Waitangi, signed by Maori chiefs with the British in 1840. The most notable example occurred in the late 1990s and involved the Tainui nation, and assets given by the government as compensation for breaches of the treaty dating back to the 1860s. The compensation was in both cash and land. The Tainui management body, however, invested in assets including a contentious sporting franchise.[4] As a result, considerable internal conflict ensued over control of the assets, generating negative publicity.

The public perception is that bad financial management, revealed in audited accounts and often accompanied by allegations of corruption and nepotism, has led to the squandering of legitimate settlements using state assets. This is matched by the view of some of the intended beneficiaries of these organisations that their own leaders deprived them of resources. Although some of these allegations were well founded, there have been few cases where criminal charges were actually pressed.

Given growing public concern, the government has taken steps to address the issue by introducing financial management training, beginning in January 2005, for community service organisations which receive state funds to deliver services, or as compensation for treaty breaches. Since the beginning of 2005 there has also been greater emphasis on the importance of government departments assessing the organisations' management capability before funds and land are released.

Promoting integrity in the public sector

Legislative moves to promote integrity in the broader public sector received less media attention, but brought about significant changes. The legislation amending four existing acts of parliament, passed in December 2004, widens the remit of the State Services Commission in monitoring government agencies.

In New Zealand, there are three main areas in the public sector: the core public service consisting of traditional departments such as health, education, police, foreign affairs and statistics; service and advisory agencies, funded by parliament with boards of directors appointed by the government (covering a diverse range of roles, from administering New Zealand's no-fault accident compensation legislation, to separate agencies that ensure road, air and maritime safety); and state-owned business enterprises, such as New Zealand Post, which provides postal services and operates a retail trading bank.

Previously, the heads of all these departments reported to the State Services

Commissioner, a public servant appointed in a strictly non-partisan manner. The commissioner is effectively the employer of all heads of government departments, and has personal contracts with each departmental head. These individuals are personally responsible to the commissioner on employment and performance matters, as well as setting standards for integrity, which is included in their contracts.

Under the amended legislation, the government-appointed boards of directors of other non-core state agencies (the second and third groups described above) will also have to report to the commissioner. Non-core state agencies now have clear lines of responsibility for setting standards and cultivating an ethos of integrity. The State Services Commissioner will now be able to ensure that these agencies, which are often powerful, are obliged to promote integrity. According to the new legislation, the commission also has to monitor how these agencies fulfil their obligation to promote integrity, and any reports regarding this matter will be available to the general public.

Since the economic reforms initiated in 1984, many observers felt that serving public interest and honesty, once considered the distinguishing features of New Zealand's public sector, were in danger of being lost. The reforms aimed to promote a more competitive society and a more flexible public service by doing away with government intervention in many areas of the economy. Agency heads had fixed-term contracts and their performance was evaluated by set criteria with an emphasis on efficiency, a factor highly valued by the private sector, upon which public sector management was being increasingly modelled. No comparable emphasis, however, was placed on the proactive inculcation of ethical standards.

In 1999, the newly elected government established a special body, the State Sector Standards Board (SSSB), to review the public sector; former senior public sector executives, state sector union leaders and senior private sector executives were its members. They presented two reports to the government, which emphasised the loss of a cohesive sense of public interest service since the reforms of the 1980s. The SSSB's first report to the government in 2001 concluded that 'an over-emphasis on economic efficiency as an outcome and performance measure has distorted behaviours and undermined trust and support from the public and employees'.[5] Board members highlighted similar concerns in their second report. The new legislation seems to have addressed the SSSB's concerns by extending the commissioner's responsibilities for the promotion of ethical standards to the broader public sector.

Promoting transparency abroad

New Zealand has made no substantive progress in implementing the legislation enacted in 2001, in response to the OECD Anti-Bribery Convention. Little knowledge of the foreign bribery law exists among exporters and the government has made no effort to generate awareness of the legal liabilities. Only one reference to the new law was made in a speech by the Trade Minister while out of the country.[6] No investigations or prosecutions have resulted from the legislation.

While there is little evidence of New Zealand companies paying bribes overseas, it is thought to occur on a minor scale and some companies lobbied against the legislation when it was first drafted. The scale of bribery is largely a reflection of the size of the country's exporters, which are overwhelmingly small businesses. Moreover, New Zealand has opted out of the WTO Government Procurement Code, due to the compliance costs that would arise, since its procurement system is currently deregulated.

Yet, together with Australia, New Zealand has stepped up joint efforts to promote better governance and transparency within the broader Pacific region. This has been achieved through a multitude of programmes, many of which are coordinated via the Pacific Islands

Forum, the core regional body representing the 14 independent island nations of the South Pacific, as well as New Zealand and Australia.

New Zealand's international aid agency, NZAID, has expressed mounting concern about standards of governance in Pacific Island countries. Support for governance reforms to combat corruption is now a top priority of NZAID and it has provided assistance to civil society actors in the region. NZAID also backs efforts by Pacific Island governments to improve governance and financial management, and has played a major role in supporting the development of the Pacific Plan that was initiated by the members of the Pacific Forum. The Pacific Plan emphasises governance reform in the region. However, surveys by the Fiji-based Pacific Islands Forum Secretariat have found that previous regional commitments to standards of good governance have been largely ignored by the Pacific Island signatory nations.[7]

Shane Cave (TI New Zealand)

Further reading

John Henderson, Shane Cave and Murray Petrie, *New Zealand's National Integrity System* (Wellington: TI New Zealand, 2003)

Alan Webster, *Spiral of Values: The Flow from Survival Values to Global Consciousness in New Zealand* (Hawere: Alpha Publications, 2001)

Reports of the State Sector Standards Board: www.ssc.govt.nz/display/document.asp?NavID=196

Notes

1. www.sfo.govt.nz (see Info. Bulletins and Alerts – 4 November 2003).
2. tvnz.co.nz/view/news_politics_story_skin/459577?format=html
3. *Hansard* (New Zealand's parliamentary record), 15 February 2005.
4. See commentary on the Kingi Michael Porima case in the *Maori Law Review*, September 2000, available at www.bennion.co.nz/mlr/2000/sep.html
5. www.ssc.govt.nz/display/document.asp?navid=196&docid=2330&pageno=2#P29_1346
6. Author's interview with trade ministry officials.
7. www.forumsec.org.fj/docs/FEMM/2002/femv04.pdf

Nicaragua

Conventions:

OAS Inter-American Convention against Corruption (ratified May 1999)
UN Convention against Corruption (signed December 2003; not yet ratified)
UN Convention against Transnational Organized Crime (ratified September 2002)

Legal and institutional changes

• Article 68 of the Constitution, which exempts the media from paying import duty on supplies, was revoked in March 2005. The measure is expected to have an adverse effect on the **media's ability to report on corruption**.

• A flawed **Judicial Career Law**, which the National Assembly ratified in September 2004, was due to enter into effect in September 2005. The law establishes competitive examinations for judges, but leaves open the possibility that judges will be appointed without competing for their positions. It also fails to separate the Supreme Court's administrative and judicial functions, and assigns responsibility for oversight of the judicial career processes to a commission formed of Supreme Court judges, rather than an independent body.

- In March 2005, the Partido Liberal Constitucionalista (PLC) tabled a bill that, if passed, would grant an **amnesty** to anyone accused of a crime against the public administration during the past 20 years. This includes the PLC leader and former president, Arnoldo Alemán, who was sentenced to 20 years under house arrest in 2003 for money laundering, embezzlement and fraud (see below).

Rival parties' stranglehold over government stymies anti-corruption efforts

President Enrique Bolaños' anti-corruption efforts had a promising start when he decided to press charges against his political mentor, former president Arnoldo Alemán, who is currently serving a 20-year sentence under house arrest for fraud, money laundering and embezzlement (see *Global Corruption Report 2005*). But the fight against corruption has since stagnated as the two main parties in the National Assembly collude to block prosecutions and exploit Bolaños' weaknesses by promoting legal action for alleged campaign funding abuses.

Investigations against former officials have been shelved and, with the exception of Alemán, no member of the former government has been imprisoned for corruption. Nor are they likely ever to spend time in prison, thanks to a five-year statute of limitations that applies to their crimes. The time period for prosecuting members of the former government for corruption could expire even sooner if an amnesty bill peddled by the Partido Liberal Constitucionalista is approved.

Emblematic of the failure to act decisively against corruption is the case against Byron Jerez, the former director general of income and Alemán's close associate. He was exonerated in five separate trials in 2004–05 and in the one case in which he was convicted, the sentence was overturned even though there was 'ample and convincing' evidence against him, according to attorney general Alberto Novoa. Novoa is in the process of recovering seized assets, including the beach house allegedly built with money diverted from Hurricane Mitch relief funds.

Bolaños, who came to power at the helm of an alliance of five political parties, lost the support of his party, the PLC, in 2002 when his government prosecuted Alemán, head of the PLC, who had originally picked him as presidential candidate. Since then, the PLC and the main opposition party, the Frente Sandinista de Liberación Nacional (FSLN), which together control over 90 per cent of the National Assembly, have gradually tightened their hold over the institutions of state, making it practically impossible to act against corruption.

The two parties' leaders, Alemán and Daniel Ortega, reached an informal pact in 2000 to push through a constitutional change that enhances their control of institutions and grants Alemán an automatic seat in the National Assembly and therefore parliamentary immunity. The pact has since widened in scope and plays a critical role for their political survival since both face high rates of disapproval within their parties and externally, and are being investigated for corruption in Nicaragua and third countries.[1] They are both unpopular with the US government, and featured on a list of high-level party officials who have been denied entry visas to the United States on the grounds of corruption.[2]

Control of the legislative branch has enabled the two parties to steer through several laws that make it more difficult to tackle corruption. They have ended tax concessions for media companies who complain that the move was motivated by a desire to crack down on freedom of expression. Another controversial move saw the passing in September 2004 of a judicial career law that allows the Supreme Court to continue to exercise responsibility for both the administration and dispensation of justice. This went directly against recommendations of several civil society organisations. The law allows judges and other court staff to be hired and promoted without participating in competitive processes.

The law also ratified existing judicial positions, which effectively amounted to the PLC's approval of the appointment of judges whom it had denounced a year before for 'working for' the FSLN.

The PLC has shifted power to the FSLN in other ways as well, most significantly by handing it the presidency of the National Assembly, marking the first time in two years that a member of that party has held a senior post in the legislature. The apparent quid pro quo for the numerous concessions made by the PLC to the FSLN is support for Alemán's release.

A rash of lawmaking in mid-November 2004 saw 14 laws adopted in four days (when none had been approved in the previous six months) many of which helped to shift the balance of power from the government to the legislature. Both the Central American Court of Justice and the Organization of American States have criticised the new laws for eroding the powers of the executive.[3]

Among the new legislation is a law that grants the National Assembly the power to ratify or dismiss nominees to ministerial and diplomatic posts, and reduce the number of legislators required to reject a presidential decree. The National Assembly was also granted power not only to accept or reject the budget, but also to modify it. Another law places a number of new institutions under Assembly control, including the supervisory bodies for the public services, social security and private property claims.

A strong legislature is important and a decade ago it was wide-ranging presidential powers that were cause for concern. But the worry now is whether the balance has shifted too far, leaving insufficient counterweights granted to the executive or other institutions. This is especially worrying given Nicaragua's weak democratic tradition. Although political parties are required by law to select candidates using the most democratic method available,[4] this stipulation is almost universally ignored. Party grandees do not hold primaries, but rather draw up closed lists of their favoured candidates to fill the powerful National Assembly. These same favoured candidates also end up filling key positions within the judicial, electoral, audit and other institutional bodies.

The political duopoly is becoming entrenched through laws and practices that make it difficult for opponents to compete, or for state institutions to gain independence. The legal framework ushered in by the two main parties since 2000 makes it next to impossible to create new parties,[5] while the lack of internal party democracy means that reformists within the two main parties are consistently blocked. Though Alemán and Ortega are unpopular within their parties and amongst the electorate, at least one of them – and perhaps both – will run in 2006. In the past, with involvement from politicised state institutions, popular candidates Pedro Solórzano and José Antonio Alvarado had their electoral ambitions derailed (in 2000 and 2001, respectively). Now, the same fate threatens popular candidates Herty Lewites (FLSN) and Eduardo Montealegre (PLC) in the run-up to the 2006 general election.

The control exerted by the two main parties over the Supreme Electoral Council (CSE), the body charged with monitoring electoral activity, has prompted fears that the CSE is too disinterested to act neutrally in the 2006 elections, and that the elections will not be free or fair.[6]

Even if an outsider were to win the presidency, however, the increased authority granted to the National Assembly, and the firm grip Alemán and Ortega have over it, all but guarantee them enough power to continue to pose a serious obstacle to efforts to fight corruption.

Roberto Courtney (Grupo Cívico Etica y Transparencia, Nicaragua)

Further reading

G8 countries and the Government of Nicaragua, 'G8/Nicaragua Partnership Compact to Promote Transparency and Combat Corruption: A New Partnership Between the G8 and Nicaragua', June 2004, www.whitehouse.gov/news/releases/2004/06/20040610-35.html

Universidad Centroamericana, 'Tercera encuesta sobre Percepción de la población sobre la corrupción' (Third Survey on the Population's Perceptions of Corruption), April 2005, www.uca.edu.ni

Grupo Cívico Etica y Transparencia (TI Nicaragua): www.eyt.org.ni

Notes

1. Accounts opened under Alemán's name have been frozen in Panama, where investigations into alleged money laundering are under way. US authorities are investigating similar charges.
2. US authorities have refused entry visas to at least 13 Nicaraguan state or party officials, including two Supreme Court judges, an electoral court judge and the state supervisor for public services 'for suspicions or investigations related to terrorism or corruption'.
3. The OAS has sent a number of missions to evaluate whether the reforms and the stalemate between the executive and the legislature represent a 'rupture of the democratic order'. Nicaraguan analysts are consistent in their criticisms of the reforms, which they argue affect the balance and independence of powers.
4. Article 63 of the electoral law.
5. See *Global Corruption Report 2004* and *2005* for an analysis of the impact of the 2000 electoral law.
6. The civil society electoral monitoring groups Grupo Cívico Etica y Transparencia and el Instituto para el Desarrollo y la Democracia (IPADE) declared a state of 'yellow alert' in March 2005, citing the high level of risk of electoral fraud and the failure of the state to tackle the problem even after the EU, the OAS and the Carter Center criticised the legal framework and the performance of the electoral authorities in the 2001 elections. Electoral monitors discovered irregularities in the 2004 municipal elections, which they argue is evidence that the problems have not been rectified ahead of the 2006 general elections: voters encountered difficulties in acquiring or renewing the ID cards mandatory for voting, or did not appear on the electoral list, despite having registered; electoral authorities overturned the result in Granada, the country's third largest city, giving victory to the FSLN in place of the APRE (Alliance for the Republic) on grounds that critics have called fictitious.

Panama

Conventions:
OAS Inter-American Convention against Corruption (ratified October 1998)
UN Convention against Corruption (ratified May 2005)
UN Convention against Transnational Organized Crime (ratified August 2004)

Legal and institutional changes

- Executive Decree No. 335, issued on 1 September 2004, the day President Martín Torrijos Espino took office, derogates Executive Decree No. 124 of May 2002 which regulated the transparency law. The 2002 decree was issued under former president Mireya Moscoso and was an obstacle to **accessing information** since it restricted official information to any interested person with a 'direct relationship to the information requested'. The Supreme Court had rejected many habeas data writs by appealing to the earlier decree.

In May 2004, the Supreme Court voted that some of the most restrictive articles of the earlier decree were illegal.

- When the new government took office in September 2004, Minister of the Presidency Ubaldino Real promised to publicise how the president utilised his **discretional budgetary allocations** and to reduce the amount from US $25 million per year to less than US $5 million. Both promises have been fulfilled. Information is available at both the president and ombudsman's websites.[1] The amount approved in the first year of the current administration was US $3.9 million. The auditor general has prepared draft regulations for the use by future presidents of the funds, which tended in the past to be used to cover personal expenses, or to benefit family and friends. The two websites and investigations by the newspapers *La Prensa* and *El Panamá América* reveal details of numerous allegations of misuse of funds to buy jewellery, artwork, clothes, to pay for entertainment and bribe journalists during the administrations of Ernesto Pérez Balladares (1994–99) and Mireya Moscoso (1999–2004).

- In December 2004 a **code of ethics** was issued that forbids public servants from: soliciting or accepting gifts or other benefits; maintaining relationships or entering situations in which their personal, economic or financial interests could be in conflict with their ability to carry out their work properly; directing, managing, advising, endorsing, representing or providing services (paid or voluntary) to people who manage or exploit state concessions or privileges, or who have contracts with the state; and maintaining links, benefits or obligations to bodies that are directly supervised by the body employing the public servant. The code states that public servants should refrain from appointing relatives to public positions. Sanctions for violating the code range from a verbal dressing-down to dismissal. Each government body is responsible for enforcing the code, however. There are no external monitoring mechanisms as yet.

- Executive Decree No. 179 of October 2004 created the **National Council for Transparency against Corruption**, a consultative body that provides advice to the executive branch of government on matters relating to transparency and corruption prevention. In January 2005, its members were named as the Minister of the Presidency, the attorney general, the attorney for administrative matters, the auditor general, the ombudsman and one representative each from the private sector, unions, civil society, the church and the media. The council, which works on a voluntary basis, has been tasked with drawing up a working plan whose implementation will be supported by US funds (see below).

- In January 2005, the newly appointed attorney general, Ana Matilde Gómez, appointed a **new anti-corruption prosecutor**, taking the number of such prosecutors to three.

- In March, the government signed a 'State Pact for Justice' that created a special commission with six months to analyse and propose **improvements to the judicial system**. The Supreme Court has been the subject of particular scrutiny since a number of its judges have accused one another of corruption. Civil society organisations have demanded the resignation of all judges and a revision of the procedure for selecting them in order to eliminate all possibility of political interference (see below).

National Council for Transparency against Corruption

Corruption and the high level of impunity for people implicated in it are major concerns in Panama, second only to unemployment, according to recent surveys.[2] The administration of President Martín Torrijos Espino took office with a pledge to promote greater transparency and to clamp down on corruption. He promised to appoint a National Council for Transparency against Corruption; derogate a decree that limited the effectiveness of the transparency law; disclose the use of discretionary funds; professionalise the civil service; introduce a general salary law; introduce policies to make public contracting more transparent; and select a new attorney general. Torrijos has taken steps to fulfil most of these pledges, though their impact on corruption levels has still to be demonstrated.

Most of the legal changes have been tabled, if not adopted, and Ana Matilde Gómez was named attorney general in January. One of her first tasks was to investigate progress in some of the country's more scandalous corruption cases. On releasing her report she said she would open further investigations, including one into alleged illicit enrichment involving allies of former president Mireya Moscoso. The government has so far filed a number of complaints against illicit enrichment, but many are stalled in the Supreme Court.

The National Council for Transparency against Corruption (NCTC) was created by decree on 27 October 2004 and was intended to fill a perceived gap in anti-corruption strategy by focusing on prevention. Former public prosecutor Cristóbal Arboleda was named its first executive secretary for a period of four months. On taking up his post, he said he would only investigate allegations of corruption made in the media, and with an administrative, rather than criminal, process.

Nepotism has also been alleged in certain institutions, but the anti-corruption secretary failed to respond. One such allegation concerned the appointment to the Panamian consulate in the Dominican Republic of Sandra Noriega, daughter of the jailed former president Manuel Antonio Noriega, in spite of the fact that she had been barred from holding public office for 10 years following a conviction for abusing public funds in 1996. The anti-corruption secretary again failed to comment, though

the government had specifically identified 'due levels of competence and integrity of appointees for the diplomatic and consular corps' as one of its priorities.

The civil society representative on the NCTC wrote to Arboleda in February 2005 asking him to request all public institutions to investigate possible cases of nepotism and to sanction any proven cases in line with the new code of ethics for public servants. The letter featured in the national television and print media. The following day Arboleda offered his resignation, which President Torrijos accepted. In March, Alma Montenegro de Fletcher took over the position. She was attorney general for administrative affairs from 1994 to 2004 when she created a public ethics network. She is now pushing for support at each of the public offices under her jurisdiction in order for the council's work to be more effective.

There is much scepticism about the value of the executive secretary and the NCTC, though the first steps have been taken to develop an anti-corruption plan with short-, medium- and long-term objectives. The council is well aware that it must show results soon.

Among its goals is a plan to reform Law 59, which regulates asset declarations, so that they can be properly audited. Another priority is to reform the administrative career law so that appointments are based more on merit (Panama was ranked bottom alongside El Salvador on this issue by the Inter-American Development Bank). Other possible activities are the development of whistleblower protections and citizens' complaints mechanisms.

Recently, the NCTC has required public bodies to provide information about their compliance with the government's 16 anti-corruption targets. Five of the 16 goals have been attained so far, according to research by TI Panama. Without any real reform of the justice system, however, the council's efforts are unlikely to improve domestic or international perceptions of corruption in Panama.

Pact for Justice

Panama's institutions have been in a state of crisis since January 2002 when Congressman Carlos Afú announced that he and several of his colleagues had been bribed to vote in favour of a contract between the government and a private consortium to build a Multi-modal Industrial and Service Centre (CEMIS) in the Colón Port area. Afú's colleague from the ruling Partido Revolucionario Democrático (PRD) party, Balbina Herrera, had earlier told the National Assembly plenary that he had received a US $1.5 million bribe from high-level government officials to break ranks and vote for two of Mireya Moscoso's nominees to the Supreme Court (one was a minister at the time, the other a congressman: both belonged to the Partido Arnulfista, which was then in power). Since then, various organisations have been pushing for the two judges to resign and for the congressmen who took bribes to be prosecuted. This has not happened to date.

The court closed the CEMIS case on the grounds that the congressmen had immunity when the investigation was initiated. On 30 March, the Commission for Oversight of Credentials and Judicial Affairs in the National Assembly decided not to investigate a further complaint, first aired in the media and repeated at a press conference by Judge Adán Arnulfo Arjona, who alleged that one of his colleagues consistently ruled in favour of drug traffickers.

In an attempt to retrieve the Supreme Court's crediblity, the government called together the heads of the legislature and judiciary, the two attorney generals, the ombudsman, the president of the national college of lawyers, and the civic society NGO Alianza Ciudadana Pro Justicia, to sign a 'Pact for Justice'. The pact creates a Commission of State for Justice, with 180 days to present recommendations for restructuring and modernising the judiciary and public prosecutions service. Civil society organisations and the public were given the opportunity to submit their proposals.

Some of the most important areas to be revised are:

- changes to the organisational structure, and procedures and regulations to increase the independence, efficiency and competence of the judiciary and public prosecution offices;
- improved transparency in the selection process for Supreme Court judges;
- accountability mechanisms and evaluation processes for judges, magistrates, public attorneys and public prosecutors in order to ensure that the judiciary and public prosecution budgets are properly used;
- drafting of a legal reform bill that simplifies judicial processes and makes the judicial system easier to use.

The public's attitude to the pact was initially negative because what it wanted most was concrete action, not another commission of inquiry. The proposal that generated most interest involves the selection and removal of Supreme Court judges. According to the proposal, a pre-selection committee of five civil society NGOs would send a shortlist of 15 candidates to the president, who would then select the winner. The proposal was criticised for providing too many candidates. A final draft was to be presented in September 2005, along with the commission's other proposals.

Once drafted, the reforms will still need National Assembly approval if they involve legal or constitutional reform. While the commission ponders, the complaints against the two Supreme Court judges are on hold. A report that fails to propose the deep-rooted reforms that civil society hopes for, or that meets with resistance from the government or legislature, will probably result in the two cases being reactivated – and possibly wider protest.

Angélica Maytín Justiniani (TI Panama)

Further reading

Alianza Ciudadana Pro Justicia, 'Audito ciudadano del Caso CEMIS' (Citizens' Audit of the CEMIS Case), 2004, www.alianzaprojusticia.org.pa
Fundación para el Desarrollo de la Libertad Ciudadana, 'Propuestas para fortalecer las instituciones que investigan y previenen la corrupción en Panamá' (Proposals to Strengthen Institutions that Investigate and Prevent Corruption in Panama), 2004, www.libertadciudadana.org

TI Panama: www.libertadciudadana.org

Notes

1. See www.presidencia.gob.pa and www.defensoriadelpueblo.gob.pa
2. TI Panama, 'Corruptómetro', www.transparency.org/tilac/herramientas/2001/dnld/cap03/ corruptrometro_panama.pdf

Papua New Guinea

Conventions:
UN Convention against Corruption (signed December 2004; not yet ratified)
UN Convention against Transnational Organized Crime (not yet signed)

ADB-OECD Action Plan for Asia-Pacific (endorsed November 2001)

Legal and institutional changes

- A private members' **bill to protect whistleblowers** has been drafted, but by mid-2005 had yet to be submitted to parliament for debate by its sponsor, the MP Kimson Kare. There is limited support in government for the bill.

- Parliament passed the **Proceeds of Crime Bill** in July 2005. The legislation provides measures against money laundering, including the confiscation of illegally gotten gains.

- Attempts to establish an **independent commission against corruption** (for which the *Global Corruption Report 2003* argued strongly) have again come to nothing. Despite statements of endorsement by all leading government politicians, a sponsor for the bill supporting the creation of the commission has yet to be found. The bill was tabled under the Bill Skate government, but lapsed after the demise of his administration in 1999.

- Amendments to the Forestry Act 1991 have been announced. The original act was introduced in response to the widespread corruption and **abuse in the country's timber sector** uncovered by the Barnett Commission of Inquiry. The Forestry Amendment Bill 2005 is ostensibly aimed at updating and eliminating inconsistencies in the earlier act, but there are concerns that it might generate increased opportunities for corruption. There are concerns that it concentrates authority for awarding logging permits in the forestry minister and makes it more difficult for the public to gain access to information about permits and licences. Transparency International Papua New Guinea (TI PNG) is currently monitoring the sector to see if these concerns are valid.

- The government agreed in July 2004 to create the National Anti-Corruption Alliance (NACA), a loose alliance of all the government agencies with responsibility for monitoring and fighting corruption.[1] Comprising the auditor general, the solicitor general, treasury department financial inspectors, the ombudsman commission, the police fraud squad, the public service inspectorate and provincial affairs inspectors; the alliance is intended to bring greater efficiency to the fight against corruption in public services. The NACA had a successful beginning when it visited Western Province and uncovered massive fraud in the provincial government. Seventeen provincial officials, including the governor, were successfully prosecuted as a result.

- NGOs concerned with corruption have widened their activities to cities other than the capital, Port Moresby. Representatives of the Media Council, TI PNG and the Ombudsman Commission travelled to Lae in late 2004 with a view to establishing a branch of the Community Coalition against Corruption (CCAC) there. The CCAC is a coalition of churches, youth groups, women's groups, NGOs and citizens, and claims to represent about 2 million of the country's 5.7 million population.

Audit of by-elections uncovers need for strengthening elections machinery

Detailed monitoring of three by-elections held in mid-2004 by civil society groups and the Electoral Commission has shed light on weaknesses in the legislative framework and problems in the financing of political parties.[2] These need to be addressed ahead of the 2007 general elections.

The audit was launched in response to concerns about the capacity of the electoral authorities to manage the electoral process. Some of the key worries are the influence of private funding on the election process and the transition from a first-past-the-post system to a system of limited preferential voting.

The report followed on from the findings of a team of electoral observers from TI PNG, who noted that the by-elections were in the main conducted successfully, but that their high cost cast doubts over the financial sustainability of future elections. The costs of security including a policing bill of €3.5 million (US $4.5 million) or 70 per cent of the total election cost, and of counting and administering the electoral roll were considered especially high.

The audit looked at the by-elections in greater detail, and questioned the integrity of various aspects of the election process. The electoral roll was found to contain a number of fictitious voters. In Chimbu, for example, 40 per cent more votes were counted than the entire total population for that area, according to the 2000 National Census.

The introduction of the limited preferential voting system under the 2001 Organic Law on the Integrity of Political Parties and Candidates (OLIPPAC)[3] was deemed to have successfully reduced the ethnic polarisation of voters and ensuing violence, which had become a hallmark of elections in Papua New Guinea.[4]

Administrative complexity and low voter awareness remain a concern. In terms of corruption in the financing of politics, the OLIPPAC is important in that it provides for registration of political parties and public funding of registered parties, and sets limits on contributions to parties from local and foreign sources.

Enforcement of the law has been poor, however. The Office of the Registrar of Political Parties has statutory responsibility for monitoring and enforcing the OLIPPAC, including oversight of annual returns from both individuals and parties that outline their funding sources and powers to scrutinise returns for accuracy. But the office lacks the resources needed to successfully perform these tasks. To date, a large majority of candidates and parties fail to comply with these requirements.

The Electoral Commission was a core partner for the audit, and has taken on board the findings outlined in the audit report. The government has since established a task force to reform the electoral system ahead of the 2007 elections.

Police chiefs told to curb corruption

The Internal Security Minister has given the Commissioner of Police and his senior officers until the end of 2005 to introduce a series of reforms aimed at reducing incidences of mismanagement of funds and corruption, as well as improving leadership within the police force. Failure to adopt the suggested reforms could result in disciplinary action against the police chiefs.

The reform proposals resulted from the first-ever internal review of the Royal Papua New Guinea Constabulary (RPNGC),[5] which took place between February and September 2004. The report was coordinated by a review committee made up of representatives of the Ombudsman Commission, the Chamber of Commerce, the police union, the attorney general's department and a women's representative. An external opinion was provided by a former commissioner of the Australian Federal Police.

The committee took written submissions and toured the country, taking oral submissions from police as well as the general public. It toured neighbouring Pacific Island nations and Arnhemland in northern Australia to gain first-hand knowledge of policing in comparable environments. The report was tabled in parliament and a monitoring task force is to be set up to ensure that the recommendations are not ignored.

A key finding of the report was that internal disciplinary mechanisms within the RPNGC have almost completely collapsed. Unprofessional and unethical conduct by members of the RPNGC has gone largely unpunished.[6] This has led to the loss of confidence and trust that once existed between the government, the wider community and the RPNGC.

The report called for the government to increase its support for the RPNGC, with funds as well as in official rhetoric. Progressive disinvestment by the government has left the RPNGC in a fragile state.[7] The quality of managerial leadership within the RPNGC is poor, and the report recommended setting up an Office of the Inspector General of the Constabulary to strengthen internal discipline, monitor effectiveness and audit performance across the whole of the RPNGC.

More wide-ranging recommendations addressed the need for more police officers: at present there is one police officer per 1,121 inhabitants[8] and consequently the police force draws heavily upon reserves and auxiliaries. Undisciplined and violent, the actions of poorly trained reserves and auxiliaries have cost the government dearly, in legal fees and loss of trust in the police.

Finally, the committee called for the implementation of an immunity process whereby police officers would be able to admit to less serious past misdemeanours, including acts of corruption, without the risk of prosecution for these offences. This, the committee argues, will allow police to perform their duty and enforce discipline without fear of being reported for a previous indiscretion.

Transparency International Papua New Guinea

Further reading

Steven Gosarevski, Helen Hughes and Susan Windybank, 'Is Papua New Guinea Viable?' in *Pacific Economic Bulletin* 19(1), 2004, peb.anu.edu.au/pdf/PEB19-1Hughes-policy.pdf

Helen Hughes and Susan Windybank, *Papua New Guinea's Choice: A Tale of Two Nations* (St Leonard's, NSW: Centre for Independent Studies, 2005), www.cis.org.au/IssueAnalysis/ia58/IA58.pdf

Albert Mellam and Daniel Aloi, 'National Integrity Systems TI Country Study Report, Papua New Guinea, 2003', www.transparency.org/activities/nat_integ_systems/dnld/pap_new_guinea_25.09.03.pdf

Mekere Morauta, 'The Papua New Guinea–Australia Relationship', *Pacific Economic Bulletin* 20(1), 2005, peb.anu.edu.au/pdf/PEB20-1morauta.pdf

TI Papua New Guinea: www.transparencypng.org.pg

Notes

1. www1.oecd.org/daf/asiacom/pdf/refpro_2impcyc_papuanewguinea1.pdf
2. The audit was conducted by TI PNG, the Institute of National Affairs (PNG), the Institute of Policy Studies of New Zealand and the PNG Electoral Commission.
3. This change of voting systems was just one of a number of important changes brought in by the OLIPPAC, which was aimed primarily at reducing post-election 'horse trading' and vote-buying in the legislature.
4. www.thenational.com.pg/0607/nation2.htm
5. *The Age* (Australia), 19 November 2004. Full report available at www.inapng.com/Police%20R eview%20Report%20final.pdf
6. The review was not mandated to investigate individual cases of unprofessional and unethical conduct, and thus did not pursue them beyond its own terms of reference.
7. The review stated explicitly that the low salaries were an issue for police misconduct. The minister responded in early 2005 by raising police salaries by an average of about 10 per cent.
8. The UN recommended police:population ratio is 1:450. Police:population ratios for other jurisdictions are: Fiji, 1:550; Solomon Islands, 1:500; Queensland 1:475; and Northern Territory of Australia 1:280.

Peru

Conventions:

OAS Inter-American Convention against Corruption (ratified June 1997)
UN Convention against Corruption (ratified November 2004)
UN Convention against Transnational Organized Crime (ratified January 2002)

Legal and institutional changes

- Reforms to the **penal code and code of criminal procedures** were approved in July 2004 and will enter into force in February 2006. They make it easier for prosecuting judges to prepare their final reports and broaden the instances in which preventative detention can be used to include complicated cases where more than 10 people are implicated (thus reducing the number of suspects implicated in the drawn-out corruption cases benefiting from house arrest or release under bail). Sanctions for public officials found guilty of corruption have been increased and a clear difference established between those who propose or extort a corrupt transaction – who will receive on average four years more than under the previous sanctions regime; and those who carry out the corrupt act – who face a sentence of two years more than before. Sentences for illicit enrichment are also increased to 8–18 years for senior public officials.

- A new law on **state contracts and acquisitions** was adopted in July 2004 and secondary regulations implementing it entered into force in December. The law contains details of an online system of state contracts (SEACE) that has been in development since 2002. It clarifies which bodies come under the law's jurisdiction; creates a national register of providers; broadens the list of grounds for disqualification from state contracts; increases the 'cooling-off' period for former public officials who wish to enter into contracts with the state; declares void any contracting processes that are not included in the annual purchasing plans of state institutions; and clarifies which supply contracts qualify as 'urgent', and therefore can be issued without tenders, because the institution would be paralysed without them. The main flaw is that there is no need to prove what kind of situation qualifies as 'urgent'.

- The law governing the **Financial Intelligence Unit** (UIF) was modified in July 2004, and grants it new powers to request any information from any public institution (previously it could only request information about suspect transactions). The modification also increases its sphere of operations to include the prevention and detection of financing of terrorism, and increases cooperation with international organisations and other domestic public institutions. The reform was criticised for reducing the UIF's independence, however, because the head of the body will now be directly responsible to the cabinet and not the superintendent for banking and insurance (SBS), which is constitutionally independent. The body's financing has been restricted to funds provided by the treasury, funds recovered from the Fujimori regime (which are limited) and fines imposed by the UIF.

- The **Congressional Ethics Commission** was reformed in September 2004 in an attempt to bolster its poor performance. Since it was created in March 2003, it had failed to find fault with a single MP in spite of the dozens of complaints brought to its attention. It now consists of seven MPs under a new president. Since it was reformed, the commission recommended a 120-day suspension for an MP who assaulted a government official, but Congress later reduced the sanction.

- A **commission created by Justice Minister Blado Kresalja** in May 2004 to design an anti-corruption programme (see *Global Corruption Report 2005*) collapsed in July, following the minister's resignation in opposition to a new media law that allows up to 40 per cent foreign ownership of Peru's radio and television stations.

- A complaints and redress commission for corrupt acts committed by teachers, school directors or officials related to the **education sector in Lima** was created in February 2005.

Attempts to dismantle Fujimori's machinery foiled

After four years of legal and political struggle against the criminal mafia led by former president Alberto Fujimori and his close adviser, Vladimiro Montesinos, there have been some important achievements, albeit partial ones. By September 2004, 201 cases had been opened involving more than 1,400 suspects, and US $175 million had been recovered. The investigation has now entered a second, crucial stage, focusing on the state's ability to sanction those responsible. Successful convictions at this stage would go a long way towards overcoming the widespread public perception that impunity is the rule in Peru, not the exception.

The government's reluctance to tackle the roots of corruption was confirmed during the course of investigations led by Luis Vargas, who headed the Fujimori–Montesinos inquiry, when he discovered clear links between a member of President Alejandro Toledo's inner circle and a leading figure in the organisation that looted so much of Peru's wealth in the 1990s. The investigations revealed that César Almeyda, Toledo's friend, adviser and former lawyer, had had communications with former general Oscar Villanueva, also known as Montesinos' 'treasurer'. The evidence supplied was a recorded conversation in which Almeyda allegedly offered Villanueva improved prison conditions in exchange for information that could be used against Toledo's political enemies. Villanueva committed suicide when this recording was made public in September 2002. The conversation implicated those at the highest levels of power and Toledo was unable to prevent Almeyda's subsequent arrest. However, the case didn't stop there.

Vargas wanted to take charge of the new investigation to determine how far the tentacles of the Fujimori–Montesinos network had penetrated the current administration. The government expressed its trenchant opposition, arguing that the special investigator's office had been created solely to deal with events from 1990 to 2000 and that its remit should not go beyond that period. The auditor general, public prosecutor and head of the legal defence council all supported the government's position, but Justice Minister Baldo Kresalja was reportedly in favour of widening the terms of reference initially, though he later changed his mind.

Relations between the investigating team and the government deteriorated further after the media revealed in July 2004 that Perú Posible, the ruling party, had allegedly falsified hundreds of thousands of signatures in order to register as a new party in time for the 2001 general elections. This had apparently been achieved because of the party's close links to the Oficina Nacional de Procesos Electorales (ONPE), the electoral body, which was still under the control of Fujimori and Montesinos (see below).

Vargas' term of office was due to expire in October 2004, though officials had already suggested he be replaced during a smear campaign that had belittled the results of his inquiry, and his failures to secure more convictions or extradite Fujimori from Japan.[1] Vargas' term could easily have ended there and then were it not for a large public demonstration and several opinion polls that showed most Peruvians wanted him to stay. Public opinion won

through, but his contract was renewed for only three months, after which Antonio Maldonado was appointed the new special investigator.

A number of Vargas' team resigned in protest, citing their concern that Maldonado would not tackle in sufficient depth either the Almeyda case or the allegation of signature faking, because they involved the investigation of highly placed politicians.

The conviction that the corrupt enjoy immunity from prosecution is strong among the population, as evidenced by the annual opinion poll conducted by the anti-corruption NGO, Proética, which found that 79 per cent of respondents believe that corruption charges do not lead to any form of sanctions, and 83 per cent think corruption will be as bad or worse in five years time.

With its reputation tarnished by alleged links to the Fujimori regime, the government is caught dangerously off-balance. Torn between the desire to protect the president and his party, and a public commitment to punish corruption, it chose to emasculate its special investigation team, rather than risk opening itself up to further enquiry.

Toledo's reaction to the case of the 'signature factory'

The Toledo government's precarious popularity with voters (his approval rating at the time of writing hovered at 10 per cent) was further damaged by news that signatures had been falsified to qualify the ruling party to fight the 2001 election.

Among the methods allegedly employed by Perú Posible was the creation of a 'signature factory', staffed by personnel hired by the party chiefs who were charged with 'manufacturing' the 500,000 signatures required by law to register a new party.

Since July 2004, a string of further revelations has come to light. A key witness appeared, then disappeared in a mysterious manner; retracted his original statement; then later accused politicians of involvement in his disappearance, implicating a number of officials along the way. While this saga continued, other witnesses stepped forward with contradictory statements and another signature factory was discovered, linked to Congressman Rafael Rey and his Code-Renovación party. Rey was well known for his pro-Fujimori stance in the 1990s, but claims to have severed links with the regime.

This last revelation created the impression that the majority of parties engaged in falsifying signatures and other forms of corruption to compete in the election. Indeed, Fujimori and Montesinos were both reported to control the electoral commission, the ONPE and the national elections jury (JNE). This view was reinforced when Heriberto Benítez, one of five members of a parliamentary commission set up to investigate the signature factories, proposed a blanket amnesty for all parties implicated in order to avert a crisis in the political system. Housing minister Carlos Bruce accepted that Perú Posible had falsified signatures, but defended it on the grounds that the ends – defeating the Fujimori regime – justified the means.

The commission had made little progress by the time it presented its conclusions in May 2005. The members agreed that the leaders of Perú Posible, including President Toledo, were responsible, but failed to agree on what sanctions to impose. One of the commission's aims had been to question President Toledo, but the request was denied. He eventually did agree to attend on condition that the meeting was not recorded, a decision that confirmed to many his unwillingness to collaborate with the commission. The case has now been sent to the public prosecutor's office.

The case – and Congress' failure to punish those responsible – can only contribute to the low regard in which the electorate holds political parties in Peru. A poll by Lima University in 2003 showed that 81 per cent of citizens do not trust political parties.

Samuel Rotta Castilla and Leonardo Narvarte Olivares (Proética)

Further reading

Beatriz Boza, *Acceso a la información del Estado: Marco legal y buenas prácticas* (Access to State Information: Legal Framework and Good Practices) (Lima: Fundación Konrad Adenauer, 2004)

Defensoría del Pueblo, 'Índice de Buen Gobierno. Resultados del IBG aplicado a los Gobiernos Regionales en el Perú: enero 2003–junio 2004' (Good Governance Index: Results of the Index Applied to the First Six Months' Administration of the Regional Governments in Peru: January 2003–June 2004) (Lima: Defensoría del Pueblo, 2004)

Instituto Prensa y Sociedad (IPYS), *Acceso a la Información de las Entidades del Sector Salud* (Access to Information in Health Sector Bodies) (Lima: IPYS, 2004)

Felipe Portocarrero S. (ed.), *El Pacto Infame. Estudios sobre la corrupción en Perú* (The Infamous Pact: Studies on Corruption in Peru) (Lima: Red para el Desarrollo de las Ciencias Sociales en el Perú, 2005)

Proética, 'III Conferencia Nacional Anticorrupción' (Third National Anti-corruption Conference), Lima, 2005, transcripts of proceedings published at www.proetica.org.pe/Descaragas/Conclusiones%20Finales%20TALLERES%20III%20Conferencia.doc

Proética (TI Peru): www.proetica.org.pe

Note

1. See *Global Corruption Report 2004*. At the time of writing, the Japanese authorities were examining an extradition request filed in late 2004. Analysts expected the request to be rejected since Fujimori holds Japanese citizenship and Japan does not extradite nationals. While banned under the constitution from standing in the next election, Fujimori has said that he is still considering a political role.

Poland

Conventions:
Council of Europe Civil Law Convention on Corruption (ratified September 2002)
Council of Europe Criminal Law Convention on Corruption (ratified December 2002)
OECD Anti-Bribery Convention (ratified September 2000)
UN Convention against Corruption (signed December 2003; not yet ratified)
UN Convention against Transnational Organized Crime (ratified November 2001)

Legal and institutional changes

- Parliament adopted an **amendment to the law governing MPs and senators** in January 2005 that came into force in mid-May. Under new provisions, parliamentarians who have been arrested or imprisoned will automatically be deprived of their rights and obligations as representatives, including remuneration. There is a right of appeal. The amendment was introduced following a series of criminal cases and scandals involving MPs (see below).

- In a bid to eliminate **corruption in the courts**, the Sejm (lower house) approved a bill in September 2004 giving citizens the right to lodge a complaint against drawn-out proceedings in criminal, civil and administrative cases. The provision was adopted after Polish claims at the European Human Rights Tribunal in Strasbourg rose to a record 5,784 in 2004, mostly as a result of tardy court processes. Poland's old-fashioned case registration system gives poorly paid court clerks wide discretionary power to influence the order of proceedings.

- An **act on freedom of economic activity** was passed in August 2004 limiting tax officials' ability to exploit their power for bribes. Business start-ups now require fewer permits to commence trading and the law prevents tax offices from conducting more than one audit at a time, unless an official investigation is in progress.

- An amendment to the law preventing assets from illegal sources from entering the financial system, which was passed after the 9/11 terrorist attacks, entered into force in July 2004, **further tightening financial regulation**. Financial institutions, the National Deposit of Securities, the lottery, the postal system, public notaries, real estate agents and others are required to register any transaction exceeding €15,000 (US $19,000) with the authorities and to notify the General Inspector of Financial Information on a monthly basis of any suspicious deals.

- By December 2004, all provincial police forces had established **specialised anti-corruption departments**. The first was established in Silesia in 2000. The units provide police with a set of new tools for combating corruption, including aiding whistleblowers, for example through 'controlled bribery' (when, under a court order, police provide whistleblowers with marked banknotes, a tape-recorder or camera to catch a public official extorting a bribe). The new methods may have already begun to have an impact. In the first quarter of 2005, police initiated 1,664 investigations of corruption, compared to 2,825 throughout 2003.

Lay judges tamed, but still powerful

The judiciary has been criticised for many years for its lengthy proceedings and perceived corruption. Files went missing, cases were barred before entering the docket and verdicts were delivered on the basis of false evidence. The judges were not exclusively to blame. Public attention has recently focused on dishonest court experts who falsify evidence and corrupt lay judges who are available for hire. Lay judges are members of the panels that preside over the criminal, family and labour courts. In the three-person panel system used in Polish courts, the two lay judges exert a decisive influence. According to the 2001 law that defines their conditions, any citizen of 'impeccable character', who has lived for a year in the place where the court presides, is qualified to become a lay judge. 'Organisations', trade unions, presidents of courts or groups of 25 citizens can all put forward a candidate who must prove that he or she does not have a criminal record. *Gmina* (municipality) councils elect lay judges for a four-year term of office.

The current regulations concerning lay judges, based on those of the communist legal regime, are seriously deficient. For a start, the existing law does not adequately define the term 'organisation', with the result that political parties nominate their own candidates to administer local justice. In some *gminas*, councillors from different parties agree on the quota of judges each will appoint. They or their family members can also assume this influential post, as do people against whom penal proceedings are pending in other districts. According to the presidents of Poland's district courts, as many as 135 criminal court proceedings had been completed or were in progress against lay judges in March 2004.

Though irregularities in the election of lay judges have been commonplace since the early 1990s, the issue rarely captured the public's interest. This changed after the last election in late 2003. In June 2004, the administrative court in Łódá declared that the appointment of lay judges by the city council of Łód was against the law. The Administrative Court in Cracow overruled one election in July 2004 on the grounds that not all the elected lay judges had the appropriate police recommendations. In July 2004, the administrative head of Mazowieckie region overruled a resolution in Legionowo because political parties had recommended the judges for election (though the law does not actually prohibit this).

The question of lay judges' political affiliations became the focus of media attention in the same year. As a result, the government prepared a draft amendment to the law on the structure of the common courts that was submitted to parliament in March 2005. Under this bill, lay judges, like professional judges, will henceforth be apolitical. The draft amendment also limits the participation of lay judges in the administration of justice. They will not participate in cases related to social insurance and their involvement in family cases will be much reduced. Candidates for the post will have to provide a statement to the effect that no criminal proceeding is underway against them. The draft provisions also require that candidates have attained a secondary education, at the very least.

The adoption of the amendment is expected to improve the situation, as will a justice ministry instruction in August 2004 that bars councillors from standing as lay judges. Opinion varies from wanting to abolish lay judges entirely to arguments that politicians should not be responsible for the election of lay judges for fear of nepotism and cronyism.

Tackling the log roll

In May 2005, the Sejm adopted an amendment to the acts on the civil service and on local government aimed at ending the widespread practice of 'log rolling' whereby every election is followed by a major turnover of personnel at every level of state and local hierarchies. The basis of recruitment is often kinship, party affiliation and ties of friendship with those in power. This nepotism in the administration produces a lower quality of public service and makes the oversight of office operations difficult.

Under new regulations, information about vacancies in the civil service and local administration must be published, specifying the requirements of any given position and the relevant dates of the recruitment procedure. The list of candidates meeting the criteria must also be published, along with the name of the winner and a justification for why he or she was selected. The procedures are binding on all government institutions.

The amendment is a step in the right direction, but more decisive legislation is required if the forced rotation of experienced personnel is not to impact on the quality of administration and even the economy. The new law does not provide sufficient safeguards against the detrimental practice of awarding public tenders to companies owned by relatives of local officials. Further measures are required to restrict another harmful log rolling of reserving top managerial posts in state or municipally owned companies for members of the winning party.

Some local governments have begun to understand that good governance is also a route to political success and are introducing transparent standards of operation on their own initiative, despite the dearth of official regulations. In 2004, the head of the administration of Pabianice introduced competitive procedures to the recruitment of public officials. At the end of 2004, two competitions to fill vacancies in the administration were announced and the requirement details were published on the Internet and the local bulletin board.

In early 2005, the Pabianice administration issued six more regulations to align its policy with EU standards. In addition to the competitive recruitment process, the district now possesses formal rules for performance assessment, remuneration and career advancement, and an ethical code for its officials. Similar changes are being introduced by a group of *gminas* in Wielkopolska, in collaboration with TI Poland.

MPs above the law

A number of high-profile cases involving Polish politicians have come to light. Zbigniew Sobotka, former deputy minister of internal affairs and administration, Henryk Długosz and Andrzej Jagiełło, both senior officials in the regional organisation of the ruling Democratic Left Alliance (SLD), were sentenced in January 2005 to three and a half, two, and one and a half years in prison respectively for leaking information of an organised raid to a criminal ring in Starachowice which the police had targeted. Another MP and former leader of the SLD's Łódzkie chapter, Andrzej Pęczak, was arrested in 2004 on charges of corruption. Court proceedings are underway against Renata Beger, a deputy from the radical Samoobrona party, and Józef Skowyra, from the right-wing League of Polish Families. Both Beger and Skowyra were charged with forging signatures on lists supporting their candidatures for the elections. MPs' involvement in crime opened a debate on the need to limit their rights, which remain largely intact even after imprisonment. Following public pressure, parliament adopted an amendment to the law on the performance of MPs and senators in January 2005. The new provisions strip arrested or imprisoned MPs of their obligations and rights, including their salaries. However, the amendment does not apply to sentenced MPs who are still eligible for appeal. This legislation did not therefore affect the three MPs arrested in the Starachowice case, who carried on as usual. Furthermore, even after the arrest and imprisonment of an MP, they still retain their mandate and immunity. Under the constitution, fresh charges can only be brought with the approval of the Sejm.

The criminal scandals swirling around Polish MPs led to calls for a ban on anyone with a criminal record from standing for parliament. A group of MPs from the left-wing Polish Social Democrats tried to change the constitution in March 2005 by adding a clause excluding from parliament anyone sentenced for intentional crimes and crimes prosecuted ex officio. The initiative failed due to the lack of the required number of signatures. The Sejm's legislative committee took another approach to the problem. It proposed giving courts the power to deprive a sentenced person of the right to stand for parliament. This initiative also failed to win the necessary support. MPs are now discussing a third possibility in the form of a legal obligation to publish information if a candidate for parliament has been logged in the register of convicted persons.

Julia Pitera (TI Poland)

Further reading

EU Acccession Monitoring Programme of the Open Society Institute, *Korupcja i polityka antykorupcyjna. Raporty krajowe. Polska* (Corruption and Anti-corruption Policy) (Warsaw: EU Accession Monitoring Programme, Open Society Institute, 2002)

Maria Jarosz, *Władza, przywileje, korupcja* (Power, Privileges and Corruption) (Warsaw: Wydawnictwo Naukowe PWN, 2004)

Wojciech Krupa, Marzena Rogalska and Maciej Wnuk, *Elementy korupcjogenne w wybranych przepisach prawnych regulujących funkcjonowanie samorządu gminnego* (Corruption-generating Elements in Selected Legal Provisions Regulating the Functioning of *Gmina*-level Self-government) (Warsaw: TI Poland, 2003)

Celina Nowak, *Dostosowanie prawa polskiego do instrumentów mi dzynarodowych dotycz cych korupcji* (Adaptation of Polish Law to the International Instruments Concerning Corruption) (Warsaw: Fundacja Batorego, 2004)

TI Poland: www.transparency.pl

Romania

Conventions:
Council of Europe Civil Law Convention on Corruption (ratified April 2002)
Council of Europe Criminal Law Convention on Corruption (ratified July 2002; Additional Protocol ratified November 2004)
UN Convention against Corruption (ratified November 2004)
UN Convention against Transnational Organized Crime (ratified December 2002)

Legal and institutional changes

- An 'urgency ordinance' in February 2005 waived the **immunity protections of members of the former government** in line with the recommendations of the Council of Europe's Group of States against Corruption (GRECO), paving the way for prosecution of past corruption crimes (see below). But there are categories of people who still benefit from immunity. Under a modification to the law on the legal profession in June 2004, lawyers cannot be prosecuted or indicted without the approval of the general prosecutor of the court of appeal where they are registered.

- A law on the **protection of whistleblowers**, passed in December 2004, improves safeguards for public employees who disclose breaches of the law inside the institutions where they work. It guarantees whistleblowers disciplinary and administrative protection in the event of retaliation by their administrative superiors or colleagues, and introduces an inverted burden of proof whereby a whistleblower is legally presumed to be in good faith, requiring the accused to bring evidence to rebut the allegations made. Critics have pointed out that this might make the law a platform for frustrated civil servants to denounce or harass their superiors. Another strong point of the law is that whistleblowers can report to a wider array of public and private authorities than is usual in most Western whistleblower acts.[1] The law's effectiveness will depend on raising awareness of its existence and raising the level of trust among civil servants.

- An amendment to the law on the **prevention, disclosure and punishment of corrupt acts**, passed in November 2004, closes an important gap in the criminal law framework. Before the amendment was adopted, criminal law treated certain acts of corruption as crimes of abuse, which were often converted in court into crimes of negligence and sanctioned with fines rather than imprisonment. For example, if a civil servant took or refused a decision to grant an authorisation or a lease against the rules, incurring damage to a party, it would be treated as a crime of abuse, irrespective of the personal benefits obtained by the civil servant or a third party. The sanction for these crimes will now be 3–15 years in prison, as in bribe-taking cases.

- An amendment of the Criminal Procedure Code, passed in November 2004, widens the **plaintiff's litigation guarantees** by introducing the mandatory motivation and communication of all prosecutorial decisions in a case. This gives the plaintiff legal backing to attack any prosecution decision that runs counter to law. The modification is particularly relevant for situations in which the prosecution refuses to start, drops or suspends criminal proceedings on unjustified grounds, allowing criminals to escape prosecution.

- A law published in July 2004 provides a **new legal framework for gifts** received by dignitaries, magistrates and civil servants during the course of their duties. All goods received in 'protocol activities' must be declared to the head of the relevant department within 30 days of receipt. When their value exceeds €200 (US $240), the beneficiary can either surrender them to a special commission or keep them, having first reimbursed their cost. Any gifts worth less than €200 may be retained. The law does not provide similar provisions for services of protocol which may include trips, bursaries, and events and so on, that may amount to important sums of money. Nor does it provide a mechanism for monitoring or sanctioning false declarations or the potential refusal to declare gifts.

- A law on the running of the Superior Council of Magistracy (CSM) was adopted in July 2004 as part of a package intended to meet the EU accession requirement of an **effective and independent judiciary**.[2] The amendments mainly targeted the career path and disciplinary responsibility of magistrates, which were placed definitively under the auspices of the CSM. Other responsibilities formerly held by the justice minister and now transferred to the CSM include decisions on the establishment or dissolution of courts; acts regarding the organisation of the judiciary; and the budgets of courts and prosecutors' offices. The CSM has financial autonomy[3] and may initiate draft laws that relate to the functioning of the judiciary (see below).

- The National Anti-Corruption Prosecution Office (PNA) continued to draw fire for its performance in 2004. A **23 per cent increase in personnel** (prosecutors, judicial police and other experts) authorised in April 2004[4] was offset by the decision to simultaneously broaden the PNA's mandate to include smaller acts of corruption.[5] This stretched the agency's capacity to breaking point. By the end of 2004, the government intervened with another ordinance that restored the bribe threshold to €5,000 (US $6,000), still well above its original level. Under the judicial reform package outlined above, PNA does not answer to any state authorities (see below).[6]

EU membership depends on anti-corruption drive

Romania's hopes for accession to the EU in 2007 depend on it discovering remedies to its deep-seated problems of corruption and the rule of law. The judicial reform package, adopted in July 2004, alleviated some concerns over the independence of the judiciary, but qualms remain as to whether the new government of President Traian Basescu will implement its framework on time. The anti-corruption programme is on much thinner ice as debates in the European Parliament showed in December 2004. Recent strategy has been designed to secure signature of the EU Accession Treaty, which it did in April 2005, but the lack of convincing progress in the fight against grand corruption could trigger a 'delay clause' that puts back EU entry for one year.

MEPs' doubts about Romania's fitness to join the Union were encapsulated in the *Report on Romania's Progress towards Accession*, presented by parliamentary rapporteur Pierre Moscovici in December 2004. He noted the low rate of successful high-level corruption prosecutions and urged Romania to resume its campaign. More critical voices could be heard in the chamber after accession negotiations ended two days later. One MEP submitted a motion for the reopening of negotiations on the grounds that Romania was incapable of tackling its problems by the date of the treaty signature.[7] The motion was rejected.

The newly elected government took office later that month with a mission to resolve these concerns. President Basescu paid calls on all the authorities responsible for combating corruption – the CSM, PNA, intelligence services – to insist on their full and effective cooperation, and warned that

corruption was now a threat to national security.[8] He stressed his support for the independence of the magistracy and appointed a non-political figure to head the justice ministry as a sign of that support.[9] Basescu's get-tough approach contrasted sharply with that of his predecessor, Ion Iliescu, who was characterised as a 'passive' president surrounded by controversial associates. After this, heads began to roll in the police force and elsewhere in the administration, a move that the opposition Social Democratic Party (PSD) called 'political dismissals'. Another significant decision was to waive immunity for crimes committed by former ministers while in office (see above). Concurrently, a spate of arrests, investigations and prosecutions scooped up a number of high-level figures in the business and administrative world related to the former and present governments.[10]

In February 2005, the justice ministry ordered an independent audit of the first National Anti-Corruption Strategy (2001–04) as part of a pledge to the EU to provide a future basis for anti-corruption measures in the run-up to accession.[11] Its findings broadly reflected those reached by the EU's parliamentary rapporteur, but it reserved particular scorn for the PNA, which it called inefficient, and the previous administration, which it accused of influencing the judiciary in its fight against corruption. The report was well received by the public, the government and EU institutions alike, but officials from the institutions it targeted and the PSD criticised its 'lack of professionalism'.

In March 2005, the government approved a new anti-corruption roadmap focusing on three fronts – prevention, sanctions and institutional cooperation – with measures ranging from the strengthening of freedom of information legislation to restructuring the CSM and PNA, to tightening anti-money laundering laws. The strategy also envisions the creation of a new agency to check asset declarations and conflicts of interest and to monitor the implementation of the law on the protection of whistleblowers. The government's plan of action was unveiled amid considerable fanfare and against a backdrop of intense public discussion about corruption and the future of Romania.

On the day the government approved the anti-corruption strategy, the Romanian president stated that he was backing reform of an 'inefficient and corrupt' judiciary.[12] This statement marked a new turn in the president's attitude towards public authorities, in particular the judiciary, and raised eyebrows among advocates of judicial independence.

President Basescu has indicated a change of direction, but has yet to start to turn the corner. Time is short for Romania, but the goal of a speedy EU accession should not be grounds for riding roughshod over the judiciary or the existing legal framework.

Romania's infrastructure nightmares

There are roughly 200 km of highways in Romania which has a similar surface area to Italy, where there are 6,000 km of highways. Among its EU commitments, Bucharest must build some 1,500 km of highways under the 'Pan-European Corridor IV' that links Germany with Turkey through the Czech Republic and Hungary at a total cost of €2 billion (US $2.4 billion). Under the programme, Romania is due to build a highway from Arad in the west to the Black Sea port of Constanta by 2015.

Despite these commitments, the previous government decided to invest in a highway running parallel to the 'Pan-European Corridor' from Oradea to Brasov, in the centre of the country. In late 2003, it announced the signature of a contract with US company Bechtel, at a cost of roughly US $2.5 billion. However, there was no public procurement

bid for the tender,[13] even though it was the largest motorway project in Europe. Moreover, the contract was signed a few months before Romania was given the green light for entry into NATO in March 2004.[14]

After signing the Bechtel deal, the government embarked on a raft of contracts without orthodox procurement procedures. One of the most controversial was with the Franco-German-Spanish consortium European Aeronautic Defence and Space (EADS) to secure the national borders at a cost of around €1 billion (US $1.2 billion). The contract was classified as secret and awarded without a public tender.[15] The EADS contract was signed in August 2004, a few months before Romania needed to close the EU accession negotiations under very difficult conditions. Smaller contracts followed, including one with French company Vinci, also signed without a public tender, to build a motorway between Bucharest and Brasov.

After the elections in November 2004, the new government rescinded all contracts signed outside normal procurement regulations by the previous administration. After the contractors complained, the government agreed to renegotiate terms with Bechtel and EADS so as to make conditions fairer for Romania.[16] Both companies accepted this compromise, which raised questions about the soundness of the original contracts.

The government has made an effort to bring in those responsible for the questionable contracts. In June 2005, the administration and interior minister, Vasile Blaga, announced that he had launched a criminal investigation against several heads of the police, within the ministry, for a suspected breach of the basic requirements of public procurement legislation.[17] Prime Minister Tariceanu in turn announced an investigation would be initiated against the former transport minister, Miron Mitrea, to probe irregularities in the Bechtel contract.[18] Both contracts have been criticised by EU officials for breach of procurement requirements. At this writing, the investigations were still ongoing and no prosecutions had been made. But the lifting of former ministers' immunity in early 2005 (see above) opened the way for prosecutions.

The stakes are indeed high: the renegotiation of past contracts that flouted the rule of open, competitive bidding, the initiation of criminal investigations against officials in charge of shady contracts and a marked improvement in the handling of future contracts will be critical if Romania is to receive a green light for EU entry.

Adrian Savin (TI Romania)

Further reading

Freedom House, 'The Anti-Corruption Policy of the Romanian Government: Assessment Report', (Washington, DC: Freedom House, 2005), available at www.gov.ro/engleza/presa/documente/200503/FH_Audit_EN_16_031.pdf

Government of Romania, *National Anti-Corruption Strategy* (Bucharest: Government of Romania, 2005), available at www.just.ro/files/lupta_anti_coruptie/Lupta%20anticoruptie/National%20Anticorruption%20Strategy.htm

Transparency International Romania, *Raportul Naţional asupra Corupţiei 2005* (National Corruption Report – 2005) (Bucharest: TI Romania, 2005), www.transparency.org.ro/doc/rnac2005_ro.pdf

TI Romania: www.transparency.org.ro

Notes

1. These authorities include the immediate superior, head of institution, disciplinary commissions within the institution, public prosecutions bodies, parliamentary commissions, the media, NGOs, unions, professional associations and employers' associations.
2. The other two laws in the judicial reform package were on the statute of magistrates and the organisation of the judiciary.
3. The CSM elaborates its own budget in consultation with the finance minister.
4. The institution's capacity to fight corruption was hampered from the outset because it employed fewer than 100 prosecutors for the entire country.
5. The bribe 'threshold' that mandates a PNA investigation was lowered from €10,000 (US $13,000) to €3,000 (US $4,000).
6. Amendments to the law on the judiciary passed in July 2005 altered this. PNA must now present an annual report to the Superior Council of the Magistracy and justice ministry, giving them more authority over the institution. The justice ministry can also forward the report to parliament for further discussion.
7. www.euractiv.ro, 2 March 2005.
8. www.euractiv.ro, 29 December 2004.
9. Before being appointed Minister of Justice, Monica Macovei was executive director of the Association for the Defense of Human Rights, Helsinki Committee.
10. *Ziua* (Romania), 30 March 2005.
11. The audit report was written by Freedom House (see 'Further reading').
12. See www.gov.ro/engleza/presa/afis-doc.php?idpresa=4712&idrubricapresa=&idrubricaprimm=&idtema=&tip=&pag=1&dr=
13. *The Economist* (UK), 15 April 2004.
14. *Financial Times* (UK), 2 February 2004.
15. *Financial Times* (UK), 23 February 2005.
16. Prime Minister Calin Popescu Tariceanu was quoted as saying the renegotiation with EADS saved the budget about €150 million (US $180 million), according to ProVest TV, 26 June 2005.
17. Press release of the Romanian Ministry of Administration and Interior, 15 June 2005.
18. *ZiarulFinanciar* (Romania), 27 June 2005.

Serbia

NB: This report does not cover developments in Montenegro or Kosovo

Conventions:
Council of Europe Civil Law Convention on Corruption (signed April 2005; not yet ratified)
Council of Europe Criminal Law Convention on Corruption (ratified December 2002)
UN Convention against Corruption (signed December 2003; not yet ratified)
UN Convention against Transnational Organized Crime (ratified September 2001)

Legal and institutional changes

- After considerable delay, parliament adopted the **law on access to information** in November 2004.[1] The law introduces the public right to any information held by the government, local authorities, public enterprises and all other agencies or organisations financed by the state, unless it can be legally shown there is an overriding interest in not disclosing the information. Statutory exemptions include the protection of life, health and security of persons, the judiciary, national security, public safety, economic welfare and classified information. Even in such cases, grounds for denying access must be cross-checked against a clause in the law that requires that the interest in question could not be otherwise protected in accordance with the standards of a 'democratic society'. The law also provides for fines for violations and the creation of the post of Commissioner for Information of Public Importance as a decision-making and appeals body (see below).

- The **Board for Resolving Conflict of Interest**, envisaged under legislation adopted in April 2004, was assembled in December 2004 through a combination of judicial appointments and parliamentary votes. Given that most of the April law could not be implemented without a full board, critics suspected that the delay in filling the nine-member panel was not mere negligence or poor pre-session negotiation between parliamentary groups, but rather a sign of a lack of political will to see the law implemented. Despite lacking premises and funding, the board produced its first significant output in March 2005 with new regulations for implementing the law and detailed forms for public officials' property and income disclosure (see below).

Anti-corruption laws: lip service or business as usual?

Serbia's law on access to information largely survived its passage through parliament, though the right of appeal against decisions of the 'highest state authorities' (such as the president, government, parliament, Supreme Court, and so on) concerning access and provisions to protect whistleblowers was absent. It also fails to apply to the institutions of the Serbia and Montenegro State Union, though they are almost entirely financed from Serbia's budget.[2] However, the essence of the original, drafted by an NGO, the Centre for Advanced Legal Studies, remains. In addition to guarantees of free access to any information held by the executive, legislature, judiciary, local government, public enterprises and other institutions financed by the state or local government – with the usual exemptions – the law obliges the relevant authorities to publish an annual directory containing the most important data on their activities, and encourages them to publish data on the Internet.[3] With all its imperfections, the law represents a significant addition to the statute book and a potential blueprint for root-and-branch reform of public administration and the government–citizen relationship.

Given the international community's interest in Serbia's institutional evolution, legislation is often introduced more to comply with external pressure than to meet domestic needs. The implementation of laws adopted under these conditions is often weak. This applies equally to the information law and much of the anti-corruption legislation adopted in recent years.

Early evidence of this comes from the fact that parliamentary discussion of the draft law on information was chiefly confined to disputes between two opposition parties, the Serbian Radical Party and the Democratic Party. MPs from pro-government parties, by contrast, mainly abstained, either because they did not wish to unsettle relations in the coalition, or because they never considered the effects of the law and were thus uninterested in its details.

Since the law's entry into force in November 2004, the authorities have done little to make it function smoothly. No funds were allocated to implement it in the 2005 budget although Rodoljub Sabic, vice-president of the Social Democrat Party, one of the ruling coalition members, was elected to the post of commissioner in December 2004 (he resigned from the party after his nomination). No office was assigned to Sabic until April 2005 and he had to pay the cost of his official stamp himself. Though neither corruption nor obstruction was necessarily to blame for depriving the new law of 'teeth', its neglect certainly pointed to a lack of strategy and care.

According to research undertaken by TI Serbia during the first quarter of 2005, only 65 per cent of ministries, 33 per cent of public enterprises and 19 per cent of local governments responded to requests for information about the measures taken to implement the law by the end of March.[4] The percentage of those that had appointed staff to deal with public requests for information was far lower.

Salaries of public officials: between populist policy and need to prevent corruption

Over the past four years, political discussion has often turned to the need for an appropriate level of salary to ensure the integrity of officials entrusted with power over decision-making. The existing system is anchored in a 'basic' wage, established by the government or National Assembly, supplemented by 'coefficients' based on the responsibility of the post, level of education, working conditions and job complexity. This works out to an average public sector salary of around €190 (US $230) per month, which is no disincentive to bribery or other forms of corruption.[5]

The coalition government that ruled after the overthrow of Slobodan Milošević in 2001 opted to pay its members modest, uncompetitive salaries out of deference to public sensitivity. Attitudes to salary have altered since the new coalition government assumed power in March 2004.[6] Ironically, the law on the prevention of conflict of interest, in force since July 2004, is partly to blame since it eliminated the legal means whereby officials boosted their salaries by barring them from working for private companies, consultancies or managing their own enterprises. In October 2004, 205 of the 250 MPs sought a salary increase through a new law, only to encounter a furious reaction from the public that led to the withdrawal of what was otherwise a necessary piece of legislation. A few months later, the government discreetly – but significantly – increased the salaries of its own officials in a manner that is legally problematic.[7]

In February 2005, the MPs followed suit through a legitimate parliamentary procedure.[8] Again there was tumult in the media. President Boris Tadić, who heads the opposition Democratic Party, distanced himself from the award, but the majority argued that higher salaries were an 'anti-corruption preventive measure'[9] and dismissed the president's statement as 'populist'.[10] Minister of Finance Mlađjan Dinkić said in March 2005 there were insufficient funds to pay the increase.

Few would claim that higher salaries will eliminate corruption or even ensure better work by MPs, but there are other reasons to take the issue seriously. Under a Constitutional Court ruling in May 2003, MPs are ultimately 'masters' of their mandate even when elected from a party's list, rather than directly. When MPs 'cross the floor' to join other parties, they remain the representatives of their constituencies. In 2003, the defection of MPs to parties defeated in the elections led Dr Vladimir Goati, a political analyst at the University of Belgrade, to refer to Serbia as an example of 'non-elective parliamentarism'. Even if they accept bribes to vote for a law or join another party, MPs are not liable for corruption since, under Serbian law, there is nothing that representatives 'should or should not do in the scope of their authorisation'.

Doubtful effects of conflict of interest legislation

Conflict of interest legislation was adopted in April 2004 and dealt with duties in the public and private sector, gifts, and the declaration of assets and incomes.[11] Public officials, including some 1,000 people in the central government and at least 10,000 in lower levels of administration, were obliged to comply with two deadlines. The first, due in July 2004, was to cancel all consultancy arrangements, to resign from management jobs and to transfer any managerial roles in private enterprises. The second was to file property and income declarations for themselves and their immediate family after the launch of the Board for Resolving Conflict of Interest.

The board was envisaged as an independent, autonomous body, but in reality it suffered a number of hindrances.

The procedure for nominating members was long-drawn-out, the government did not provide enough resources for it to function by the deadline of May 2004, and nor did it benefit from the 2005 budget. Such oversights obstructed the law's intent since the deadline for submission of disclosures was set to coincide with the board's creation, and no other agency existed to verify and punish violations. By the first deadline, the government announced on its official website, www.srbija.sr.gov.yu, that all 'officials appointed by the government have complied with their prescribed duties', but there was no agency in place to check. The media quickly detected two prominent cases of non-compliance.

Bogoljub Lazić, then deputy minister of capital investment, came to his job from the Mobtel telephone company which he was also investigating as part of a commission responsible for determining the extent of the state's holding in it. When appointed, Lazić 'froze' his position in Mobtel in line with the legislation valid at the time, but failed to terminate his contract as required under the new law. The government removed him from his post in September 2005. A weightier conflict of interest issue concerned Lazić's manager, the Minister of Capital Investment, Velimir Ilić. The media pointed out that Ilić, who is president of the New Serbia party, which also has close relations with the Force of Serbia Movement (FoSM), is inevitably linked with Bogoljub Karić, who is both head of the FoSM and effective owner of Mobtel. Since Ilić's ministry is partly responsible for regulating Serbia's telecoms industry, this posed a serious conflict of interest. The second victim was Oliver Bogavac, former head of the money-laundering prevention unit in the Ministry of Finance. The media reported that Bogavac had agreed to act as a consultant for the state-owned enterprise Belgrade Airport in 2004 and had not cancelled his contract.[12] The government dismissed him from the post in February 2005.

Events passed more smoothly with regard to the second deadline but its overall success was limited. Most central and provincial post holders submitted disclosures by 1 April, but officials in local governments and public enterprises largely ignored the requirement. The board's next task is to follow up the names and assets of those who failed to respond. But members of the public, who might have more precise information about the wealth of individual officials, are denied access to the contents of the disclosure files, cutting off a huge resource of information for the board.

Nemanja Nenadic (TI Serbia)

Further reading

Ivana Aleksić and Srećko Mihajlović, *Korupcija u Novim Uslovima* (Corruption in a New Environment) (Belgrade: Centre for Policy Studies, 2002)
Boris Begović, *Corruption in Customs: Combating Corruption at the Customs Administration* (Belgrade: Centre for Liberal-Democratic Studies, 2002)
Vladimir Goati, Nemanja Nenadić and Predrag Jovanović: *Financing the Presidential Electoral Campaign in Serbia 2004 – A Blow to Political Corruption or Preservation of Status Quo?* (Belgrade: TI Serbia, October 2004), www.transparentnost.org.yu/english/PUBLICATIONS/index. html#financing

TI Serbia: www.transparentnost.org.yu

Notes

1. A nearly identical version of the bill was submitted to parliament in 2003 but was soon withdrawn by the former government (see *Global Corruption Report 2005*).
2. These include five ministries, including the Ministry of Defence and Ministry of Foreign Affairs.
3. Article 39. Among other information, the directory will include: description of powers, duties and in-house organisation; data on budget; procedures for submitting requests for access to information or complaints against decisions made; overview of requests, complaints and other measures undertaken by interested parties; data on the manner, medium and place of storing information; and type of information held.
4. See www.transparentnost.org.yu/english/ACTIVITIES/ACCOUNTABILITY/2001-e05.html
5. See www.srbija.sr.gov.yu/vesti/vest.php?id=13926
6. The coalition, headed by Prime Minister Vojislav Kostunica, is comprised of the Democratic Party of Serbia, G17 Plus, the Serbian Renewal Movement and New Serbia, supported by the Socialist Party of Serbia.
7. The basis for calculating salaries in the executive branch was changed through a 'conclusion' of the government, which is not published in the official gazette and therefore not public, contrary to new laws on access to information and conflict of interest. Moreover, the ruling establishes a different 'basic wage' for various categories of officials, although their level of responsibility is already mirrored in the different 'coefficients' assigned to different posts.
8. www.beta.co.yu/korupcija/default.asp?st=a&str=1&p=1&lis=1&pi=1164523
9. See, for example, the statement of Zoran Andjelkovic, chair of the Socialist Party group, at www.beta.co.yu/korupcija/default.asp?st=a&str=&p=1&lis=1&pi=1114390
10. www.nspm.org.yu/PrenetiTekstovi/2005_evropa_dinkic_feb.htm
11. See also *Global Corruption Report 2005*.
12. *Blic* (Serbia), 9 February 2005.

Slovakia

Conventions:
Council of Europe Civil Law Convention on Corruption (ratified May 2003)
Council of Europe Criminal Law Convention on Corruption (ratified June 2000; Additional
Protocol ratified April 2005)
OECD Anti-Bribery Convention (ratified September 1999)
UN Convention against Corruption (signed December 2003; not yet ratified)
UN Convention against Transnational Organized Crime (ratified December 2003)

Legal and institutional changes

- In February 2005, parliament approved an act regulating the **financing of political parties**
  and electoral campaigns. From the viewpoint of corruption, it contains several principles
  that improve regulation and increase transparency of party financing, but weaknesses
  remain, most notably the monitoring of the law's implementation (see below).

- An amendment to the act on administrative proceedings, effective since November 2004,
  strengthens citizens' right of **access to information** by requiring all authorities to post
  details of their decisions on the Internet or an accessible notice board. The amendment
  requires authorities to inform the public clearly and in good time about all meetings, their
  conduct and the decisions reached that could constitute a 'subject for public interest'.

- A law on the **property of the municipality**, effective since September 2004, amended
  the previous act and offers further potential to fight corruption at the local level. The
  first of two amendments stipulates that no municipality may transfer ownership of its
  property to any employee – mayor, deputy, budget directors, or any persons or companies
  close to them – other than by public tender under the commercial code. The second
  amendment allows for a reasonable exception by stating that an apartment, a plot of
  land or a movable asset worth less than SK50,000 (US $1,600) may be transferred to an
  employee of the municipality without a public tender.

- The law on the establishment of a **special court and prosecutor to fight corruption
  and organised crime** entered into force in September 2004.[1] By December 2004, the
  prosecutor's office had investigated 416 cases, 12 per cent of them involving corruption.
  The establishment of the special court, meanwhile, was delayed. Following the failure of
  the Judicial Council (the body responsible for nominating judges) to elect the requisite
  number of special judges, its powers were temporarily delegated to the Banská Bystrica
  regional court. By June 2005 the special court had finally reached the number of judges
  required for it to begin work.

New party law plagued by loopholes

Since 1991, Slovakia has financed political
party activity partly from the national budget,
due to the poor economic situation and
the lack of a culture of private donations.[2]
However, the transparency of management
has remained low and the monitoring mechanisms created have been far from adequate.

The tendency to increase state support
continued until 2004 and politicians, irrespective of the parties they belonged to, were
the system's main advocates. In that year,
civil society NGOs warned that citizens no
longer felt adequately represented by their
parties, and harboured suspicions that their
political leaders were mired in corruption,
cronyism and conflicts of interest.

The legislation regulating party finances has changed several times. Amendments in 2000 and 2001 improved monitoring by imposing obligations on parties to publish annual accounts, lists of donors and to submit statements to an independent auditor, but the act contained defects that enabled it to be circumvented. It did not limit the amount members could contribute; it emphasised transparency in only one form of income (gifts from persons and legal entities); and it placed the onus of monitoring on a parliamentary committee, thereby effectively licensing parties to monitor themselves.[3]

In February 2005, a new act on political parties and political movements was passed, replacing the original 1991 act. It contains anti-corruption provisions, some of which were recommended by the Council of Europe and civil society groups, including Transparency International Slovakia.

The new act has both positive and negative implications. One disadvantage is that it introduces the principle of unlimited expenditure for election campaigns and increased state funding for political activities. According to the Fair Play Alliance, an NGO that monitors party finance in Slovakia, parties can expect to receive SK617 million (US \$19.9 million) in the next election and, if their showings remain consistent, they could receive SK1.2 billion (US \$38.7 million) over the period 2006–10. An increasing amount of money will flow into political parties from public funds, but that does not necessarily mean that all party funds (including those from private donors) will be open to public scrutiny. Until now, parties could invest a maximum of SK12 million (US \$390,000) in their campaigns, a restriction cancelled under the new act. The first test of the new legislation will be the elections in autumn 2006.

The new act does introduce better transparency of financial flows. Parties will only be allowed to accept gifts of more than SK5,000 (US \$160) if they sign a contract. If the gift exceeds SK100,000 (US \$3,200), the donor's signature will require verification. Parties are also required to keep records of all member contributions exceeding SK25,000

(US \$800), which are publicly accessible. This is expected to increase transparency of campaign financing, but real change will depend on the enforcement mechanism, in particular, the checks in place to ensure that records are kept and action taken if irregularities are found.

According to Pavel Nechala of TI Slovakia, the parties have left their options open with the new legislation. They are entitled to establish companies whose operations are not monitored publicly. A party, for example, could publish a book and have all the copies 'sold' to a sponsor whose identity will remain unknown.[4]

Moreover, parliamentarians could not agree on SMER's (Social Alternative for Slovakia) proposal to create a special committee to scrutinise the parties' annual accounts and monitor their management. Ján Drgonec, the MP who heads the parliamentary constitutional law committee, is convinced such regulation would prove futile. 'The parties would monitor each other', he said. 'I do not see there being an honest interest in monitoring.' Róbert Madej, a SMER MP, prepared a draft amendment of the constitution that would delegate these powers to the Supreme Audit Office, but the lawmakers turned it down.[5]

The Fair Play Alliance argues that the monitoring of parties is still not sufficient. 'It is useless to make rules stricter if nobody will strictly monitor their observance', said Zuzana Wienk who has disclosed breaches of the act in the past. In most cases, no prosecutions followed. The group proposes instead the creation of an independent authority to monitor party financing or at the very least, monitoring by a ministry, such as the Ministry of Interior. However, none of the parties agree. 'Any approval of stricter rules for themselves is difficult for them and deputies try to avoid it', said Wienk.[6]

First senior public officials tried for corruption

A spate of high-level bribery cases in early 2004 could have sparked more energetic anti-corruption measures, but the year ended without adoption of important changes in strategy. For the first time in recent history, these cases concerned the municipality level, which had been out of the public eye for a long time. The cases were spread evenly across the country and involved the representatives of several political parties, including the Movement for Democratic Slovakia (HZDS), the Christian Democratic Movement (KDH), the Slovak Democratic and Christian Union (SDKU) and the Party of Hungarian Coalition (SMK).

In March 2004, two HZDS members, MP Gabriel Karlin and Milan Mráz, who heads the administration in Banská Bystrica, were indicted on charges of accepting a SK500,000 (US $16,000) bribe in exchange for a favourable decision concerning a SK17 million (US $550,000) building contract for a local school in late 2003. Karlin was stripped of his parliamentary immunity two days after police raided his office and retrieved the cash from his briefcase. In court, Karlin maintained that the secret services had framed him and Mráz in turn claimed Karlin had framed him. Karlin was found guilty in May 2005, but is appealing and has retained his post, while Mráz was found innocent and is still head of the Banská Bystrica regional office.[7]

In April 2004, Pavol Bielik, chairman of the regional branch of the KDH in Bratislava and mayor of Bratislava-Rača, was charged with accepting a SK5 million (US $160,000) bribe for promising to deliver the approval of MPs to rehabilitate a building and construct two new ones in Rača. In May, Bielik was charged with the further offence of negligence in administering entrusted property. According to the weekly *Domino fórum*, police suspect that Bielik approved other improper allocations worth SK750,000 (US $24,000) for various projects in 1999.[8]

In August 2004, the media reported that evidence incriminating Bielik, including the record of his tapped telephone calls, had mysteriously disappeared.[9] The special prosecutor confirmed this and began an investigation into how the records were lost. Following the initial indictment against Bielik, KDH's chairman Pavol Hrušovský called for him to resign from all his party posts, which Bielik has refused to do. Though officially charged with corruption, he continues to chair the KDH regional council whose membership includes the Interior Minister Vladimír Palko.[10]

In March 2004 Eugen Čuňo, a member of the SDKÚ central council and deputy mayor of Košice, was detained for accepting a SK18 million (US $581,000) bribe for a SK180 million (US $5.8 million) contract to build 150 municipal apartments in the city. According to the Interior Minister, the bribe by construction company Kame was disguised as a loan.[11] The investigator also charged another SDKU member, Ladislav Lumtzer, mayor of a district in Kosice, and Maroš M, a Kame employee who had been helping the police to entrap Čuňo. Kame allegedly issued invoices for works that were never executed; Lumtzer approved them and ordered their settlement; and Maroš M, as construction supervisor, signed them off.[12] As a result of the scandal, construction of the housing was halted and the SDKU suspended Čuňo and asked Lumtzer to resign as mayor. Čuňo insists on his innocence and several prominent individuals from Kosice support him. At the time of writing, the case was still open.

These and other scandals appear to illustrate a 'decentralisation' of corruption in imitation of the fiscal decentralisation that has taken place in Slovakia. One proposal to stem its further spread is to give the Supreme Audit Office the right to control local government expenditure. This requires an amendment to the constitution, which was approved by the cabinet in June 2005 and at this writing was still awaiting adoption by the parliament in September 2005. But the measure is very unpopular among local government officials, some of whom are members of parliament.

Emilia Sičáková-Beblavá (TI Slovakia)

Further reading

E. Sičáková-Beblavá, 'Transparentnos' a korupcia' (Transparency and Corruption), in M. Kollár and G. Mesežníkov (eds), *Súhrnná správa o stave spoločnosti* (Global Report on the State of Society) (Bratislava: Institute for Public Affairs, 2004)

E. Sičáková-Beblavá (ed.), *Korupcia a protikorupčná politika na Slovensku 2004, hodnotiaca správa* (Corruption and Anti-corruption Policy in Slovakia, Evaluation Report) (Bratislava: Transparency International Slovakia, 2005)

TI Slovakia: www.transparency.sk

Notes

1. For more details, see *Global Corruption Report 2005*.
2. In 2000, the government introduced a contribution of SK500,00 (US $16,000) per National Council deputy, complemented by two other forms of subsidy: a contribution for votes, paid at SK60 (US $1.90) per vote to each party which obtained over 3 per cent in the previous election); and a contribution for activities, paid at a quarter of a qualifying party's contribution for votes.
3. Z. Wienk, 'Financing of the Political Parties in 2004', in E. Sičáková-Beblava (ed.), *Corruption and Anti-corruption Policy in 2004* (Bratislava: Transparency International Slovakia, 2005).
4. *Hospodárske noviny* (Slovakia), 7 May 2005.
5. *Hospodárske noviny* (Slovakia), 7 February 2005.
6. *Sme* (Slovakia), 5 February 2005.
7. *The Slovak Spectator* (Slovakia), 16 May 2005.
8. *Domino fórum* (Slovakia), 19 May 2004.
9. *Sme* (Slovakia), 19 August 2004.
10. *Sme* (Slovakia), 13 September 2004.
11. *Sme* (Slovakia), 12 March 2004.
12. Ibid., and *Sme* (Slovakia), 19 July 2004.

South Africa

Conventions:

AU Convention on Preventing and Combating Corruption (signed March 2004; not yet ratified)

SADC Protocol against Corruption (ratified May 2003)

UN Convention against Corruption (ratified November 2004)

UN Convention against Transnational Organized Crime (ratified February 2004)

Legal and institutional changes

- The Division of Revenue Act came into effect in April 2005. Its objective is to promote **transparency and equity in the allocation of resources** to municipalities and provinces, and to promote accountability by ensuring that all allocations are reflected in their budgets. Corruption is rife at local government level, with serious backlogs of service delivery in many poorer areas. The act is an attempt to improve public expenditure management, although the Financial and Fiscal Commission has raised concerns over the conditionalities introduced through the act in the allocation of funds.

- The Financial Services Ombud Schemes Act 2004 was signed into law in February 2005. The act provides for the recognition of **financial services ombudsman schemes**; outlines minimum requirements for them; promotes consumer education; and empowers the Ombud for Financial Services Providers to act as a statutory ombudsman in certain cases. Though many providers have been members of voluntary complaints schemes; unscrupulous, non-member institutions have in the past sold inappropriate products, given inadequate advice or otherwise duped naive, less-literate citizens.

- The Companies Amendment Act, signed into law in October 2004, aligns company law with the Prevention and Combating of Corrupt Activities Act of April 2004. The amendment empowers the Registrar of the Court to **debar directors and other company officers** who have previously been convicted of fraud or other criminal activities in the operation of a company, and to maintain a public register of their identities. Such naming and shaming is intended as a deterrent against fraud.

- The Second National Anti-Corruption Summit in March 2005 resolved to include **ethics education** in school curricula to raise awareness among young people. The summit also asked the Law Commission to investigate the Protected Disclosures Act regarding the inadequate **protection of whistleblowers** and to report to parliament by the end of the year (see below).

- The Johannesburg Securities Exchange **Social Responsibility Index** launched in 2003 was revised in October 2004 in an attempt to implement the recommendations of the government's 2002 'King 2' report on corporate governance. The index includes a requirement that companies report on their political donations. The index is voluntary, but it sets a standard and is thought to be the first of its kind in the developing world.

MPs incriminated in 'Travelgate' scandal

MPs are issued with vouchers each year to defray travel expenses between their constituencies and the parliament in Cape Town. Allegations of misuse of the vouchers first surfaced in 2003, leading to an investigation in which more than 100 MPs and seven travel agencies were questioned in 2004.[1] The alleged frauds included the exchange of vouchers for cash; use of vouchers by family and friends; use of airfare vouchers for accommodation and vehicle hire; and MPs holding shares or receiving financial benefits from the travel agents involved. When two of the travel agents involved were closed down, 40 MPs entered plea bargains with the elite Scorpions investigation unit.[2] The first five MPs were convicted in March 2005, with sentences ranging from R40,000 (US $5,800) or one year's imprisonment, to R80,000 (US

$12,000) or three years in prison.[3] Under the constitution, an MP can only lose a seat if sentenced to more than 12 months' imprisonment, without the option of a fine. South Africa now finds that nearly a quarter of its legislators have been incriminated in questionable behaviour.

The confidential report of the investigation, undertaken by PricewaterhouseCoopers (PwC), recommended new investigations and legal action. Parliament appointed a special task team to consider its findings and the National Prosecuting Authority (NPA), which oversees the Scorpions, South Africa's elite crime unit, is also investigating. The report points out that the entire system for processing air tickets for MPs was overseen by a single employee, whose work was never checked by her superiors. The PwC report says there was insufficient accounting information available to determine whether MPs were party to the fraud, what the extent of the fraud was and whether MPs received undue benefits from travel agents.[4]

Smuts Ngonyama, spokesman for the ruling African National Congress (ANC), noted that the party will initiate 'relevant organisational disciplinary processes' against its MPs and the opposition has called for convicted MPs to 'do the honourable thing and resign'.[5] In June 2005, the ANC announced that five of the convicted MPs had resigned, while three more who had plea-bargained are no longer in parliament. Another 21 current or former MPs are expected to stand trial in July 2005.

The fallout from Travelgate has been varied. On the one hand, it showed that the anti-corruption bodies and judiciary have a fair degree of independence and are able to carry out their functions without hindrance, even when high-ranking members of the ANC were involved. On the other, there have since been moves to 'muzzle' the Scorpions by incorporating the unit into the regular police force. A judicial commission of inquiry has been convened to determine the Scorpions' future. That decision could signal the strength of the government's commitment to fighting corruption at the highest levels.

Deputy president removed for alleged bribery

The US $5 billion arms purchase of 2000 came under intense scrutiny in 2003 when former NPA head Bulelani Ngcuka announced that, although the Scorpions had found prima facie evidence of corruption against Deputy President Jacob Zuma, the state would not prosecute because the case was 'not winnable'.[6] Some interpreted the trial since October 2004 of Zuma's financial adviser, Schabir Shaik, as a trial of Zuma by proxy. When Justice Squires found there was a 'generally corrupt relationship' between Shaik and Zuma, President Thabo Mbeki removed Zuma from his post in June 2005. The NPA announced plans to indict Zuma, whose first court appearance was scheduled for 29 June. Zuma maintains he is innocent, retains the deputy presidency of the ANC

and enjoys wide grassroots support among trade unionists and youth, who claim that he was framed. The judge found that Shaik had solicited a bribe on Zuma's behalf from French defence company Thomson-CSF (now renamed Thales) to protect it from the investigation into the arms deal.[7] The trial also investigated questionable loans totalling more than R1 million (US $146,000) from Shaik to Zuma.[8]

The consequences for the former deputy president and the country's oversight institutions are far-reaching. Zuma has refused to comment on whether he will enter the race to succeed President Mbeki, but his supporters maintain that the Scorpions' investigation and Shaik's trial were designed to discredit Zuma and stall his presidential ambitions. The trial highlighted weaknesses or abuse in oversight mechanisms in parliament, the director of public prosecutions, the public protector and the auditor general. The Joint Investigation Team (JIT), which first looked into the arms deal in 2001, found that although there was some corruption, it did not significantly influence the contracts.[9] Since the JIT included investigators from all the above oversight bodies, the court verdict calls into question the rigour of their enquiries.

There have been allegations of extensive executive interference in the auditor-general's report.

The opposition Democratic Alliance (DA) has called for the former defence secretary, Pierre Steyn, to testify before the Parliamentary Standing Committee on Accounts (SCOPA). Steyn had resigned from his post, questioning the legality of the arms deal and arguing that the procurement process was irregular.[10]

The fact that the JIT deliberately bypassed SCOPA prevented it from exercising its oversight role. Some commentators feel that this whole episode has weakened SCOPA, transforming it from a rigorous and non-partisan regulator into an arena for political manipulation. DA MP Eddie Trent stated: 'The challenge now is for parliament to ensure both the executive and the Auditor-General are made to account for their conduct in the arms deal.'[11] The Shaik trial highlighted Zuma's alleged failure to declare his loans from Shaik to parliament's Public Accounts Committee.[12]

The Shaik trial also shows up the responsibility of multinational corporations for the 'supply side' of international bribery. The OECD's 1999 Anti-Bribery Convention could mean increased scrutiny for Thales and other companies implicated in the arms deal.

Whistleblower law found wanting

In March 2005, the deputy director-general in the justice department, Michael Tshishonga, brought a R2 million (US $292,000) defamation lawsuit against former justice minister Penuell Maduna, alleging that Maduna had called him a 'dunderhead' and 'a relic from the Bantustans' in a televised statement in October 2004. Tshishonga has recently been reinstated as managing director of the Master of the High Court after Maduna suspended him on grounds of contravening the Public Service Code of Conduct.[13]

The office of the Master of the High Court is responsible for the appointment of liquidators of insolvent estates. Tshishonga went public in October 2003 with allegations of corruption and nepotism involving Maduna, insolvency practitioner Enver Motala, and a senior official in the Master's office.[14] Tshishonga accused Maduna of maintaining a corrupt relationship with Motala that had earned the latter fees of R50 million (US $7.8 million) over a period of two years from appointments he received from Leon Lategan of the Master of the High Court's office. Tshishonga had initially reported his concerns about Motala to the then director general of justice, Vusi Pikoli. When nothing happened, he blew the whistle. Tshishonga was then hauled before an internal disciplinary hearing and Maduna suspended him.[15]

The internal hearing stemmed from the Public Service Code of Conduct, which states

'that an employee must use appropriate channels to air his or her grievances or to direct representations'. The hearing concluded in July 2004 that Tshishonga's statements were protected under the Protected Disclosures Act (PDA) of 2000, the legislation that protects whistleblowers.

However, the justice department refused to reinstate Tshishonga on the grounds that it 'is still studying the findings of the disciplinary hearing and will decide on the course of action to take once this process is complete'. He took the department to Labour Court, which ordered his reinstatement as of February 2005.[16] Detectives arrested Motala on 2 July 2004 on charges of fraud and corruption, together with eight other people. Lategan has been redeployed to 'training and evaluation' pending the outcome of the investigation. South Africans are now waiting to see if Maduna will be prosecuted or will be allowed to walk away. Will Pikoli, recently appointed national director of public prosecutions, be called upon to explain his failure to take action after Tshishonga, then his deputy, informed him of the irregularities? What message is being sent to potential whistleblowers?

Though well intended, the PDA appears to have failed whistleblowers in several instances, not only because it sets out exactly to whom disclosures are to be made, but also how the informant wishes to claim its protection. The act specifies that a whistleblower must make what is referred to as a 'protected disclosure' to a specified group of persons if he or she wishes to avoid suffering 'an occupational detriment'. The manner in which the disclosure is made is also regulated. Government employees, of whom Tshishonga was one, are free to register grievances as long as a prescribed procedure is followed. It was his apparent failure to follow procedures that resulted in disciplinary action being taken against him. The disciplinary offence – and the legal confusion – derives from the public service regulations, and what they proscribe in terms of communicating, especially outside the public services. There is therefore a tension between the regulations and the PDA.

The jury is still out on the effectiveness of the PDA, as many potentially successful attempts to blow the whistle are likely to go unreported; the act is up for review by parliament in late 2005. But this case highlights the difficulty of implementing the legislation and the extent to which there is resistance to sanctioning senior officials.

Ayesha Kajee (TI South Africa)

Further reading

John Daniel, Roger Southall and Jessica Lutchman (eds), *State of the Nation: South Africa 2004–2005* (Cape Town: HSRC Press, 2004)
Hennie van Vuuren, 'National Integrity Systems: South Africa' (Johannesburg: Transparency South Africa, 2005)

TI South Africa: www.tisa.org.za

Notes

1. *Sunday Times* (South Africa), 1 August 2004.
2. *Mail and Guardian* (South Africa), 28 January 2005.
3. *Mail and Guardian* (South Africa), 18 March 2005.
4. *Mail and Guardian* (South Africa), 4 March 2005.
5. *Mail and Guardian* (South Africa), 18 March 2005.
6. *Sunday Times* (South Africa), 24 August 2003.
7. *The Witness* (South Africa), 29 June 2005.
8. *Mail and Guardian* (South Africa), 26 November 2004.
9. Government of South Africa, 'Joint Investigation Report into the Strategic Defence Procurement Packages', November 2001.
10. *Pretoria News* (South Africa), 31 March 2005.
11. *Pretoria News* (South Africa), 31 March 2005.
12. *Business Day* (South Africa), 15 March 2005.
13. www.iafrica.com/news/sa/237039.htm
14. www.armsdeal-vpo.co.za/articles07/pickle.html
15. www.info.gov.za/speeches//1999/9911091035a1017.htm
16. www.info.gov.za.speeches/2004/04080408151007.htm

South Korea

Conventions:
OECD Anti-Bribery Convention (ratified January 1999)
UN Convention against Corruption (not yet signed)
UN Convention against Transnational Organized Crime (not yet signed)

ADB-OECD Action Plan for Asia-Pacific (endorsed November 2001)

Legal and institutional changes

- The Amendment on Anti-Corruption Act, proposed by the Korean Independent Commission Against Corruption (KICAC) in November 2004, is currently under review by the Legislation and Judiciary Committee. The act only applies to corrupt practices in the public sector. The broad thrust of the amendment is to expand its coverage to the private sector so as to root out bribe payers, as well as bribe recipients. Among the proposed changes is the **extension of existing whistleblower protection** to employees in the private sector to encourage more of them to come forward.

- In December 2004, the government submitted a draft that provides for the creation of the post of **Citizen Ombudsman** at local government level in order to increase the protection of citizens' rights. One of the main points of debate is whether to make the post mandatory. Some civil society leaders suggest it should be introduced gradually so as to minimise the resistance it is expected to encounter from members of local councils who feel the post threatens their own duties. Another point at issue is the ombudsman's degree of seniority. Since they must be independent, autonomous and neutral from government, it is important to set their credentials and authority high enough for them to be effective, but low enough to be realistic.

- In November 2004, the State Council passed a bill establishing the Corruption Investigation Office (CIO) for **investigating high-ranking public officials** suspected of corruption. The CIO will be created under the KICAC as an independent agency responsible for investigating corruption cases of high-ranking officials, members of the National Assembly, mayors, governors, judges and public prosecutors. At the time of writing the National Assembly still had to debate how the agency will operate, but one of its unspoken aims will be to provide a counterweight to the Prosecutor's Office, the only organisation with power to indict. Proponents argue that complaints to KICAC have decreased because it lacks investigative powers. Moreover, greater efforts are needed to tackle corruption amongst senior government officials who, according to KICAC's annual survey on perceived corruption, are considered most in need of reform. Many experts are sceptical as to whether the body, if established under the presidential KICAC, will be free from political intervention.

- In April 2005, the **Council for the Pact on Anti-Corruption and Transparency** was incorporated under the Korean Pact on Anti-Corruption and Transparency (K-PACT) signed a month earlier. Its mission is to raise the level of cooperation among participants and enforce agendas of inspection, evaluation, dissemination and renewal. Initiated by Transparency International Korea, the K-PACT is a national alliance of representatives from civil society and the public, private and political sectors committed to improving transparency. Encouraging citizens to sign up to a 10-point Citizen's Charter will be the Council's most important task, because the K-PACT will not have much tangible impact without widespread public support (see below).

K-PACT: a people's compact against corruption

A total of 120 leading figures attended the signing of the Korean Pact on Anti-Corruption and Transparency on 9 March 2005. The event was remarkable for the range of participants, but also because it was the culmination of six months' work to ensure that the K-PACT is a collective effort, involving the private sector, civil society and government. The rationale behind the K-PACT is that while South Korea has many corruption prevention measures in place, cases of corruption continue to recur. The K-PACT's organisers, including TI-Korea, argue that corruption could be reduced if the population were involved in building a more transparent society, and that public pressure can be an effective deterrent against corruption.

In January 2005, the K-PACT's civil society proponents met in Ankook-Dong and asked the government to join the movement for a social agreement on transparency under the slogan, 'Together! Cleaner!' After the participants delivered the proposal to President Moo-Hyun Roh, chairman of the National Assembly Won-Ki Kim, the Federation of Korean Industries and the Korea Chamber of Commerce and Industry, a number of intersectoral steering committees were formed to discuss the K-PACT in detail, and to divide the workload between the four participating sectors.[1]

As a result, the public sector has effectively undertaken to: adjust the responsibilities of South Korea's anti-corruption agencies; improve local government transparency; expand public participation; reform the Information Disclosure Acts; strengthen anti-corruption awareness; and improve the transparency of public corporations. The political sector agreed to impose limits on immunity; strengthen the National Assembly Ethics Committee; introduce the blind trust system (see below); and eradicate illegal political funding and lobbyism. The private sector proposes to improve corporate ethics; reduce subcontractor corruption; strengthen the function of audit committees; protect whistleblowers; enhance information disclosure; and ensure the professionalism of outside directors. Civil society committed its efforts to improving the accountability of civil society and introducing the post of Citizen Ombudsman. To prevent the recurrence of corruption, the K-PACT contains a provision to limit the power to grant amnesties to criminals convicted of corruption.

The K-PACT is only likely to be effective if it captures the imagination of South Korea's citizens. The 10-point Citizen's Charter, which includes statements of intent on aspects of corruption from tax evasion, money laundering and bribery to information on corruption and whistleblower protection, provides some guidelines for popular participation and awareness raising. The K-PACT also includes a Code of Ethics for Citizens as a standard for implementing principles designed to overcome corruption. Citizens can participate indirectly by signing up to the charter and code, or actively as inspectors to oversee the implementation of the K-PACT. Civil society and the political, public and private sectors have pledged to organise regular inspection groups to evaluate their performance and to publicise progress in implementing the K-PACT.

Political observers and citizens' groups are doubtful that the K-PACT will make much difference to the level of corruption in South Korea, though they hope it will. The Council for the K-PACT, established in April 2005 to ensure cooperation between its participants, is reliant for financial support from the very sectors that it was set up to police, narrowing its room for manoeuvre. Much depends on a sense of popular vigilance as a campaigning tool that carries more weight in Asia than in other regions of the world. Koreans are generally aware of the K-PACT's existence and purpose, though they are perhaps less certain of how to participate. The council's primary mission in the short-term, therefore, must be to 'advertise' what Koreans can do to help.

Preventing government officials' conflicts of interest

The problem of conflicts of interest at senior government level has been a focus of attention over the past few years, following a series of allegations that private businesses are influencing policy making, either by donating money to political parties and expecting policy favours in return, or because politicians have private interests in particular companies' fortunes. Amendments to ethics codes for elected officials and public servants, including a requirement that high-ranking appointed officials put their stocks into a blind trust during their tenure in office, have been tabled in an effort to address the problem.

There is public pressure for reform. The 2003 JoongAng-EAI poll demonstrated that one in three people pointed to anti-corruption reform as an immediate social reform need, while on the political agenda, 'collusion between politics and business' (41.3 per cent) topped the list of concerns.

Since 2003, a code of conduct for maintaining the integrity of public officials has regulated conflicts of interest for civil servants, though not elected officials. This code, enacted by presidential decree, specifies the standards of conduct to be observed by both state and local public officials. It covers areas related to the prevention of conflict of interest, the prohibition to use public office for private purposes, and the obligations of neutrality and impartiality. It also regulates the legitimate acceptance of gifts from persons related to public duties. This is a matter of particular importance given that the presentation of gifts forms an integral part of the national culture. But compliance with the code has been weak and KICAC is only looking now at establishing a procedure for handling money, or expensive items received in violation of the code.

The Public Service Ethics Act, a separate document, focuses mainly on the asset disclosure of high-level officials and does not have any provisions regarding conflicts of interest. A draft amendment submitted to the National Assembly would incorporate conflict of interest mechanisms within the act, including a blind trust system.

The purpose of this amendment, submitted to parliament in May 2005, is to require public officials with stock holdings that exceed a certain value to either sell or place the excess stock into a blind trust, unless the relevant commission rules that the stockholding is not related to the work of the official. High-ranking public officials would be prohibited from trading stocks or influencing stock prices with information acquired while in office, thus enabling them to concentrate on their duties as public servants.

The commission for blind trust assessment will be established under the Ministry of Government Administration and Home Affairs, to examine whether those who are required to disclose details about their property hold stocks connected to their work. The commission will be comprised of nine members, appointed by the president from a shortlist nominated by the National Assembly and Chief Justice of the Supreme Court. Once a contract with a blind trust is entered into, those required to disclose details of their property, as well as other concerned parties, will not be able purchase stocks until the contract terminates.

While the blind trust system is a positive development, it is unlikely to do much to assuage fears that some politicians use their positions of power for personal gain. Indeed, the government's messages on the need to separate political and business interests have not been entirely consistent. In May 2005, President Moo-Hyun Roh decreed an amnesty for business people incriminated in an illegal party funding scandal in the run-up to the 2002 presidential elections.[2] The president – who earlier promised to resign if it were demonstrated that his campaign had received more than 10 per cent of the illegal funds received by his opponent – argued that the amnesty, effective from 15 July, would protect the economy from recession. A number of civil society organisations argue that the private sector's support for the K-PACT was in order to improve the likelihood of an amnesty. Article 6 of the K-PACT states: 'Government should set up systematic mechanisms to limit the presidential power to grant amnesty.'[3]

Geo-Sung Kim (TI South Korea)

Further reading

TI Korea (South): www.ti.or.kr

Notes

1. For full text, see www.ti.or.kr/k-pact/
2. www.koreafocus.or.kr/chronology.asp?vol=40
3. www.ti.or.kr/k-pact/

Spain

Conventions:

Council of Europe Civil Law Convention on Corruption (signed May 2005; not yet ratified)

Council of Europe Criminal Law Convention on Corruption (signed May 2005; not yet ratified)

OECD Anti-Bribery Convention (ratified January 2000)

UN Convention against Corruption (not yet signed)

UN Convention against Transnational Organized Crime (ratified March 2002)

Legal and institutional changes

- A number of **corruption-related initiatives** have been adopted under the framework of the Plan of Economic Reactivation presented by the Economy and Finance Ministry in March 2005. The Council of Ministers has approved the plan, which includes steps to tighten laws regulating the public sector, improve public access to information, the regulation of contracts for public–private partnership schemes and the adoption of a code of conduct for public contracting.

- The Ministry of Public Administration approved a 'programme of actions for good government' in February 2005 which, if it passes the legislature, will regulate **conflicts of interest** by elected MPs and high-level bureaucrats (see below).

- In February, an expert group advising the government on the reform of **mass media laws** called for public television to be 'fully independent from the government' with mixed funding and content of public service quality. One of the purposes of the group is to limit the political incumbents' abuse of state media in their re-election bids.

Zapatero tries to clean up governance

Spain's first socialist administration since Felipe González lost power amid a series of corruption scandals in 1996 came to office in April 2004. Prime Minister José Luis Rodríguez Zapatero promised to deliver clean government and to distance his Socialist Party (PSOE) from its past misdeeds. Zapatero lacks an absolute parliamentary majority and needs the support of other parties to push through the laws tabled by his government.

At the heart of Zapatero's governance programme is a committee of experts, which has proposed measures that would, if applied, help obviate the risks of corruption. Among the most important measures are: the clarification of rules on conflicts of interest, and the monitoring of incompatibilities by an independent body; the declaration of assets and income by politicians and senior officials; reform of party financing laws, including a ban on company donations and caps on campaign spending; the creation of a national agency to evaluate public policy; a law on access to information; and greater independence for RTVE, the state-owned broadcaster, whose programmes will be monitored for political bias.

Two draft laws approved in early 2005 went some way toward meeting the first two items on this agenda. These were the law on conflicts of interest and a code of good governance. The law on conflicts of interest amends a 1995 regulation that had little effect. The only sanction for breaching it was a note in the official gazette. The body responsible for investigating alleged misdemeanours was hampered by its structural dependency on the central government and usually failed to carry out its tasks. The PSOE had acknowledged the need to reform the law and several draft bills were presented to parliament, without success. The bill currently before parliament reflects recommendations by the OECD, the UN and the Council of Europe.

Though an important step, the draft bill could yet be modified by parliament. Its weakest point is enforcement: the body charged with sanctioning conflicts of interest is subordinate to a ministry and likely to receive low priority. The most important features of the legislation are: a ban on officials taking second jobs in the public or private sectors; a two-year moratorium on officials taking private jobs related to their work for government; the declaration of assets by ministers, secretaries of state and senior officials; and the creation of a new Office of Conflicts of Interest in the Ministry of Public Administration. Where a conflict of interest involving a state contractor is discovered, it will be investigated and published in the official gazette. Those found guilty of breaching the law will be dismissed, lose the right to compensation and be asked to repay any money lost as a result of their actions. A contracting company that hires a high-level public official during the two-year 'cooling-off' period loses the right to bid for public contracts during the same amount of time. Officials who infringe the law will be barred from competing for public posts for between 5 and 10 years.

The second piece of anti-corruption legislation, the new code of government, became effective in March 2005. Successive reports by international bodies, notably the damning report in 2001 from the Council of Europe's Group of States against Corruption (GRECO), pushed for the elaboration of codes of conduct for public officials. Laws exist to proscribe the criminal behaviour of public servants, but what was needed was a set of guidelines to orient public employees when they navigate the greyer areas of their work, such as conflicts of interest.

Under the new code, one of Zapatero's electoral pledges, senior officials will be required to: provide timely public information on the performance of their departments; keep copies of their documents for oversight by subsequent governments; refrain from accepting jobs that infringe upon their commitment to government work; refrain from improper use of power; reject any gift, favour or service that affects the performance of their duties.

The code has a number of weaknesses, however. There is no clear mechanism for legally sanctioning infringements of the code. Moreover, it does not apply to more junior public officials or other state employees, although a complementary code for public servants is at the initial drafting stages.

Property is a corruption host

On 10 March 2005, police mounted a series of raids on a money-laundering network in the resort town of Marbella, the culmination of an 18-month investigation involving police in seven countries. At its nerve centre was the law firm of Fernando del Valle, alleged to have set up hundreds of shell companies through which multimillion-dollar investments were channelled from groups linked to organised crime. Most of the money had been funnelled into the property sector on the Mediterranean shore, which European police have long recognised as a capital of organised crime.

Police estimate that more than €600 million (US $770 million) may have been laundered through the del Valle firm's offices, fuelling a phenomenal boom in the construction industry. Half of all new construction projects in Spain take place on the southern coast, around Malaga, a city with one of the highest unemployment rates in the country. They suspect that many more law firms along the coast are involved in money laundering.

The so-called 'Operation White Whale' marks the first time police have established a direct link between organised crime and Spain's construction and real estate industries. Where it exists, corruption at the local government level, where decisions over land use and ownership are taken, makes the sector an ideal vehicle for laundering money.

A 2003 report by Malaga University's Andalusian Criminology Institute points to a tight relationship between construction magnates and town halls; some of the latter raise much of their municipal funds from issuing licences to the former.[1] Real estate deals require landowners to make payments to local governments that are often above the amount required by law, particularly if the owner wants to develop the property.

A study in 2004 found that almost every mayor in the coastal region was in favour of development agreements as a way of obtaining income.[2] Such agreements leave plenty of room for 'negotiation'. In Majorca alone, municipalities modified agreements on 227 separate occasions. There is little supervision of illegal construction or planning alterations, and sanctions almost never lead to demolition. A report by *La Vanguardia* newspaper suggests that there are tens of thousands of properties in Marbella that fail to comply with building regulations, including some 1,600 properties in Marbella that are illegal because they were built on parkland.[3]

Marbella tops the list of town halls that have suffered corruption scandals in recent years. Two former mayors, Jesús Gil and Julián Muñoz, were banned from holding public office. Gil approved a zoning plan for Marbella that was illegal and was being investigated on 15 counts of corruption and links to Italian and Russian mafia bosses when he died in 2004. The Andalusian government announced plans in early 2005 to overhaul the Costa del Sol's urban planning process. The new plan would take away zoning and licensing powers from local authorities that consistently fail to implement the appropriate building regulations and laws.

Catalonia has also been in the headlines for corruption involving real estate. In the so-called '3 per cent case', investigators uncovered a connection between corruption in the construction sector and political party financing. In February 2005, the president of Catalonia accused the former government of charging a 3 per cent commission on public works contracted out during its period in office. The sum was allegedly used to finance the coalition that has dominated power for more than 20 years. In March 2005, Catalonia's parliament established a commission to investigate irregularities in public works between 1995 and 2005 that contributed to the collapse of houses in the Barcelona neighbourhood of Carmelo, due to errors in building a metro tunnel. The commission will also look at possible violations to political financing laws.

Suggestions of a link between corruption in the construction industry and party financing were raised in the Marbella scandal as well. No substantive changes have been made to the institutional and legal framework governing party financing in recent years, however, despite the prominent scandals of the 1990s and many electoral campaign pledges.

Manuel Villoria (King Juan Carlos University, Madrid)

Further reading

Roberto Blanco Valdés, *Las conexiones políticas* (Political Connections) (Madrid: Alianza, 2002)

Carlos Jiménez Villarejo, 'La delincuencia financiera, los paraísos fiscales y la intervención de los bancos' (Financial Crime, Tax Havens and the Intervention of Banks), mimeograph, 2004

Fernando Jiménez and Miguel Caínzos, 'Political Corruption in Spain', in Martin Bull and James Newell (eds), *Corruption in Contemporary Politics* (London: Palgrave, 2003)

J. M. Maravall, *El control de los políticos* (The Control of Politicians) (Madrid: Taurus, 2003)

TI Spain: www.transparencia.org.es

Notes

1. José Luis Diez Ripolles et al., *Prácticas ilícitas en la actividad urbanística. Un estudio en la Costa del Sol* (Illicit Practices in Urban Activity: A Study of the Costa del Sol) (Valencia: Editorial Tirant, Instituto Interuniversitario Andaluz de Criminología, 2004).
2. Antonio Vercher, 'La corrupción urbanística' (Urban Corruption), *Claves de Razón Práctica* 139, January–February 2004.
3. *La Vanguardia* (Spain), 17 March 2005.

Sri Lanka

Conventions:

UN Convention against Corruption (ratified March 2004)
UN Convention against Transnational Organized Crime (signed December 2000; not yet ratified)

Legal and institutional changes

- After a three-month delay in appointing a new chairperson and two new commissioners, the **Commission to Investigate Allegations of Bribery and Corruption** became operational once again in March 2005. Its agenda includes awareness-raising programmes and training on corruption issues for 30,000 graduates recently admitted into the public services. It is also developing a curriculum to train investigative officers in financial auditing, investigations related to control systems, areas of corruption, and analysis of evidence and technique. Certain key reforms are still needed within the commission if it is to develop into a useful tool in fighting corruption. It needs to recruit more investigators with experience in the practice of law, while reducing its dependence on the police for its personnel needs. Another important step would be to allow the commission to initiate investigations on its own accord. The commission's financial status is also problematic since the Treasury may not release the funds allocated by parliament. Finally, a recruitment criterion that all three commissioners must be recruited from among retired judges, police or audit inspectors eliminates the prospects of younger, more dynamic anti-corruption campaigners leading the commission.

Tsunami aid and transparency

The tsunami that struck 13 of Sri Lanka's 25 provinces on 26 December 2004 affected 1,000 km of the island's coastline. By early February, it was calculated that 30,974 people had died, 4,698 were still missing and 558,287 displaced. Nearly 100,000 private houses were destroyed and 45,000 partially damaged.[1]

As in other affected countries, it was an unforeseen catastrophe requiring the immediate attention of a large number of international and local actors with no precedent to fall back on for guidance. A flood of donor aid overwhelmed the country's financial and institutional structures, leading to administrative lapses that paved the way for corruption. On the one hand, the weakness of the accountability framework highlighted the need for intensive public participation to ensure transparency in the use of post-tsunami reconstruction funds. On the other, the lack of a freedom of information law, weak parliamentary oversight and an attenuated anti-corruption body left Sri Lanka in particularly poor shape to monitor funds correctly.

A multitude of allegations concerning unethical behaviour or misappropriation of relief funds has emerged. In April 2005, a local newspaper revealed how World Food Programme volunteers recruited for disaster relief activities were the spouses or relatives of existing staff members with no relevant expertise, but who were accommodated in five-star hotels.[2] Another case highlighted how supplies allocated to the inhabitants of Batticaloa allegedly ended up in Polonnaruwa district through the relief arm of the ruling coalition partner, People's Liberation Front (JVP). Once in Pollanaruwa, the local JVP MP stored the supplies privately and distributed them to party supporters in Giritale, which had been unaffected by the tsunami.[3] In Rambukkana, police seized goods from houses belonging to employees of the social services department that were reportedly stolen from supplies intended for refugees in the Kalmunai area. They included clothing, toys, plastic mats and 5,000 kg of lentils.[4]

Other criticisms focused on the 'task forces' set up to handle the distribution of relief. President Chandrika Kumaratunga appointed several in the immediate wake of the tsunami, but the main coordinating role was given to the Task Force for Rebuilding the Nation (TAFREN). Given the urgency of the disaster, TAFREN members were appointed outside normal parliamentary procedures. A civil society group, the Alliance for Protection of National Resources and Human Rights, expressed concerns that they lacked disaster relief expertise and alleged that private sector

delegates on the task force were politically aligned. At the same time, the government announced it would establish a statutory body to handle all operations in relation to post-disaster activities, sparking criticism that it would be riddled with nepotism and become another 'white elephant', unless a strong legal framework were introduced. To date, the government has given no indication that it will present the proposed law to the public before sending it to parliament. A special Parliamentary Select Committee for Natural Disasters was also formed, although its mandate is restricted to investigating the island's lack of preparedness and recommending steps to minimise damage in the event of a recurrence.

Instead of opening one central account to handle the inflow of funds, the government set up several, raising fears over accountability, lack of coordination between departments and possible duplication of effort. Sri Lanka's limited freedom of information provision played an important role in stimulating these concerns. A draft freedom of information law was due to go to parliament in 2004, but no steps have been taken to proceed.[5] The current disempowerment of citizens and communities affected by the tsunami is not helped by the absence of legislation on disclosure and whistleblower protection that would have gone some way towards rolling back corrupt practices during the earliest phase of disaster relief. Nor did the government consult tsunami victims when the first damage and needs assessments were made. As a result, the reconstruction programme gives the impression of being a top-down, one-size-fits-all affair. Civil society made suggestions for more appropriate reconstruction interventions, but has received little response to date.[6]

The state-controlled media painted a far rosier picture of the success of the reconstruction process than researchers on the ground. A case in point is the allegedly uneven distribution of aid to districts inhabited by Sinhalese and Tamils, particularly in the north-east which is controlled by the rebel Liberation Tigers of Tamil Eelam (LTTE). A ceasefire three years ago ended the civil war between the LTTE and government, but the post-tsunami relief effort surfaced new tensions. The LTTE asked to receive relief funds directly, citing the government's poor record on corruption as justification, but was refused. Political parties in the south raised the issue that LTTE might use the money to fuel the separatist war. To defuse the situation, the two sides agreed on the formation of a joint mechanism, known as the Post-Tsunami Operational Management Structure (PTOMS), to ensure the equitable allocation of funds to all affected areas. The move was the subject of great controversy in parliament where it met resistance from the Party of Buddhist Clergy, the Muslim parties and the JVP, which claimed the PTOMS 'legitimised' the LTTE (the JVP later quit the coalition over the issue).[7] Under the agreement, all communities are expected to share the nearly US $3 billion in aid pledged, and will divide responsibility for reconstruction in the Tamil-dominated north and east.[8] The funds are to be channelled through the government, with the World Bank to serve as custodian. The PTOMS ran into further trouble in July 2005 when its constitutionality was challenged in the Supreme Court.[9] The court issued an interim order freezing the process until the conclusion of the case.

Although earlier independent and government reports tended to confirm the swifter pace of reconstruction in the south compared to the north, those most affected by the nightmare wave are generally excluded from the debate on aid relief, due to the lack of investigative capacity in the print and electronic media.[10]

Slow road to parliamentary fiscal oversight

Corruption was certainly not introduced to Sri Lanka by the tsunami. The lack of accountability and transparency is pervasive, starting with the scrutiny of public funds. Two standing parliamentary committees are responsible for carrying out the legislature's oversight duties. The Committee on Public Accounts (COPA) reviews the accounts of ministries, departments and local authorities, while the Committee on Public Enterprises (COPE) deals with state-owned corporations and the government's other ventures. Contrary to practice in most Commonwealth countries, Sri Lanka does not have a budget or estimates committee to deliberate the national budget.

Legislative scrutiny of public funds is poor because the committees meet in camera, to the exclusion of the media, general public and even fellow MPs. 'The government is not required to respond to the recommendations of these committees within any stipulated period of time', according to one civil society observer. 'This leaves the accountability loop open.'[11]

Nor do the committees have the adequate technical capacities or incentives to enforce accountability. A positive move occurred in September 2004 when the membership of COPA and COPE was increased to 19, widening participation in the monitoring process. The two committees also have longer, uninterrupted sittings. This has had little visible impact upon accountability, however. Provisions were made in September 2004 for COPA and COPE for the creation of sub-committees to handle different tasks simultaneously, but they have yet to be appointed and, in addition, they would suffer from inadequate secretarial provision and the absence of a filtering process for prioritising items for discussion. To help address these issues, the World Bank and UNDP initiated a capacity-building programme in early 2005, based on reports prepared by Ernst and Young. Two consultants have been recruited to provide COPA and COPE members with advanced training, financed by the Treasury.

Another problem is the large proportion of ministers and deputy ministers to MPs; at this writing it stood at 81, out of 225 parliamentarians. One by-product of such concentration of MPs in office is that it dramatically dilutes legislative scrutiny of executive activities. Provisions were made in the parliamentary period January

2002–February 2004 for both committees to be headed by an opposition MP, but the chairman elected to COPE, Rohitha Bogollagama, defected to the ruling United Peoples Freedom Alliance (UPFA) in November 2004. He is now technology minister, but continues to serve as chairman of the Parliamentary Oversight Committee, raising concerns about his independence – and possible lack of scrutiny in his own ministry.

A number of diagnostic studies on parliamentary oversight mechanisms and the auditor general's department were conducted in recent years, leading to the drafting of a new Audit Act at the end of 2003 that aims to strengthen the powers and independence of the auditor general, and make the position an 'officer of parliament'.[12] Discussions with the strong union in the auditor general's department are continuing, while the finance ministry and cabinet have still to approve the draft before it is submitted to parliament. Thus, contrary to Commonwealth practice, the auditor general remains a public officer and subject to the administrative control of the executive.

The auditor general's reports are customarily referred to the two oversight committees for review and proposed recommendations. In the past, delays in submission meant the reports were usually outdated by the time they came up for consideration with the result that committees could not deal with issues in a timely manner. In addition, their contents were not debated in parliament. In September 2004, the auditor general began forwarding preliminary findings to the committees to facilitate a more updated review practice. The reviews are still not very useful, however, due to the infrequency of meetings, narrow focus on excess expenditure and the lack of follow-up by the ministries concerned.

With regard to the Fiscal Management (Responsibilities) Act of 2003, the government fulfilled its duties by submitting two reports on fiscal policy and performance in 2004.[13] However, the reports were considered too technical, while public awareness of the act's provisions is minimal. Civil society has so far taken no initiative to participate in the process of scrutiny, despite the provisions made for this in the act.

Anushika Amarasinghe (TI Sri Lanka)

Further reading

Institute of Policy Studies, *Phoenix from the Ashes: Economic Policy Challenges and Opportunities for Post-Tsunami Sri Lanka* (Colombo: Karunaratne and Sons, 2005)
Institute of Chartered Accountants of Sri Lanka, *Accounting and Management Systems and Procedures for Tsunami Relief Projects* (Colombo: Institute of Chartered Accountants of Sri Lanka, 2005)
Transparency International, *National Integrity Systems Country Study 2003 – Sri Lanka* (Berlin, Colombo: Transparency International, 2004), available at www.transparency.org/activities/nat_integ_systems/dnld/sri_lanka_r.pdf
Transparency International Sri Lanka, *Report on Key High Posts* (Colombo: Vishwaleka Publishers, 2004)

TI Sri Lanka: www.tisrilanka.org

Notes

1. Figures are derived from the *Preliminary Damage and Needs Assessment* prepared for Sri Lanka 2005 Post-Tsunami Recovery Programme by the Asian Development Bank, Japan Bank for International Cooperation and the World Bank, 1–28 January 2005.
2. *Sunday Leader* (Sri Lanka), 10 April 2005.
3. *Sunday Leader* (Sri Lanka), 12 June 2005.

4. *Daily News* (Sri Lanka), 13 June 2005.
5. See 'A Critique of the Draft Freedom of Access to Official Information Bill 2003', published by the Commonwealth Human Rights Initiative (New Delhi: CHRI, 2004), available at www.humanrightsinitiative.org/programs/ai/rti/international/laws_papers/srilanka/foibill-critique-v2-feb04.pdf. See also *Global Corruption Report 2005*.
6. www.tisrilanka.org/tsunamiedited/tsunami.html
7. *Daily Mirror* (Sri Lanka), 13 June 2005.
8. *BBC News* (UK), 27 June 2005.
9. *Sunday Leader* (Sri Lanka), 3 July 2005.
10. See statement from the conference 'After the Tsunami: Human Rights and Vulnerable Populations' (3–4 June 2005, Bangkok, Thailand), sponsored by the University of California, Berkeley's Human Rights Center; the University of Hawaii's Globalization Research Center; and the East–West Center, available at www.eastwestcenter.org/events-pr-detail.asp?press_ID=383
11. Asanga Welikala, Research Associate, Centre for Policy Alternatives (Sri Lanka), in Transparency International, *National Integrity Systems Country Study 2003 – Sri Lanka* (Berlin/Colombo: TI, 2004).
12. See *Global Corruption Report 2005*.
13. www.eureka.lk/fpea/

Switzerland

Conventions:

Council of Europe Civil Law Convention on Corruption (not yet signed)
Council of Europe Criminal Law Convention on Corruption (signed February 2001; not yet ratified; Additional Protocol signed June 2004)
OECD Anti-Bribery Convention (ratified May 2000)
UN Convention against Corruption (signed December 2003; not yet ratified)
UN Convention against Transnational Organized Crime (signed December 2000; not yet ratified)

Legal and institutional changes

- A new **law on freedom of information** entered into force in April 2005. Until then, the principle of non-disclosure was paramount, every document was considered confidential and people had to give reasons for seeking access to records. The list of exemptions to the new law includes limits to protect public or private interests, such as commercial and industrial information; the contents of penal proceedings; and information related to internal or external security. The authorities are required to stipulate the legal context of any official denial of access.

- In March 2005, the National Council (lower house of parliament) passed a law requiring companies quoted on the stock exchange to **disclose the salaries** paid to individual members of their boards and the total amount paid to management. The same principle will apply to other executive benefits, such as bonuses, stock options, loans, profit sharing plans, assisted mortgages and all other components of payment. The bill is aimed at protecting shareholders by increasing transparency. The law passed the Council of States (upper house of parliament) in June 2005.

Switzerland 'redefines' money laundering

Instant transactions make all financial centres vulnerable to playing host to money launderers, but Switzerland is particularly at risk since around 30 per cent of all internationally invested private assets are managed from there.[1] Recent legal proposals, however, include a selective definition of the underlying criminal activity required for a transaction to be categorised as 'money laundering' that could be seen as an incentive to certain kinds of illegal operations.

Switzerland is a signatory nation of the OECD's Financial Action Task Force (FATF), the main forum against international criminal money flows, and international cooperation has helped in its fight against money laundering. However, the financial authorities have some way to go. A recent OECD report recommended that Switzerland strengthen its money-laundering oversight, specifically calling for greater transparency, the independence of the intermediaries and a tighter deadline for reporting suspicious transactions.[2] In January 2005, the finance ministry launched a consultation round that is hoped will produce new legal measures to ensure full compliance with the 2003 revision of FATF's 40 recommendations. The proposals extend the list of crimes connected to money laundering to include commercial piracy, counterfeit goods, insider trading, human trafficking and some aspects of smuggling. The list of intermediaries subject to due diligence will be extended to include dealers in art, precious stones and precious metals, and property managers.

In March 2005, the Council of States (upper house of parliament) accepted the Federal Council's draft proposal to bring into Swiss law the Council of Europe Criminal Law Convention on Corruption. While this was a positive step, dangerous loopholes are built into the draft. Corruption involving private entities (for example, a Swiss firm that bribes a foreign firm to buy its goods or services) is categorised as a simple offence (punishable by fines or imprisonment of up to three years) and not a crime (sanctioned with imprisonment of up to 20 years). This has serious consequences because, under the Swiss criminal code, the money must have derived from a crime for laundering to have occurred. Thus, funds transferred and traceable to an offence – such as bribery among companies or the case of cigarette smuggling mentioned below – are not considered money laundering under Swiss law. The same problem arises with funds arriving in the country with the purpose of evading another jurisdiction's tax system. Tax evasion has proven to be a very effective means of detecting money laundering crimes, but the Swiss authorities cannot respond to foreign requests for information about suspected evasion because of domestic banking secrecy regulations and the narrow definition of 'crime'. Finally, with regard to domestic oversight of money laundering, when an intermediary accepts money arising from private corruption, the intermediary is not required to report it under Swiss law. Transparency International Switzerland views this situation as seriously deficient and hopes that the National Council (lower house of parliament) will recategorise private corruption as a crime in autumn 2005, when it is scheduled to discuss the draft law.

A positive development came in November 2004 when finance minister Hans-Rudolf Merz approved a plan to bring the oversight of money laundering under a single regulator, provisionally entitled the Federal Financial Market Authority (FINMA). Originally proposed in 1998, the project was delayed due to the standard, lengthy consultation with other official agencies and private interest groups that accompanies any legislative reform in Switzerland. It is now due to be implemented in two years. Responsibility for oversight of money laundering is split between the finance ministry, the Swiss Federal Banking Commission, the Federal Office of Private Insurance, the Swiss Federal Gaming Board and 11 self-regulating bodies supervised by the finance ministry. According to the finance minister, the new entity will allow the regulator to deal better with the wide scope of transactions and improve communications between the various anti-money-laundering agencies.

The Money Laundering Reporting Office Switzerland (MROS) is the Swiss version of a financial intelligence unit. The organisation's function is to insulate the prosecution and enforcement agencies from intermediaries while simultaneously protecting their client–banker confidentiality commitments. Under the Money Laundering Act of 1997, intermediaries (including banks, lawyers and accountants) must file a suspicious transaction report with the MROS whenever they perceive one, or risk losing their licence. The number of reports actually filed is low compared to other major financial centres, suggesting widespread non-compliance within the country's 7,000-strong financial services sector, and the ultimate sanction has never once been imposed. MROS referred 821 suspicious transactions for further investigation in 2004, compared to 863 a year earlier. Significantly, with just eight permanent staff responsible for oversight in one of the world's largest financial centres, the MROS is vastly understaffed.

According to MROS, 11 per cent of the 821 cases filed for criminal investigation in 2004 involved sums larger than 1 million Swiss francs. The outcomes of the ensuing investigations are less widely publicised. The judgment in March 2002 against Pavel Borodin, currently State Secretary of the Union of Russia and Belarus, resulted in a fine of just US $177,000, or the equivalent of 0.3 per cent of the funds he is alleged to have siphoned out of Russia, according to an investigation by a Swiss judge. The lack of cooperation from the Russian authorities proved to be the case's undoing.[3] The crucial role of international cooperation is also indicated by the fact that referrals outnumber domestic requests by two to one: suspicious transactions referred onward after foreign requests amounted to 1,701 in 2004, compared to 821 from domestic sources. In 2002, the finance ministry returned US $77 million of laundered funds to the government of Peru from accounts belonging to former intelligence director Vladimir Montesinos after it was determined that they had resulted from criminal activities. Another important case involved the fortune accumulated by the late Nigerian dictator Sani Abacha. The Supreme Court ruled in February 2005 that US $458 million were illegally obtained and ordered the amount returned to Nigeria (in addition to US $200 million returned in 2003).

Not all the money-laundering news has been positive. The problem of legal interpretation resurfaced when a court in 2001 gave a suspended sentence to an Italian who had smuggled 1,000 tonnes of cigarettes a month in defiance of EU rules and laundered the proceeds in Switzerland. Under existing law, laundering criminal assets from smuggling is only a fiscal offence, rather than a crime. The MROS annual report for 2004 provided for the first time an account of the cases it has referred for prosecution since the law entered into force in 1998. Of the 2,708 transactions reported, only 47 convictions were obtained and 1,397 cases are still in the courts. More worrisome is the fact that there is an unknown number of cases that have not been reported to MROS.

Switzerland has made progress in devising legislation and designing institutions to combat money laundering, but international cooperation is essential to improve the number of convictions, and since two crimes must be proven (the predicate crime and money laundering), this is an especially difficult task. What is also required is more insistent pressure on intermediaries to report suspicious transactions, and to overcome their tendency to report cases by new customers, rather than by established clients. MROS is to be congratulated for reporting the status of cases referred in the past, but the numbers show a disturbing trend toward the suspension of investigations before they get to court. The rate of successful prosecutions must also be increased if Switzerland is to gain a credible reputation as a foe of money laundering.

Above all, the National Council must be encouraged to consider private corruption a crime. If the current draft law is allowed to stand, some cases of money laundering will continue to be ignored due to the narrow categorisation of the crime under the Swiss penal code.

Political finance in the spotlight

The principle that politics is voluntary and unremunerated is paramount in Switzerland. Parties do not benefit from government funding, apart from small contributions to party factions, and politicians work on a voluntary basis, while supporting themselves through other jobs. Initiatives to professionalise parliament have tended to fail because of the prevailing opinion that politicians choose their profession through conviction, rather than for financial gain. As a result, Swiss politicians finance their own election campaigns and find their own sponsors. Nor is there any requirement to declare the source or amount of any financial aid they receive. This makes Switzerland's party funding system one of the murkiest in Europe.

Since 1 December 2003, a new law on the Federal Assembly has introduced a little more transparency. Parliamentarians are now required to declare their membership of administrative boards and all consultant activities to prevent conflicts of interest arising. If they fail to publish the information, they are subject to removal or exclusion from their positions for a period of six months. But watchdog groups, including TI Switzerland, point out that the new law does not go far enough since it does not address the question of parliamentary sponsorship. The existence of this loophole was highlighted by last year's 'donation scandal'.

In summer 2004, it was alleged that Anita Fetz and Roberto Zanetti, both Socialist Party MPs, had not declared their membership of the board of Pro Facile, a foundation that runs investments. This left them open to disciplinary action, but the case blew into a scandal because the foundation had been applying the controversial methods developed by hedge-fund manager and socialite Dieter Behring to the 'donations' it received. His system promised investors a return of 8 per cent, half of it accruing to the foundation. This fell way beyond the conventions of good foundation management. In October 2004, Behring was arrested on suspicion of investment fraud involving hundreds of millions of francs.[4] Behring had allegedly been a major backer of Fetz's political ambitions, giving large sums to her re-election campaign. Behring later went to prison for six months before being released on bail in April 2005,[5] and Fetz resigned from office after the media broke the story.

For the notoriously discreet Swiss, the 'donations scandal' was a *grande affaire*. Why had Fetz, previously considered of open and honest character, not declared her membership of Pro Facile in the first place? As board member of two respected banks, why had she not resigned immediately instead of waiting for the media to expose the foundation's alleged fraudulent practices? Why had she not admitted that Behring was her election sponsor?

The scandal also focused attention on the flaws of Switzerland's existing system of political financing. Until there are regulations that require politicians to declare donations and other support, the space for irregularities and corruption will persist. Until parties are obliged to account for their use of funds and disclose the identities of their donors, it will be impossible to decide if they are acting according to their own principles or in the interests of their sponsors. It would be naive to believe that no return service is expected for the large sums that sponsors invest in politicians' election campaigns.

In spite of the damage to their profession caused by the 'donations scandal', not one of the major parties has come up with proposals to increase the transparency of private money in the political system. This, no doubt, reflects a reluctance to disclose their own funding sources.

Jeffrey Nilsen, Anne Schwöbel and Stefanie Teickner (TI Switzerland)

Further reading

Tiziano Balmelli and Bernard Jaggy (eds), *Les Traités internationaux contre la corruption. L'ONU, l'OCDE, le Conseil de l'Europe et la Suisse* (International Anti-Corruption Treaties: The UN, the OECD, the Council of Europe and Switzerland) (Lausanne, Berne, Lugano: Edis, 2004)

Othmar Hafner, *Korruption und Korruptionsbekämpfung in der Schweiz. Eine Übersicht von Transparency International – Schweiz* (Corruption and the Anti-corruption Fight in Switzerland. An Overview by Transparency International Switzerland) (Bern: TI Switzerland, 2003)

Daniel Jositsch, *Das Schweizerische Korruptionsstrafrecht. Art. 322ter bis Art. 322octies StGB* (Anti-corruption Criminal Law in Switzerland) (Zürich: Schulthess, 2004)

Ivo Kaufmann, 'Länderexamen Korruption – die Schweiz im internationalen Vergleich' (An International Comparison of Corruption: Report on Switzerland), *Volkswirtschaft* 78, March 2005.

Mark Pieth and Gemma Aiolfi (eds), *A Comparative Guide to Anti-Money Laundering, A Critical Analysis of Systems in Singapore, Switzerland, the UK and the USA* (Cheltenham, UK, and Northampton, USA: Edward Elgar Publishing, 2005)

TI Switzerland: www.transparency.ch

Notes

1. The Swiss Financial Centre (Bern: Swiss Federal Department of Finance, June 2003).
2. 'Switzerland: Phase 2, Report on the Application of the OECD Anti-Bribery Convention' (Paris: OECD, December 2004), www.oecd.org/dataoecd/43/16/34350161.pdf
3. www.albionmonitor.com/0203a/swissbankrussialaunder.html
4. *Neue Zürcher Zeitung* (Switzerland), 5 March 2005.
5. *Neue Zürcher Zeitung* (Switzerland) online, 12 August 2005.

Uganda

Conventions:
AU Convention on Preventing and Combating Corruption (ratified August 2004)
UN Convention against Corruption (ratified September 2004)
UN Convention against Transnational Organized Crime (ratified March 2005)

Legal and institutional changes

• The government issued a White Paper in October 2004 recommending that the Inspector General of Government (IGG) be given more latitude to arrest and prosecute persons involved in **corruption or abuse of public office**. This would amend sections of the Leadership Code Act of 2002 to bring it in line with the 1995 Constitution, which grants the IGG prosecutorial powers. A previous constitutional ruling in May 2004 trimmed the IGG's powers. To strengthen the institution, the White Paper proposed the creation of an anti-corruption tribunal to try cases. The agency was re-energised after the appointment in January 2005 of a new IGG, Justice Faith Mwondha, and her deputy, Raphael Obudra Baku. They instructed all MPs and political leaders to declare their wealth before the end of March 2005 and warned that those who did not comply would face legal action (see below).

• In July 2004, the Directorate of Ethics and Integrity (DEI) launched a four-year **strategy to combat corruption and rebuild integrity in public office**. The programme, due to run from 2004 to 2007, aims to improve the enforcement and coordination of existing law and to ensure that the public is actively involved in the fight against corruption. The DEI has drafted whistleblower protection legislation that will be submitted to parliament after the presidential and parliamentary elections in March 2006. The DEI is also reviewing the Prevention of Corruption Act 1970 with a view to presenting a new version to parliament.

Institutional failure looms

Despite an extensive legal framework and ample opportunity for participation by media and civil society, the lack of political will to curb corruption has led Uganda to the brink of institutional failure. Corruption by politicians and officials is one of the biggest challenges facing the country.

One case involved Major Roland Kakooza Mutale, a senior adviser to President Yoweri Museveni who made a major contribution to his re-election in 2001. A May 2003 report by the Inspector General of Government recommended that Mutale be sacked for refusing to declare his wealth under the 2002 Leadership Code Act. He was relieved of his post as adviser soon afterwards.

This was the start of a widening rift between the IGG and the government. Senior officials were already disgruntled to find their wealth and possessions published in the media in 2002. Mutale took the matter to court and got President Museveni to swear an affidavit in his support, effectively condoning his refusal to comply with the law.[1] By March 2004, a constitutional court ruling in Mutale's favour had contrived to render entire sections of the Leadership Code Act null and void. This duel between the IGG and the government is a clear demonstration of a flagging institutional system in Uganda. It also exposed a weakened judiciary that is unable to temper the powerful executive.

A second incident occurred in May 2004 when the solicitor general refused to surrender files on the James Garuga Musinguzi case when asked by the IGG. The IGG had expressed alarm at the amount of compensation awarded by the government to Musinguzi, a city tycoon and rancher. Musinguzi was due to receive UShs13 billion (US $7.4 million) as compensation for the confiscation and redistribution of his ranches in Rakai. The case was handled out of court through an 'amicable arrangement' between the solicitor general's office and Musinguzi.[2] When the solicitor general refused to hand over the file, the ombudsman ordered his arrest. Mutale promptly mobilised a platoon of soldiers to protect him.[3] This interference in the execution of the IGG's duties was a serious breach of the 1995 constitution which states that the IGG 'shall be independent in the performance of its functions and shall not be subject to the direction or control of any person or authority and shall only be responsible to parliament'.[4] The fact that Mutale could carry out such an operation without legal or political backlash indicates how cosmetic the government's commitment is to implementing the rule of law. It also raises questions about the IGG's survival.

Another negative milestone was passed in August 2004 when the High Court nullified a report into allegations of corruption at the Uganda Revenue Authority.[5] A petition was issued by two members of the commission of inquiry after a disagreement with the chairperson over sections in the report. Instead of allowing further inquiries to be made regarding the contested passages, the court decided to expunge the document altogether. The decision reflected a failure of the court's moral responsibility to bring acts of corruption to justice; it also meant that no further legal action could be taken against those implicated. Following cases like these it is no surprise that, according to various auditor general reports from 2001 to 2003, more than UShs2 billion (US $1.1 million) is lost to corruption every year.

A further setback nearly occurred in September 2004 when the cabinet proposed to the Constitutional Review Commission that the offices of the Ombudsman and the Human Rights Commission be merged, a move that would have stripped the latter of its powers of prosecution. The proposal was dropped after protests from public and civil society organisations questioning the government's commitment to fighting corruption.[6]

Uganda's institutions are facing challenges of a systemic nature, making them subject to the whims of politics. The constitution of 1995 is a case in point: while clearly providing for presidential term limits and the question of succession, parliamentarians voted to scrap term limits in July 2005, paving the way for President Museveni to seek re-election in March 2006. The decision to amend the constitution sets a bad precedent that a hallowed document can be altered to suit the political climate.

Corruption 'decentralised' along with government functions

Political corruption at local government level has increased since 1996 when the new government ushered in a process of decentralisation of governance to local councils under the 1997 Local Government Act. Uganda's local governments have responsibility for revenue collection, planning, resource allocation and service delivery, including primary education, primary health care, water and sanitation, rural roads and agriculture. Such weighty responsibilities combined with weak legislation, lack of oversight, poor remuneration, costly campaign bids and an electorate that expects favours from politicians, rather than transparent government, provide ample opportunities for corruption.

In some cases, local politicians have virtually taken over the award of tenders, especially for the construction of schools, dams and health units, usurping the mandate of district tender boards. In a tender for electrical installations for the Kasaali maternity ward in Rakai district in 2003–04, the only pre-qualified firm, Kamungolo General Services, was not awarded the contract, which went instead to a firm that had not even put in a bid.[7] In Kabira sub-county in 2004, the construction of teachers' residences for Bukaala Primary School was awarded before a call for tenders was issued, making it effectively futile for other contractors to bid.[8]

Decentralisation was aimed at offering citizens increased participation at the local level. But a detailed study of corruption in local government found that people's confidence has been eroded, and the quality of public infrastructure and services is deteriorating.[9]

The main channels of political corruption in Uganda's local government bodies are: influence peddling; diversion of resources; giving contracts and jobs to supporters and family members; presenting bogus allowance claims; colluding with civil servants to embezzle resources; bribery; presenting false documents in order to qualify for elected or competitive positions; using public vehicles for personal work; and political interference in decision-making.

The position deemed most corrupt by the general public is that of district chairman, which wields so much power that it has virtually usurped local boards, commissions and civil servants, including tender boards and public accounts committees, in deciding resource allocations. Residents of Baitambogwe and Buwaya in Mayuge reported that many politicians and council or board members have new properties and expensive lifestyles, yet they have no other clear sources of income to back up such wealth. Politicians feel pressure to amass wealth before leaving office so that re-election bids can be financed, and so they can survive if not re-elected.

The health and education sectors are worst hit by local-level corruption. The Muggi Health Centre II in Buwaya sub-county, Mayuge district is one example. There, the local MP halted construction of the health facility in 2002 because he wanted it built at Kasutaime – just two kilometres from an existing health centre – an area where he was seeking to bolster his political support. Also in Mayuge district, local councillors interfered in the selection process for 30 nursing assistants in 2003,[10] handpicking their favourites regardless of whether minimum qualifications were met. In the education sector, there are many examples of sub-standard construction across the districts studied, and of scholarships going to relatives of members of the district bursary commission, or district councillors.

An important causal factor is that local government positions are poorly paid and there are few institutional and legal constraints to prevent politicians from embezzling money. Indeed, the Local Government Finance and Accounting Regulations and the Local Government Act 1997 exempt politicians from accounting for public resources. Civil servants must account for the budgets they control, but politicians who may have influenced or pressured civil servants to misuse funds cannot be held liable. This problem is further compounded by a weakness of the Local Government Act, which gives politicians authority over civil servants, including recruiting them.

The private sector, as main supplier of goods and services to local government, further fuels corruption. The fact that much of the private sector is informal makes it difficult to tackle bribery. Public sector and donor-sponsored programmes aimed at improving performance, sensitising the private sector to the problems of corruption and improving the regulatory framework have had little effect.

There is a clear need to fight corruption and break a cycle of despondency in which voters are reluctant to 'waste time' holding politicians to account, rather than demanding immediate, if piecemeal, returns for votes or support.[11] Initial steps must include improving the legal and institutional framework so that politicians do not hold sway over civil servants, and civil servants cannot determine outcomes of tendering process or other resources allocation mechanisms that are vulnerable to corruption. Politicians must also respect the rule of law and declare assets before and after taking up office.

Charles Mubbale and Paul Onapa (TI Uganda)

Further reading

Directorate of Ethics and Integrity, *National Strategy Document to Combat Corruption and Rebuild Ethics and Integrity in Public Office, 2004–2007*, Kampala, 6 April 2005
Human Rights and Democratisation Programme of DANIDA, 'Anti-Corruption Manual for Civil Society in Uganda' (Kampala: DANIDA, unpublished)
Transparency International Uganda (TIU), *The Impact of Political Corruption on Resource Allocation and Service Delivery in Local Governments in Uganda* (Kampala: TIU, 2005)

TI Uganda: www.transparencyuganda.org

Notes

1. *New Vision* (Uganda), 24 September 2003.
2. *The Monitor* (Uganda), 2 June 2004.
3. *The Monitor* (Uganda), 1 June 2004.
4. Article 227 of the 1995 constitution.
5. *New Vision* (Uganda), 17 August 2004.
6. *The Monitor* (Uganda), 4 September 2004.

7. Transparency International Uganda, *The Impact of Political Corruption on Resource Allocation and Service Delivery in Local Governments in Uganda* (Kampala: TIU, June 2005), and author interview with district councillors.
8 Transparency International Uganda, *The Impact of Political Corruption*.
9. Ibid. Research took place in 2004–05 in four districts: Kampala, Mayuge, Ntugamo and Rakai.
10. Author interview in 2003 with District Service Commission of Mayuge district.
11. Survey respondent from Rakai district, Transparency International Uganda, *The Impact of Political Corruption*.

Ukraine

Conventions:
Council of Europe Civil Law Convention on Corruption (ratified March 2005)
Council of Europe Criminal Law Convention on Corruption (signed January 1999; not yet ratified; Additional Protocol signed May 2003; not yet ratified)
UN Convention against Corruption (signed December 2003; not yet ratified)
UN Convention against Transnational Organized Crime (signed December 2000; not yet ratified)

Legal and institutional changes

- Although delayed, plans to set up an independent body, the **National Bureau of Investigation**, remain a top priority. In March 2005, the government set up a working group on the development of a concept for the bureau, which will focus on fighting corruption. It remains to be seen, however, how the creation of this agency will complement existing anti-corruption bodies.

- In April 2005, an **anti-smuggling programme** was approved by cabinet to address the problem of bribing to avoid customs duties and import taxes. A 'single window' concept was introduced with instant dismissal for anyone reported demanding or receiving a bribe (see below).

- In May 2005, the president issued an edict regarding the liberalisation of entrepreneurial activities and state support of entrepreneurship. The aim is to review laws, in order to eliminate conflicting regulation, licensing and other procedures that affect **business activities**. These are often so confusing and uncertain, in terms of relevance, that the only way to satisfy all the requirements one is presented with is to employ an intermediary 'expert' who will pay an inevitable bribe. It is therefore hoped that this new edict will help curb corruption.

- In June 2005, the government approved an action plan for 2005 for the **adaptation of Ukrainian legislation to that of the European Union**. This includes a series of policy commitments to uphold European norms and values in the political, social and economic spheres, all of which would be instrumental in reducing corruption (see below).

- In July 2005, the president issued an edict regarding the **dissolution of road traffic police** structures, after months of frustration at the lack of obvious progress in reform and several public warnings (see below).

Yushchenko's new anti-corruption measures: the first six months

In January 2005, Viktor Yushchenko was inaugurated as the new president marking the end of the 'orange revolution'. This had been initiated by widespread popular protest in response to allegations of massive corruption, voter intimidation and direct electoral fraud during Ukraine's presidential election in November 2004. In the former regime, despite the fact that corruption was endemic, existing legislation appeared to support the hypothesis that corruption was not a problem and any transgressions were considered to be minor. If laws were applied they were generally misused to intimidate opponents of the regime, such as opposition activists or journalists, while criticism from foreign investors was ignored. Moreover, local business people who spoke out were often harassed by state bodies, including the tax authorities. Transparency and openness were thereby discouraged and foreign investment dwindled to a mere trickle of what should have been achieved by a country with the size and potential of Ukraine. One principal driving force behind the 'orange revolution' was the sense of public outrage at the extreme methods used by the outgoing corrupt regime to remain in power.

In June 2005, one of the main themes of the roundtable conference organised by the World Economic Forum was the issue of corruption in Ukraine. Ten action steps were proposed to the president and all appeared to be accepted with enthusiasm. The first nine steps have an indirect impact on corruption, but the tenth deals specifically with corruption in the following way: blacklisting companies; basing future appointments to the civil service and judiciary on merit and not on politics; raising salaries of civil servants to reduce incentives for corruption; introducing a new system of public procurement such as an efficient online system; and disclosing salaries and business affiliations of senior members of government, judges and legislators. It remains to be seen, however, how these recommendations will be implemented concretely in the near future.

President Yushchenko now faces a huge challenge to implement successful reform, while the expectations of his electorate to address rampant corruption hang heavily on his shoulders. Various initiatives have been pursued by the new government with varying degrees of success. The most notable is a new anti-smuggling programme approved by cabinet in April 2005 to address the problem of bribing to avoid customs duties and import taxes. A 'single window' concept was introduced with instant dismissal for anyone reported demanding or receiving a bribe. This was initially reinforced by officers of the security services observing customs officers while performing their duties. In the first month of this operation, the revenue from customs reportedly doubled, but it did cause delays. Customs duties on some items have been dramatically reduced, but it is clear that all duties need to be reduced to a level that renders the payment of a bribe uneconomic.

At the June roundtable conference, President Yushchenko repeated his earlier declaration that neither he nor his government would steal from the Ukrainian people and then made a commitment to make public the financial declarations of his ministers and top officials. Many civil servants at all levels have grown accustomed to supplementing their meagre salaries through corrupt means and have assets that could never have been acquired through previously declared personal incomes. Yet no formula has been found for providing them with reasonable remuneration. However, there is a limit to what the government can afford in terms of public sector wages and other measures could also be explored. In addition, it probably needs some form of amnesty to get the declaration process going in a thoroughly honest and open manner.

In July 2005, the road traffic police was restructured, after months of frustration at the lack of obvious progress in reform and a number of public warnings. It is not yet clear how this restructuring will work out, but it seems to reflect a similar initiative taken in Georgia, where a completely new force was recruited and trained in the space of a few months and then paid appreciably more than under the previous regime.

In the meantime, the opening up of the media is currently under way, one of the most important measures a state can take to expose corrupt behaviour to public scrutiny and hold officials to account. The media operates more freely in contrast to the previous regime, when intimidation, pro-government ownership, favouritism in granting broadcast rights and frequencies, and government press guidance were the order of the day. However, self-censorship and concentrated ownership of the media are still a concern. A confidential hotline for people wishing to report instances of corruption has also been established.

Perhaps the most significant change to come out of the 'orange revolution' was a series of policy commitments to uphold European norms and values in the political, social and economic spheres, all of which could be instrumental in reducing corruption. The key document outlining this is the EU–Ukraine Action Plan, but the Ukrainian authorities have gone beyond the commitments contained in the plan and stated their intention to fulfil all the Copenhagen criteria for EU membership, with the hope of submitting an application in three years' time. This has far-reaching implications for the relationship between the state and society, for the development of democratic institutions and a democratic political culture, for the expansion of civil society and for the protection of human rights. Most studies show that these factors are strongly associated with lower levels of corruption.

Whilst Yushchenko's commitment to route out corruption is well publicised, his ability to achieve lasting change depends on whether his 'pro-reform' team will achieve a working majority in the March 2006 parliamentary elections. Currently, parliament is still dominated by powerful business groups who are quite prepared to reject government initiatives if they do not suit their interests. This is due to the fact that the different personalities with varying political agendas only came together to unseat Kuchma's previous corrupt regime. So there is frequent public controversy between MPs and it is difficult to see how the prime minister can run an effective cabinet when there is no dominating vision. Another problem is the lack of evidence that acts of corruption committed by the previous regime or during the fraudulent presidential election process will be pursued and prosecuted effectively. Unless there are exemplary prosecutions of important individuals, the public will be hard pressed to believe that any real change has taken place. Nevertheless, the authorities must avoid perceptions of political retribution so strongly associated with the previous government.

Transparency International

Further reading

TI Ukraine: www.transparency.org.ua

United Kingdom

Conventions:
Council of Europe Civil Law Convention on Corruption (signed June 2000; not yet ratified)

Council of Europe Criminal Law Convention on Corruption (ratified December 2003; Additional Protocol ratified December 2003)
OECD Anti-Bribery Convention (ratified December 1998)
UN Convention against Corruption (signed December 2003; not yet ratified)
UN Convention against Transnational Organized Crime (signed December 2000; not yet ratified)

Legal and institutional changes

- In July 2004, the Cabinet Office announced the appointment of Sir Patrick Brown, a former permanent secretary, to undertake a review of the arrangements for **senior civil servants** moving to jobs in industry, including the requirement for a cooling-off period before jobs are taken up. Sir Patrick's terms of reference require him to 'ensure that [the rules] are compatible with a public service that is keen to encourage far greater interchange with private and other sectors'.[1] His report will be published in 2005.

- The government published its updated strategy to **fight money laundering** in October 2004.[2] However, the new strategy did not address deficiencies in the UK's anti-money-laundering regime, notably the lack of supervision of trusts and company service providers (see below).

- In December 2004, the Export Credits Guarantee Department (ECGD) revised the strengthened procedures to combat **bribery and corruption** that it had adopted in May 2004. This followed lobbying by major customers and industry bodies, and has the effect of significantly weakening the provisions (see below).

- The Freedom of Information (FOI) Act came into force on 1 January 2005. It provides a general right of **access to all information** held by public authorities in the United Kingdom (though separate legislation applies to Scotland). A request for information is made directly to the public authority holding the information. There are 7 absolute and 16 qualified exemptions. Absolute exemptions include information supplied by, or relating to, bodies dealing with security matters, where disclosure would breach parliamentary privilege, and where disclosure would constitute a breach of confidence. Qualified exemptions include the need to safeguard national security; information relating to the formulation of government policy; ministerial communications and advice by law officers; and information held by public authorities with audit-related functions. There is a right of appeal against any refusal to release information to the Information Commissioner.

Too little priority given to foreign bribery and corruption

The OECD's Phase Two Evaluation of the United Kingdom's Application of the OECD Anti-Bribery Convention was published in March 2005. While it complimented the United Kingdom on some progress made, its general tenor was critical and conveyed a sense of disappointment at the low level of priority accorded to the subject of foreign bribery, reinforcing a perception that there is a lack of will in government to address the problem.

The OECD regretted that legislative changes to reform the corruption laws had not been enacted, but acknowledged an attempt to make progress in 2003 by consulting an all-party Joint Parliamentary Committee (JPC) on a draft corruption bill. The OECD found no indication, however, of when there might be sufficient time in the legislative programme for it to be enacted. The JPC strongly criticised the draft bill, arguing that it would not be 'readily understood by the police, by prosecutors, by jurors and by the public, including – especially – the business and public sector communities, and their advisers, both here and abroad'.[3] Anti-corruption laws continue to derive from ancient common law offences and statutes that were adopted between 1889 and 1916, and updated for overseas bribery offences by part 12 of the Anti-Terrorism Crime and Security Act of 2001.

In the six years since the United Kingdom ratified the OECD Convention, not a single company or individual has been indicted or tried for the offence of bribing a foreign public official, though several UK companies have allegedly been implicated. It took until February 2002 for foreign bribery to be effectively criminalised. The OECD report expressed concern that 'the very large number of investigative bodies has resulted in excessive fragmentation of efforts, lack of specialised expertise, lack of transparency both for the public and investigative authorities, and problems in achieving coherent action'. At present, initial reports of foreign bribery are channelled to the National Criminal Intelligence Service (NCIS); cases are then passed to the Serious Fraud Office (SFO) for vetting, but if the SFO does not accept a case for investigation and prosecution, it is passed to one of 43 police forces. The OECD would prefer to see a single body, such as the SFO, holding centralised responsibility for both investigation and prosecution.

The government has taken action to remedy a similar problem of fragmentation in the fight against serious organised crime – in particular large-scale drug and people trafficking – which it sees as a priority. Legislation was passed by Parliament in April 2005 to establish the Serious Organised Crime Agency (SOCA), which will absorb the NCIS, the National Crime Squad and parts of Customs and Excise. The SFO is already under-resourced, however, and there is concern that setting up SOCA may weaken its ability to pursue overseas corruption cases since both agencies draw on a limited pool of experienced personnel.

The OECD report suggests there is a lack of awareness of the OECD convention and the foreign bribery offence among law enforcement agencies, judicial authorities and UK officials involved with UK companies operating abroad. It recommends more effort to raise awareness among these groups, and also among trade unions and small- and medium-sized enterprises that do international business. It recommends measures to publicise the conditions under which parent and affiliate companies can be liable in connection with foreign bribery, and to encourage UK companies to report to the appropriate authorities any instances of foreign bribery they encounter in their operations.

The OECD report welcomed the confiscation provisions of the Proceeds of Crime Act 2002 in the context of combating money laundering and the theft of state assets. But the act requires all confiscated sums to be paid over to the Treasury, and there is no requirement for the whole of any confiscated sum (with or without a reasonable deduction for costs) to be repatriated to the country of origin. However, the United Kingdom can deal with asset sharing on an ad hoc, purely administrative basis. The Home Office has an agreement with the Treasury to return up to 50 per cent net of costs without further authority.

The OECD examiners were concerned that the lack of a clear definition of what was understood by the UK authorities to constitute a facilitation payment to foreign public officials could result in a much wider range of payments being effectively exempted than was intended by the convention. Furthermore, responsibility for investigating defence contracts where the Ministry of Defence (or the Defence Export Sales Organisation) is party to the contract rests with the Ministry of Defence police, a situation that clearly gives rise to potential conflicts of interest. Finally, the Crown Dependencies, which are seen as financial and tax haven jurisdictions, still allow the deduction of bribes for tax purposes if 'wholly and exclusively for purposes of trade' – a clear contradiction of the OECD convention and one which the UK Treasury needs to address.

Finally, in the area of money laundering, the abuse of companies and trusts for laundering dirty money is a recognised risk. Tackling this abuse requires effective regulation of the service providers, who set up and maintain these vehicles. The United Kingdom has included such service providers within its revised money-laundering regulations, but so far it has not implemented an effective supervision regime. The supervision of trusts and company service providers is under discussion in the EU in connection with the implementation of its Third Money-Laundering Directive. But the United Kingdom has already recognised the case for such a regime by pressing the governments of its overseas territories to improve regulation of company formation and management.[4] While there are now regulatory structures in place in Gibraltar, Guernsey, Jersey and a number of other jurisdictions, there is still no supervisory regime in the United Kingdom.

ECGD buckles under business pressure

In May 2004, the UK's Export Credits Guarantee Department (ECGD) introduced a number of requirements designed to guard against bribery and corruption in the business it insures. It changed procedures to include requirements for listing the names and addresses of all agents, and amounts of commission paid to them; stronger powers to inspect exporters' contractual documents; and requirements for due diligence in relation to the activities of applicants' joint venture or consortium partners.

While most ECGD customers accepted the changes, there was strong opposition from a minority of large companies, led by British Aerospace (BAe) Systems, Airbus Industrie-UK and Rolls-Royce, supported by the Confederation of British Industry (CBI). In letters to the ECGD, BAe said that the provisions were 'unduly onerous'. Airbus felt that its network of agents was part of its 'competitive advantage' and that it was inappropriate to disclose this information. The companies succeeded in obtaining a qualification of the expression 'to the best of our knowledge and belief' in relation to the due diligence required from ECGD applicants, significantly weakening due diligence requirements. Following a number of meetings between the ECGD and these parties, revised procedures became effective in December 2004.

The OECD advised that the changes could weaken the ECGD's ability to detect and prevent foreign bribery.[5] A number of the changes were criticised in the report on the ECGD of the all-party House of Commons Trade and Industry Committee, to which TI (UK) made detailed submissions.[6] The committee observed: 'Applicants for ECGD support have no longer to give the department information on the involvement of agents in the project for which support is requested; they will not be required to vouch for the honesty of third parties to the project, except for those employed directly by them; and the ECGD no longer reserves the right of audit of exporters' documents as part of the monitoring of projects.'

A further change provides that agents' commissions do not have to be disclosed if they are less than 5 per cent of the contract price, and are not covered by the credit to which the ECGD's guarantee applies. In a large contract, 5 per cent of the price could be a substantial sum, but such sums can be, and often are, funded outside the guaranteed credit. In April 2005, the chair of the committee said: 'We are not at all convinced that the changes [to ECGD's anti-bribery rules] will not seriously weaken the department's ability to contribute to the government's policies against bribery. We do not understand that, while some of the ECGD's customers felt that they could comply with the more stringent requirement, others decided they could not.'[7]

TI (UK) and The Corner House, an NGO, expressed strong opposition to the changes in the media and in discussions with ECGD. In December 2004, The Corner House instituted legal proceedings for judicial review against the government, claiming that ECGD had significantly weakened its rules without consulting interested NGOs, thereby breaching its own consultation policy. In January 2005, the government settled out of court. Although the changes to the anti-bribery rules would remain in effect, it agreed to institute a full public consultation on them, pay The Corner House's legal costs and make public the correspondence between ECGD, CBI and the three companies that led the opposition to the May 2004 changes, as well as records of the meetings chaired by the Secretary of State for Trade and Industry. The public consultation will close in June 2005, and the government intends to publish its response three months later.

The weakening of the ECGD's anti-bribery procedures contrasted with the recommendation in the Report of the Commission for Africa that developed countries should ensure they do not contribute to the problem of corruption by encouraging 'their Export Credit Agencies to be more transparent, and to require higher standards of transparency in their support for projects in developing countries'.[8] On the corruption issue, the commission also recommended that: countries and territories with significant financial centres should take, as a matter of urgency, all necessary legal and administrative measures to repatriate illicitly acquired state funds and assets; and that all states should ratify and implement the UN Convention against Corruption during 2005. If the United Kingdom is to be effective in leading international action to reduce the damage done by corruption to developing countries in Africa and elsewhere, the government must find the political will to take stronger action at home.

Transparency International (UK)

Further reading

Sue Hawley, 'Backgrounder to OECD Evaluation of UK's Record on Combating Bribery' (Dorset, UK: The Corner House, May 2005)

Robert Neild, *Public Corruption – The Dark Side of Social Evolution* (London: Anthem Press, 2002)

Anthony Sampson, *Who Runs This Place? The Anatomy of Britain in the 21st Century* (London: John Murray, 2004)

Transparency International (UK), 'Corruption and Money Laundering in the UK – One Problem, Two Standards – A Report on the Regulation of Trusts and Company Service Providers' (London: TI (UK), October 2004)

Transparency International (UK), 'Consultation on Changes to ECGD's Anti-Bribery and Corruption Procedures Introduced in December 2004' (London: TI (UK), June 2005)

Transparency International (UK), 'Preventing Corruption on Construction Projects – Risk Assessment and Proposed Actions for Banks, Export Credit Agencies, Guarantors and Insurers' (London: TI (UK), 2005), www.transparency.org.uk/ECGD/TI.PREVENTING.CORRUPTION. RISK.FUNDERS.pdf

TI (UK): www.transparency.org.uk

Notes

1. *Guardian* (UK), 16 August 2004.
2. Anti-Money-Laundering Strategy, HM Treasury, October 2004.
3. *Global Corruption Report 2005*.
4. UK Government White Paper, *Partnership for Progress and Prosperity: Britain and the Overseas Territories* (London: HMSO, March 1999).
5. OECD, 'United Kingdom: Phase 2 Report on the Application of the Convention on Combating Bribery of Foreign Public Officials in International Business Transactions and the 1997

Recommendation on Combating Bribery in International Business Transactions', www.oecd.org/dataoecd/62/32/34599062.pdf

6. House of Commons Trade and Industry Committee's Ninth Report of Session 2004–05, 'Implementation of ECGD's Business Principles', HC 374–1, published 4 April 2005.

7. Trade and Industry Committee, Press Notice PN35 of Session 2004–05, 4 April 2005.

8. Commission for Africa, 'Our Common Interest – Report of the Commission for Africa', March 2005, www.commissionforafrica.org/English/report/introduction.html

United States of America

Conventions:

OAS Inter-American Convention against Corruption (ratified September 2000)

OECD Anti-Bribery Convention (ratified December 1998)

UN Convention against Corruption (signed December 2003; not yet ratified)

UN Convention against Transnational Organized Crime (signed December 2000; not yet ratified)

Legal and institutional changes

- In February 2005, Senators Trent Lott, John McCain and Russell Feingold, and Representatives Christopher Shays and Martin Meehan, introduced the 527 Reform Act in Congress. The proposed legislation would amend the Federal Election Campaign Act of 1971 and its 1974 amendments, to require '527s', organisations created for explicit political purposes but with no formal ties to parties or particular politicians, to comply with **campaign finance laws**, including provisions requiring them to register with the Federal Election Commission (FEC), to improve their transparency and to comply with stricter reporting requirements (see below on 'Transparency in campaign finance').

- In March 2005, Congressmen Mike Pence and Albert Wynn introduced the 527 **Fairness Act**. Critics maintain it would do nothing to change the legal status of 527 groups, and would set back campaign finance reform by repealing limits on contributions to political parties and federal candidates established by the Federal Election Campaign Act of 1974.

Legislative ethics

Throughout late 2004 and early 2005, media reports alleging that some Congress members had been involved in ethics breaches and conflicts of interest affairs raised serious questions about the effectiveness of Congress' current system of self-regulation. The main focus was congressional travel funded by lobbyists or registered foreign agents in violation of ethics rules, and the increasing amount of corporate-financed congressional travel, which is permitted, but which raises conflict of interest concerns.

Attention also focused on pressure by House and Senate leaders on trade associations and other interest groups to hire members of the Republican party in order to maintain their access to legislative processes.[1]

Both the Senate and the House of Representatives have codes of ethics for their members, which are enforced by internal standing committees. Civil society organisations and the media drew attention to the system's weaknesses, including a prohibition on outside groups from making complaints. The House Committee on Standards of Official Conduct (known as the ethics committee) adopted a rules change in 1997 that prohibits outside groups or individuals from filing complaints unless accompanied by certification signed by a House member. In January 2005, another rule change made it harder to launch an investigation by requiring a majority vote of the committee, rather than a tie vote, as previously required to trigger an automatic investigation within 45 days. Because the current committee is evenly divided between Democrats and Republicans, there were concerns that political considerations would play an even larger role in decisions.

Also in January, after the ethics committee reproached Tom DeLay, who heads the Republican majority in the House, for ethical misconduct, the Speaker replaced the committee's chairman and two other members in what many considered to be an attempt to stifle criticism. The Speaker also proposed (and the House approved) additional reforms, including the automatic dismissal of an ethics charge if the committee did not take action within 45 days; the change would have effectively allowed either party to kill an investigation merely by delaying action. Previously, charges could only be dismissed by a majority vote of the committee. A second rules change would have hampered the panel's ability to collect evidence in support of an ethics investigation by allowing only one lawyer to represent the defendant and witnesses, potentially inhibiting the fact-finding process.

Objections to these reforms hindered the committee's operations, with some committee members refusing to allow the panel to meet.[2] Since the media was then airing numerous ethics and conflict of interest allegations, the ethics committee stalemate effectively prevented any investigations from taking place. Under intense public and internal pressure, the House majority repealed the new rules in late April 2005. As public scrutiny of congressional travel intensified, the Speaker proposed that any congressional trips financed by companies or special interests would require advance written approval from the ethics committee.

While the attempts to weaken the committee were ultimately defeated, questions remained about how it would function in the future. There was concern that the majority party would try to undermine the non-partisan nature of the staff.[3] These recent events demonstrate that the self-regulating system is inherently vulnerable and creates unhealthy pressure on the committee, especially when a case concerns an influential politician.

Given the inherent vulnerabilities of a self-regulating system and the weak track record in Congress, many believe that the process should be administered by an independent body of non-members with the requisite expertise and authority to investigate complaints and recommend sanctions. In the House of Representatives, the ethics rules should permit non-members, including non-governmental organisations, congressional staff and other employees, to file complaints without the support of a House member.

Consideration should be given to other reforms, including the appointment of an independent outside counsel with experience in public corruption cases to conduct initial investigations and make recommendations to the ethics committee on whether further action should be taken.

Sarbanes-Oxley update

Following the 2001 and 2002 Enron and WorldCom scandals, the US Congress enacted the Sarbanes-Oxley Act of 2002 (SOX)[4] and the Securities and Exchange Commission (SEC) issued rules to implement it. Along with recent amendments to the Federal Organizational Sentencing Guidelines, these intensified US corporate efforts at enhancing corporate compliance programmes, internal control mechanisms and accounting systems.

Many large corporations have taken the opportunity to tighten their operations and internal flow of information, recognising that enforcement of these controls can lead to more effective corporate oversight and management.[5] However, some corporations, including foreign corporations listed in the United States and smaller US companies, have expressed concern that the costs of complying with legislation related to maintenance, audit and reporting on internal control systems are too high (US $7.8 billion in 2004).[6] Concern has also been expressed about the lack of guidance and resulting rigidity or inconsistency of auditors in their interpretations of what is required under the SOX section 404 internal controls reporting requirement.

In response, the Public Company Accounting Oversight Board (PCAOB), a private, non-profit corporation created by SOX to oversee the auditors of public companies, held public hearings in April. Chairman William McDonough noted that '[I]t is clear to us that the internal control assessment and audit process has the potential to significantly improve the quality and reliability of financial reporting. At the same time, it is equally clear to us that the first round of internal control audits cost too much.'[7]

In May 2005, the SEC and PCAOB issued guidance on 'Implementation of Internal Control Reporting', noting: 'Both management and external auditors must bring reasoned judgment and a top-down, risk-based approach to the 404-compliance process. A one-size-fits-all, bottom-up, check-the-box approach that treats all controls equally is less likely to improve internal controls and financial reporting than a reasoned, good faith exercise of professional judgment focused on reasonable, as opposed to absolute, assurance.'[8]

Action in high-profile corporate governance cases also progressed this year. Though the Justice Department case against Enron executives has yet to come to trial, a jury convicted former WorldCom CEO Bernie Ebbers of fraud and conspiracy in connection with the firm's bankruptcy. He was also found guilty of seven counts of filing false documents. In sentencing Ebbers

to 25 years in prison, the jury rejected the argument that the CEO, by being unfamiliar with the details of company accounts, was therefore not responsible for falsifications made by the company. This sets a strong precedent for upcoming accountability trials, involving executives from Enron, HealthSouth, Tyco International and Qwest Communications.

Transparency in campaign finance

Since coming into force in November 2002, the Bipartisan Campaign Reform Act, also known as the McCain-Feingold bill, has outlawed 'soft money' – the unlimited, mostly unregulated cash donations to national party committees by individuals, corporations and unions. An unintended consequence of the legislation was the shift of soft money to non-party political groups, known as '527s' (named after the section in the Internal Revenue Services (IRS) tax code that defines their status). According to the Center for Responsive Politics, 527s raised and spent more than US $479 million on activities to influence voting in the 2004 presidential and congressional elections.[9]

During the 2004 presidential election, campaign finance reform groups filed legal complaints with the FEC against some 527s, alleging unlawful election campaign spending and arguing that they were virtual extensions of national parties, rather than independent advocacy groups.

There was also concern that the public's ability to monitor these organisations was limited under existing law. Currently, 527s are governed by the IRS and many are not required to register with, or to disclose expenditures to, the FEC. IRS registration does not always reveal the organisation's underlying identity and, while the IRS requires them to disclose contributions, it does not require disclosure of contributions of less than US $200, regardless of the aggregate total raised. Moreover, some have chosen to pay a penalty equivalent to 35 per cent of a contribution, rather than reveal the contributor's identity.

In early 2005, legislation was introduced in Congress that would bring such organisations under the FEC's authority. The 527 Reform Act, introduced in both the House and Senate, would oblige 527s to comply with campaign finance laws, including provisions requiring them to register with the FEC and to disclose contributions and sources.

However, the FEC needs to be strengthened to make it more effective. It lacks real enforcement authority; can only issue findings of violations in the area of campaign finance reporting; cannot investigate anonymous complaints; and can only seek court injunctions when it has exhausted its entire enforcement process. Investigations are cumbersome processes that often take years to complete and any penalties that arise occur long after the election in which the violation occurred.

Civil society organisations, including Transparency International USA, have called for the FEC to have greater political independence, and adequate funding and staff to review, investigate and hold offenders accountable. Currently, the FEC's six voting members are evenly divided between the two major parties and serve staggered six-year terms. They are appointed by the president and confirmed by the Senate. In practice, however, the congressional party leadership determines nominations to the FEC. This could result in most FEC members being party loyalists, or having some connection to the political community that the FEC regulates. Since four votes are needed to take any action, the FEC often deadlocks along partisan lines.

Public contracting

As reported in the *Global Corruption Report 2005*, the US bidding processes for contracts in Iraq raised serious concerns. While the US Federal Acquisition Regulation (FAR) permits the use of sole-source or limited competition processes, the US government relied on them extensively in the early stages of the reconstruction effort, undermining public trust.

Under pressure from the public and contractor agencies, Congress requested the Government Accountability Office (GAO) to investigate procurement in Iraq. Its report, issued in June 2004, reviewed 25 contract actions accounting for around 97 per cent of the total dollars allocated for reconstruction as of 30 September 2003.[10] It found that 14 new contracts were awarded using other than full and open competition and, out of 11 task orders reviewed ('framework agreements' in EU procurement parlance) seven did not comply with the FAR. These task orders were issued for work that went beyond the scope of the contract and should have been competitively bid for, or justified under regulations that allow for less than full competition in specific circumstances. The GAO concluded that the failings stemmed in part from 'inadequate staffing, lack of clearly defined roles and responsibilities, changing requirements and security constraints'.[11]

Under intense scrutiny from the media, Congress and civil society, the agencies responsible for post-war contracts have become more responsive to requests for information.[12]

In June 2005, the leasing of 100 Boeing KC-767A tankers to the US military entered a new phase with the publication of the Department of Defense Inspector General's (DOD IG) review of the case. The US $23.5 billion KC-767A tanker programme was cancelled in 2004 after public concern about its excessive cost and questionable need. The review found that 'the Air Force did not demonstrate best business practices and prudent acquisition procedures in developing this program, and did not comply with statutory provisions for testing'.[13] It found that there was no urgent need for the aircraft and that the Air Force failed to conduct an analysis of the alternatives to the purchasing which was required under best business practices.[14] The review concluded: 'Senior officials of the Air Force acquisition community and the Office of the Secretary of Defense were focused on supporting a decision to lease tanker aircraft from Boeing, rather than developing objective acquisition information that would have questioned, as a matter of procedure, whether such a decision was appropriate.'[15] Both the Air Force and Boeing officials were sentenced to prison in 2004 and 2005 for violating the federal conflict of interest law. Boeing is taking further remedial steps, including hiring a special compliance officer and, under its new leadership, is working to embed ethical behaviour into the company's culture.

Beyond questions raised by such high-profile scandals, other issues have caused concern. The DOD has downsized its civilian acquisition workforce by half,[16] resulting in fewer personnel who understand procurement integrity. Furthermore, contractors hired to replace some acquisition personnel are not covered by official ethics rules because they are not government employees.[17] Congress is looking at how to ensure that contractors are covered by similar ethical structures as part of their contractual arrangements.

Nancy Izzo Jackson, with contributions from Michael Johnston,
Mark Glaze, Holly Gregory and Chris Yukins[18]

Further reading

Center for Public Integrity, 'McCain-Feingold Changes State Party Spending', 26 May 2005. Available at www.publicintegrity.org/partylines/report.aspx?aid=690&sid=300

Corporate Governance-United States, Holly Gregory, Weil Gotshal and Manges, www.weil.com/wgm/pages/Controller.jsp?z=r&sz=bl&db=wgm/cbyline.nsf&d=A9A1F3CA0B59731F85256F9E00548990&v=0

Michael Johnston (ed.), *Civil Society and Corruption: Mobilizing for Reform* (Lanham, MD: University Press of America, 2005)

Office of the Inspector General of the Department of Defense, 'Management Accountability Review of the Boeing KC-767A Tanker Program', June 2005. Available at www.dodig.osd.mil/tanker.htm

Research and Policy Committee of the Committee for Economic Development, 'Building on Reform: A Business Proposal to Strengthen Election Finance', Committee for Economic Development, April 2005

United States General Accounting Office, 'Rebuilding Iraq: Fiscal Year 2003: Contract Award Procedures and Management Challenges', May 2004

TI USA: www.transparency-usa.org

Notes

1. www.bloomberg.com, 6 April 2005.
2. *New York Times* (USA), 18 April 2005.
3. The stalemate continued until late June 2005. *New York Times* (US), 1 July 2005.
4. The Public Company Accounting Reform and Investor Protection Act of 2002 (Sarbanes-Oxley Act) was enacted in July 2002.
5. See, for example, the statement by Jeffrey Immelt, CEO in General Electric's 2004 Annual Report. The internal control requirement is 'helpful' because 'it takes the process control discipline we use in our factories and applies it to our financial statements'.
6. *Wall Street Journal* (US), 14 April 2005.
7. See 'PCAOB Issues Guidance on Audits of Internal Control', 16 May 2005, available at www.pcaobus.org/News_and_Events/News/2005/05-16.aspx
8. www.sec.gov/news/press/2005-74.htm

9. The Committee for Economic Development estimates that by the end of November 2004, 69 of the 97 527 groups, whose activities focused on the November federal elections, were formed after the adoption of the McCain-Feingold bill.

10. US General Accounting Office, 'Rebuilding Iraq: Fiscal Year 2003 Contract Award Procedures and Management Challenges', June 2004.

11. Ibid.

12. Daniel Politi, 'Winning Contractors – An Update', Center for Public Integrity, 7 July 2004. See www.publicintegrity.org/wow/report.aspx?aid=338

13. Office of the Inspector General of the Department of Defense, 'Management Accountability Review of the Boeing KC-767A Tanker Program', available at www.dodig.mil/tanker.htm

14. Department of Defense Directive 5000.1.

15. Ibid.

16. Christopher Yukins, 'Ethics in Procurement: New Challenges After a Decade of Reform', *The Procurement Lawyer* 38(3), Spring 2003.

17. Ibid.

18. Michael Johnston contributed to the essay on campaign financing, Mark Glaze to the essay on legislative ethics, Holly Gregory to the Sarbanes-Oxley update and Chris Yukins to the piece on public contracting.

Vanuatu

Conventions:
UN Convention against Corruption (not yet signed)
UN Convention against Transnational Organized Crime (not yet signed)

ADB-OECD Action Plan for Asia-Pacific (endorsed November 2001)

Legal and institutional changes

- In November 2004, the government passed the Constitution (Fourth Amendment) Act 2004 which rules that **MPs who cross the floor** will lose their seats. In addition, there can be no vote of no confidence 'within 12 months of a general election ... within 12 months of the formation of any government ... or within 12 months before the end of the life of a parliament'. The amendment could halt the instability that has dogged the government's ability to implement reform or to enjoy political continuity. In 2004 alone, there were three no-confidence motions and two cabinet reshuffles to ensure that parties did not leave the ruling coalition. Instability has a flow-on effect on corruption in that anti-corruption initiatives are not effectively carried forward from one government to the next, and politicians, aware of the brevity of their tenure, are tempted to grab as much as possible before losing power. However, there is concern that the 12-month 'grace period' may have the opposite effect by encouraging politicians to act corruptly with impunity since they will be legally protected from removal (see below).

- The **Office of the Public Prosecutor** became the focus of a commission of inquiry after it attempted to arrest the then prime minister, Serge Vohor, in mid-September. The office is responsible for handling prosecutions under the Leadership Code Act and Ombudsman Act, so all anti-corruption cases were effectively suspended. This almost resulted in the discharge of a high-profile case against the former minister for forestry, fisheries and agriculture, Stephen Kalsakau, and a number of members of the Vanuatu Maritime Authority. In May 2005, the former public prosecutor left Vanuatu and an acting public prosecutor was appointed.

Bribery and MPs

In April 2004, parliament was dissolved so that then Prime Minister Edward Natapei could avoid a vote of no confidence.[1] There were rumours that candidates from various parties had won votes through bribery in the general election of 6 July. None were substantiated, but the Office of the Ombudsman confirmed it was investigating a number of bribery complaints. In May, MPs' funding allocations, which can be distributed throughout their constituencies as they see fit, were raised from 1.2 million vatu (around US $11,000) to 2 million vatu (around US $18,000). There is some control on how this money is spent, as applications must be submitted to the speaker of parliament before the money is released. However, the misuse of MPs' allocations has been the subject of more than one ombudsman's report,[2] and current controls could be strengthened. Payments from the members' allowances are perceived by some as paybacks for votes, or a way of buying votes.[3] The accuracy of this perception has not been adequately investigated, but raising allowances increased the scope for parliamentary corruption.

No one party held a clear majority after the election and it took until 29 July for Serge Vohor to form a new government. Vohor leads the predominantly francophone Union of Moderate Parties (UMP) and had been prime minister twice before. The new government was immediately challenged by a no-confidence motion. In mid-August, the coalition changed its composition to avert the no-confidence vote.[4] There were rumours at the time that various parties and politicians were bribing backbenchers to cross the floor. Vohor publicly stated: 'Any time that there is talk of motions of no confidence in parliament, then there are people in the background causing problems with their money.'[5]

By the end of November, a motion of no confidence in the prime minister was lodged. The catalyst was Vohor's decision to establish diplomatic relations with Taiwan without the consent of the Council of Ministers and despite the government's support of a one-China policy. Allegations were made by the governing and opposition factions that MPs had been bribed by Taiwan and China, either to swing the vote or support the no-confidence motion.[6] None of the allegations was substantiated.

The no-confidence vote was successful and in December Ham Lini, brother of the founding prime minister, Father Walter Lini, and leader of the National United Party, became the new head of state. Vohor kept the subject alive with media claims that the opposition intended to take some embassies to court to make them disclose payments to MPs.[7] In late January, he said he had proof of bribery and called for an inquiry into the prime minister's actions. Lini, however, shrugged off the need for an inquiry, stating that the allegations were unfounded.[8]

The sheer number of allegations of bribery of, or by, MPs in the past 12 months is of concern. Unlike other corruption-related issues, there is no grey area in respect of accepting a payment to cross the floor, or paying a voter for support. The fact that rumours to this effect circulate so freely, and seem quite plausible, suggests there is widespread belief that MPs are by and large acting in their own interests. Of more concern, perhaps, is the possibility that voters are prepared to accept an environment in which bribery flourishes in the hope they will one day benefit themselves.

The Leadership Code Act was intended to ensure greater transparency of MPs' income and expenditure by requiring them to file annual returns, but this is clearly inadequate. It was amended in 1999 to make annual returns confidential unless they were subject to an investigation or prosecution. The Office of the Ombudsman is responsible for investigations into breaches of the Leadership Code, but it can only do so after receiving a complaint or if it 'has formed the view on reasonable grounds that a leader may have breached this Code'.[9] Since returns are confidential, it is hard for a member of the public to file a complaint on the basis of an inaccurate accounting, or for the ombudsman to 'form a view' that the return contains incorrect information.

In addition to their confidentiality, many politicians simply do not even bother to file returns. This was the subject of an ombudsman's report in 2000 though no prosecutions resulted.[10] The failure of the Office of the Public Prosecutor to prosecute in this matter, when the ombudsman had provided clear evidence of breaches, suggests that its discretion in deciding whether to go forward may be another area of weakness in the Leadership Code Act. Nor is there a legal framework governing the disclosure of donations to political parties, or how parties spend those funds. This is an area that could be usefully regulated.

Political interference in boards

A common source of corruption accusations in Vanuatu is government interference in the composition of boards of state-owned enterprises. Nepotism, and the opportunities for misappropriation of funds, are usually the motivating factors. In 2005, allegations surfaced of interference in the board of Air Vanuatu, the islands' international airline. Numerous re-mergers and de-mergers of Air Vanuatu and Vanair, the domestic airline, have occurred in recent years. In 2004, the two re-merged.

In early 2005, Air Vanuatu's CEO, Jean Paul Virelala, made comments in the media about Air Vanuatu losses of 280 million vatu (US $2.6 million) in 2004 due to competition from Virgin Blue and 'political bickering amongst its directors'. Around the same time the media became aware of plans by the Minister for Public Utilities, Maxime Carlot Korman, to increase the size of the Air Vanuatu board from 17 to 28, apparently in order to make more political appointees. Few of the appointees had experience of airline management.

In January, Virelala, who had been in his post for almost 13 years, and marketing manager Joseph Laloyer had their contracts terminated. The board then launched an inquiry in order to establish why losses had been so high in 2004. Virelala and Laloyer both maintained there were political motivations behind their dismissal.[11] Virelala is a supporter of the UMP, the party led by Serge Vohor that was ousted in December 2004. Virelala suggested that the dismissals were aimed at making way for Korman's son, Manu Carlot, to be appointed marketing manager.

In early February, the government appointed a commission of inquiry to look into Air Vanuatu's affairs, but its work was delayed after the Council of Ministers decided that an internal review should take priority. This effectively means that, despite all the allegations of nepotism and mismanagement, the airline's troubles will be treated as a commercial, rather than a political, matter. Nor is there any guarantee that the findings of the internal inquiry will be made public. 'Our politicians will call it the "Melanesian Way" or *kastom*: giving favours to their supporters or their *wantoks* at the expense of the nation and the grassroots ni-Vanuatu people', observed Marie-Noelle Ferrieux, president of Transparency International Vanuatu. 'This type of irresponsible politics and selfish and self-centred leadership is one of the main reasons why Vanuatu is one of the poorest countries in the world.'[12]

For many, the Air Vanuatu saga is both too complex and too familiar to be of much concern. This apparent acceptance of corruption is perhaps the most worrying aspect of the situation. It is too simplistic to claim that people accept political interference in boards because they see it as a legitimate use of the *wantok* system. Part of the problem is the lack of timely and detailed information and good investigative journalism. Rumours of wrongdoing circulate constantly, but it is difficult, if not impossible, to form clear opinions of whether a situation is corrupt or not. In the event that an ombudsman's report or prosecution does arise, it tends to be so delayed that the original source of the rumours has long passed from public attention. 'Switching off' is perhaps the only logical response that people can have.

Anita Jowitt (University of the South Pacific)

Further reading

Edward R. Hill, *Ombudsman of Vanuatu Digest of Reports 1996–2000* (Vanuatu: University of the South Pacific School of Law, 2001), www.vanuatu.usp.ac.fj/ombudsman/Vanuatu/Digest/digest_index.html

Edward R. Hill, 'A Structural Analysis of the Ombudsman of Vanuatu', Master of Laws thesis, Vanuatu: University of the South Pacific School of Law, 2004

Anita Jowitt, 'Vanuatu Political Review', *Contemporary Pacific: A Journal of Island Affairs* (Honolulu: University of Hawaii, 2004)

Anita Jowitt and Tess Newton Cain, *National Integrity Systems, TI International Country Study Report: Vanuatu 2003* (Berlin: Transparency International, 2004), www.transparency.org.au/nispac/vanuatu.pdf

Notes

1. The events surrounding the dissolution, and the general impact of instability on corruption, were discussed in the *Global Corruption Report 2005*.
2. These reports are: 'Public Report on the Misuse of MP Allocation Fund', by MP Vincent Boulekone, 19 February 2002, and 'Public Report on the Misuse of MP Allocation Fund', by Stanley Reginald, former MP for Banks and Torres, 8 April 2003.
3. Boulekone, Public Report on the Misuse of MP Allocation Fund.
4. This is discussed further in Anita Jowitt, 'Review of Political Events in Vanuatu 2004', *Contemporary Pacific: A Journal of Island Affairs* (Honolulu: University of Hawaii, 2005).
5. *Vanuatu Daily Post* (Vanuatu), 10 August 2004.
6. Port Vila Presse online (Vanuatu), 25 January 2005, www.news.vu/en/news/politics/050125-watch-out-for-bribery-vohor.shtml
7. Port Vila Presse on-line (Vanuatu), 9 January 2005, www.news.vu/en/news/politics/050109-vanuatu-opposition-hunt-down-brib.shtml
8. Port Vila Presse on-line (Vanuatu), 25 January 2005, www.news.vu/en/news/politics/05/01/25-watch-out-for-bribery-vohor.shtml
9. Leadership Code Act 1998, section 34(1)(b).
10. Vanuatu Office of the Ombudsman, 'Public Report on Failure of Some Leaders to File Annual Returns to the Clerk of Parliament', 29 February 2000.
11. www.news.vu/en/business/Airlines/050203-changes-in-airline-alarms-Virelala.shtml
12. www.news.vu/en/news/national/050222-drama-in-vanuatu-flag-carrier.shtml

Venezuela

Conventions:

OAS Inter-American Convention against Corruption (ratified June 1997)
UN Convention against Corruption (signed December 2003; not yet ratified)
UN Convention against Transnational Organized Crime (ratified May 2002)

Legal and institutional changes

- In July 2004, the legislature approved secondary legislation that expands the powers of the post of **ombudsman** created in 1999. The new law specifies that scrutiny of abuse of power and flaws in the provision of services will henceforth be among the ombudsman's responsibilities.

- The law to partially reform the penal code entered into force in March 2005. It fails to eliminate a provision that criminalises 'offensive expressions' directed at public officials which makes it **difficult for civil society organisations to denounce corruption**. Indeed, the reform raises sanctions on those accused of 'damaging the reputation' of public officials from a previous maximum of 18 months in prison to three years. The Inter-American Press Association says the law seriously limits press freedom. In February 2005, journalist Ibéyise Pacheco was sentenced to nine months in prison for defaming a colonel in the army. The reform also penalises civil society organisations for 'giving or receiving national or foreign resources of any kind, if they are aimed at conspiring against the integrity of the territory of the republic, the institutions of state or destabilising social order'. The terms are very broad, which means that NGOs run the risk of being investigated for receiving foreign funds for pro-democracy work. The old penal code, which is less broad, was invoked against members of the NGO SUMATE, who were accused in November 2004 of 'betraying the country' for using funds received from the US organisation National Endowment for Democracy to encourage participation in the referendum on President Hugo Chávez's mandate.

- Nine new **Supreme Court justice** positions were created in December 2004 in a process that has been criticised for political interference (see below).

Lack of independence of the judicial system

An independent judiciary is vital in a democratic state and crucial to the fight against corruption. The independence of Venezuela's judiciary has been called into question since a law on the Supreme Court in May 2004 replaced regulations that had been in force since 1976. The law was approved by a simple majority in the National Assembly, rather than the two-thirds majority required under the constitution. Deans of law faculties in four of the country's universities filed a writ of unconstitutionality that sparked a nationwide debate about the judiciary's loss of autonomy.[1] One of the main concerns was that the bill was promoted by Congressman Luis Velásquez Alvaray, a pro-government politician appointed to the Supreme Court who is also president of the commission responsible for naming or removing judges.

The law's most important change was to increase the number of judges from 20 to 32. The reason given was that the additional manpower would clear the backlog of work in the Supreme Court, although they were largely up to date with their caseload, according to the judicial authorities.[2] In the event, 17 new judges were appointed since 5 more vacancies had arisen through retirement or dismissal. National and international NGOs[3] and some sectors of the opposition insisted that the real motive behind the new law was the need to stuff the judiciary with supporters of President Chávez.

A nominations committee, composed of various sectors of society, is supposed to supervise the selection of Supreme Court judges under the constitution. In this case, the nomination committee was made up of five Congressmen from pro-government parliamentary groups and six representatives of organisations known to sympathise with the government. For example, Juan José Molina Bermúdez was legal adviser for Podemos, a party that supports the government, and had filed successful writs with the Supreme Court that made it difficult for the opposition to collect signatures for a referendum in August 2004 to revoke President Chávez's mandate. Another member was Gustavo Hidalgo, who was named director general of the executive of the Supreme Court in February 2005. Civil society organisations concerned with the administration of justice felt excluded from the process, and said so publicly.

Omar Mora Díaz, the new Supreme Court president, defines himself as 'revolutionary' (which tends to mean pro-Chávez) in interviews. The day he assumed the post, he announced a purge of judges including three who had handed down sentences that were deemed favourable to the opposition. The new law relaxes procedures for removing judges if the Moral Council of the Republic (made up of the ombudsman, the prosecutor general and auditor general) considers they have committed 'grave errors'.

This loss of independence does not only affect high-level judges. According to the Supreme Court, more than 70 per cent of judges in March 2005 were provisional, meaning they can be appointed and dismissed without administrative proceedings. This weakens the autonomy of the judiciary because judges may favour the interests of those who can help keep them in their posts. The predicament became more acute in early 2003 when competitions to enter the judicial career path were suspended, contrary to the constitution. A presidential veto in November 2003 stopped the National Assembly from adopting a code of ethics for judges – also a constitutional requirement. In February 2005, Mora Díaz presented a 'plan for the revolutionary transformation' of the judiciary, which includes the widespread removal of judges and their replacement by new judges who would be intensively trained – for one month.

As well as concerns that the lack of independence may make it difficult to process corruption cases affecting government interests, there are more immediate corruption concerns. In January, days after taking up his post as head of the judiciary directorate, Luis Velásquez Alvaray dismissed all its coordinators and directors. Before taking up the post, Velásquez Alvaray had presided over a parliamentary commission that investigated judicial corruption.

Since February, a number of complaints filed by the former head of the executive directorate, Yolanda Jaimes, to the auditor general in November 2004 have been leaked to the press. One called for an investigation into overpriced training courses for judges that had been organised by the executive directorate. According to Jaimes, US $520 was paid per teaching hour, compared to US $40 charged by the most expensive company providing the same service. Another complaint involved the investment of judiciary employee pension funds in risky financial instruments.

Audited reports for the second half of 2004, made public by the new administration of the judicial directorate, indicated that 3,000 employees had been hired without authorisation and others on the payroll did not exist. There was no register of service providers or purchases, including expensive analyses by consultancy firms that were never completed. Contracting regulations were regularly breached and companies chosen that did not comply with the technical requirements for winning the contract.

Media coverage of these irregularities coincided with the announcement of a new strategic plan for the judiciary. The plan requests an additional US $47 million for the judiciary, but fails to include mechanisms to ensure greater transparency of the judiciary and of its use of funds.

Corruption at Venezuela's state oil company

The state oil company, Petróleos de Venezuela (PDVSA), is the fifth largest oil producer in the world, generating more than 40 per cent of the country's annual budget. In the first half of 2005, a series of complaints have called into question the management and transparency of 'the industry', as it is known.

The company has not presented audited financial statements since 2002, though the law requires it to do so annually. Without these figures it is difficult to monitor the health of the company and scrutinise how it uses its resources. According to the Central Bank of Venezuela (CBV), it is possible to assert that, at the end of calendar year 2004, there was a shortfall of US $3.5 billion between the money reportedly paid by PDVSA and the amount that entered the CBV. No one knows where the money went, only that it was not registered by the CBV.[4]

According to José Guerra, former manager of CBV's investigations department, PDVSA should have filed receipts for US $9.9 billion in the first quarter of 2005, but only filed US $6.4 billion. Energy minister Rafael Ramírez told a press conference in May that PDVSA produced 3.3 million barrels per day during the first quarter of 2005, but 'It is not known what PDVSA did with the US $2.4 billion shortfall.'[5] Domingo Maza Zavala, a member of the CBV's board of directors, said that the amount received by the bank in the first quarter was US $4.8 billion, which means the shortfall might be as high as US $4.2 billion.

Since August 2003, moreover, the Minister for Energy has failed to publish the annual report 'Oil and Other Statistical Figures', or PODE, which has provided vital statistics related to the petroleum sector and international companies operating in Venezuela since 1956. Since oil production was nationalised in 1976, PODE printed the monthly, quarterly and annual information supplied by PDVSA, including net receipts, daily average production, daily amount of crude processed in refineries, price of royalties and the sales price of crude and refined products. As well as violating constitutional provisions on access to information[6] and anti-corruption law,[7] these omissions deprive the public of knowledge of the real daily level of oil production (the government says production is 3.3 million barrels a day; industry sources put the figure at 2.6 million).

In terms of undue benefits, other allegations have arisen involving multi-million-dollar commissions illegally paid for export sales.[8] Hydrocarbons are increasingly sold through intermediaries who receive commissions on each operation. One example of this questionable practice is the export of hydrocarbons with no registered destination. Failure to specify where the oil is going gives the administration enormous scope to hide the real cost of transporting the oil. Another issue recently in the news was the mass dismissal of PDVSA officials for corruption, though the allegations have not been detailed and the accused not formally charged.[9] Minister Rafael Ramírez has referred to 'administrative irregularities', though not corruption, in his explanation for the dismissal in early 2005 of 30 managers and the decision not to renew the contracts of 8,000 employees in PDVSA installations in the west.[10]

The internal controls applied to the complex processes of exploitation, processing and exporting oil and its derivatives have also been relaxed. Auditor general Clodosbaldo Russián insists that since 2000 PDVSA has been externally supervised; the auditor general's branch office for the PDVSA headquarters has been closed; and auditors are only sent in 'when the case requires it'. In February, the Minister of Energy and Mines was named president of PDVSA, ending decades of formal separation between the government and the management of the oil industry. Julio Montoya, vice-president of the Commission of Energy and Mines of the National Assembly, which is investigating the above allegations, said in May 2005 that to date the company had committed 226 illegal acts.[11] At the time of writing the investigations were in full flow.

Transparencia Venezuela

Further reading

Rafael Di Tella and William D. Savedoff, *Diagnosis Corrupción* (Corruption Diagnosis) (Washington, DC: Inter-American Development Bank, 2002)

María Méndez Peña, 'Estudios y textos acerca de la corrupción. Un intento de sistematización' (Studies and Texts on Corruption: An Attempt at Systematisation), in *Revista FERMENTUM* 40, Universidad de los Andes, Mérida, Venezuela, 2004

Mirador Democrático, *II Seminario internacional Justicia y Transparencia: Perspectivas del Gobierno Judicial y la Sociedad* (Second International Seminar on 'Justice and Transparency: Perspectives from the Judicial Government and Society'), conference report, Caracas: June 2003

Pérez Perdomo Rogelio, *Corrupción y Revolución en Venezuela* (Corruption and Revolution in Venezuela, 2004) available at www.apunto.com.ve/detalle_news.php?ID=665

Transparencia Venezuela (TI Venezuela): www.transparenciavenezuela.org

Notes

1. www.derechos.org.ve/publicaciones/infanual/2003_04/17justicia.pdf
2. www.tsj.gov.ve/gestion.asp
3. Including Human Rights Watch and Provea.
4. See www.descifrado.com/articulo.php?idart=10876&cat=Gobierno
5. *El Nacional* (Venezuela), 18 May 2005.
6. Constitution of Venezuela, article 28.
7. Law against corruption. Official gazette N° 5.637, 7 April 2003.
8 *El Nuevo Herald* (Venezuela), 11 April 2005.
9. www.pequiven.pdv.com/noticias/2005/abril/050425_02a_es.htm
10. *El Nacional* (Venezuela), 8 May 2005.
11. *El Nacional* (Venezuela), 12 May 2005.

Part three
Research on corruption

9 Introduction

Robin Hodess[1]

This year's *Global Corruption Report* once again presents a selection of important studies on transparency and corruption covering a range of themes, from corruption's relation to socio-economic phenomena, to the links between policy implementation and change. Given the ever-growing number of studies and the breadth of approaches used, there is little doubt that the empirical analysis of corruption has now gained a foothold in a number of research disciplines. The challenge for policy-makers is to gain access to this information, and then to interpret and incorporate these results in their subsequent anti-corruption efforts. The research overview presented here provides a shorthand guide to the findings and how they fit into our broader understanding of the field of corruption.

Corruption trends

Although corruption's prominence on the international agenda is a relatively new development, there has been increasing interest in understanding improvements and setbacks in terms of corruption levels, since the fight against corruption began in earnest a decade ago.

The first two research pieces presented in this volume provide some initial answers to the question: is corruption getting better or worse, and if so, where? Johann Graf Lambsdorff's trend analysis of TI's Corruption Perceptions Index (CPI) – now in its 11th year – is the first rigorous effort to establish trends in the perceptions of corruption that are based on 'real' perceptions of change, and not on methodological adjustments to the CPI itself. It finds that robust trends do emerge in nearly 30 countries, of which about half made real improvement, while the other half deteriorated over time.

These findings overlap with the work of the World Bank Institute, which released the latest of its 'Governance Matters' results in the past year, presenting findings on governance indicators including 'control of corruption' covering 209 countries over the period 1996–2004. While there is little evidence that governance has improved in global terms, there is proof that it has improved (or declined) dramatically in certain countries. More important, though, is that the six governance indicators evaluated by the World Bank point to a 'development dividend' of good governance: improving governance results in higher incomes. In light of recent debates about increasing donor assistance, particularly to help achieve the Millennium Development Goals, this is a crucial finding for all those who argue that better economic outcomes are possible without improvements in governance.

Corruption trends can also be discerned at sub-national level. Using data on corruption convictions by a single federal agency in the United States, Edward Glaeser and Raven Saks show that certain characteristics within states (such as lower income and especially education levels) predict corruption. Taking their analysis one step further, they find that corruption has deterred economic growth in the worst affected states over the past 20 years at least.

The importance of transparency

In this volume, the benefits of transparency are demonstrated in empirical terms. Research undertaken by Saadia Zahidi of the World Economic Forum sheds new light on the significant impact that lack of transparency has on the likelihood and severity of banking crises, along with related phenomena, such as favouritism and lack of judicial independence. The findings support not only stronger financial sector transparency, but also tighter regulation and adherence to principles for ensuring adequate banking supervision.

Other research on transparency focuses on its prevalence in the budget process and in the revenue payments that characterise the oil and gas sector. The Washington, DC-based International Budget Project conducted a survey to evaluate public access to budget information in a range of developing and transition countries. The main finding was that while executive budgets tended to be publicly available in most countries, monitoring and evaluation was weak and there was little facilitation of public understanding of the budget. This relatively poor performance in the realm of budget transparency precludes public comprehension of policy priorities and reduces the overall accountability of government.

Building on the successes of the 'Publish What You Pay Campaign', an international campaign for increased transparency in the payment, receipt and management of oil, gas and mining revenues in developing countries, Save the Children Fund UK undertook an assessment of revenue transparency. The practices of major international oil and gas companies in both their home countries, and within the companies themselves were examined. In most cases, neither the countries involved nor the companies themselves met commitments to disclose revenue payments. Canada, where there is strong securities regulation, led the group in terms of commitment to disclosure, and was the home country of some of the best corporate performers. As in the banking sector, the core message was that regulation must be considered a policy option if transparency is to be promoted effectively.

There are also clear links to transparency in TI Mexico's study on corporate reputation. Through their research, TI Mexico sought to provide a positive incentive for companies to improve performance, by publishing the names of top performers, in a ranking of expert opinions on eight facets of good corporate practice.

Anti-corruption policies: are they effective?

Another key question currently being asked by the policy community is the kind of impact various 'standard' anti-corruption policy remedies have on corruption levels. Ranjana Mukherjee and Omer Gokcekus evaluate the extent to which asset declaration by public officials affects levels of corruption in countries around the world. They find that the longer such laws have been in place, particularly where there is a credible threat of prosecution for violating the law, and the more the information can be accessed publicly, the greater the link between asset declaration and less corruption.

In the Inhambane province of Mozambique, where tax officials suspect massive tax evasion by business and have implemented a programme of strict fines for minor transgressions, Ralf Lanwehr explores the implications of this climate of distrust. Lanwehr finds that local and foreign investors are influenced by different factors in their investment choices.

Other research has assessed the strength of public institutions based on their commitment, capacities and performance in the fight against corruption. TI Czech Republic created the V4 Index to assess the quality of public administration, as it related to curbing corruption in four Visegrád capitals – Bratislava, Budapest, Prague and Warsaw, with Budapest emerging as the clear leader.

A study of the administration of transfers of elementary school teaching funds from the federal to municipal level in Brazil reveals significant leakage. TI Brazil analysed the irregularities uncovered by federal auditors and concluded that local authorities lack the capacity to manage funds honestly and effectively, requiring stronger supervision at state level.

Corruption and health – making the empirical link

Many of the assumptions and recommendations on health presented in the thematic section of this *Global Corruption Report* are underpinned by research findings showing how much corruption in this sector costs health systems and individual patients.

TI Bangladesh uses a rich array of research tools, including household surveys, to provide evidence of corruption in the health sector. Health is considered the fourth most corrupt sector in Bangladesh, according to the national chapter's most recent poll. Of those Bangladeshis requiring hospital care, as many as 1 in 4 had to pay bribes for these services; and 9 in 10 of those who needed medicines had to pay, despite supposedly free provision.

TI's national chapter in Colombia also has a wealth of research experience to draw on and has been at the forefront in developing assessment tools of public sector entities. The results of its Integrity Index for Public Institutions reflect the findings relevant to the health sector. Nearly two-thirds of the approximately 20 health-related institutions included in the Integrity Index have high corruption risks.

In Bulgaria, Patrick Meagher led a research project that evaluated the process of drug selection for the health system, and pharmaceutical procurement by hospitals across the country. By ranking performance in these two areas, he shows that a focus on institutional integrity can be useful for identifying weaknesses, but emphasises that policy prescriptions need to be made in conjunction with a broader analysis that takes the level of capacity and resources available for change into account.

Corruption the world over: a diversity of citizen views and experiences

Several researchers, including those from TI national chapters, explored the extent to which average citizens pay bribes, particularly to public sector officials, whether to avoid problems or to receive a service they should be entitled to at no charge. While 'corruption experience' survey work is not new, some survey tools are beginning to show trends over time, complementing the global trend analysis in international survey work discussed above.

The United States Agency for International Development (USAID) recently carried out almost a dozen surveys in Latin America on perceptions of, and behaviour regarding, corruption, the latter from a corruption victimisation approach, with Bolivians ranking as by far the most victimised. The study also located bribe demands by government institutions, which showed considerable variation across the countries polled. The results pointed to a relationship between experience of corruption and declining support for democracy, a finding that has significant implications for policies of democratic consolidation in the region.

In the Palestinian territories, TI Palestine commissioned a public opinion survey focusing on types, levels and location of corruption. The survey found that Palestinians associate corruption most with *wasta*, a form of nepotism. Corruption was found to be rife in employment bodies, such as job centres, and among the police. Significant differences emerged for the West Bank and Gaza Strip; for instance, educational institutions were seen as far more corrupt in the West Bank, making these findings relevant to the policy reform process.

Looking ahead

The studies selected for this volume demonstrate a number of advances in the scope and methods used in corruption research. First, international survey analysis regarding perceptions of corruption can now be extended to evaluate change over time, a much welcome addition to this most valuable and comprehensive source of corruption data. The research community will need to continue to innovate to supply evidence of 'wins' and 'losses' in the battle against corruption, but this insight is crucial if momentum against corruption is to be sustained, or indeed increased.

Recent research also demonstrates how important and how difficult it is to achieve transparency in both public and private sector institutional practice. Further work will need to examine not only transparency commitments, but also performance. A number of research efforts also assess the effectiveness of anti-corruption policies and provisions within public institutions. This is essential as policy instruments are refined and applied in the future. More research is still needed on the sequencing of reform, and on which reform 'packages' are most effective.

Finally, empirical research on corruption continues to provide first-hand feedback from people about their views and experiences of corruption and bribery. Not only have such surveys started to document changes in public opinion over time, but they have also begun to locate corruption more accurately within particular institutions, providing ample evidence on which in-country diagnoses and remedies can be developed. The research challenge here is to better understand the gulfs that can emerge between perceptions and experiences of corruption, and their consequences for disaffection with democracy as a whole.

TI will continue to track and support this great variety of corruption research, synthesising results and bringing them into our own advocacy efforts, but also publicising findings for use by all those engaged in anti-corruption work around the world.

Note

1. Robin Hodess is director of policy and research, Transparency International.

10 Ten years of the CPI: determining trends

Johann Graf Lambsdorff[1]

Transparency International (TI) has published its Corruption Perceptions Index (CPI) annually since 1995. It is a composite index, using surveys of business people and assessments by country analysts to provide an annual snapshot of corruption perceptions in particular countries. Year-on-year changes in a country's CPI score are the result not only of changes in perceptions of a country's performance, but of changes in survey samples and methodology and alterations in the list of sources that constitute the index. Changes in sources have made it difficult to derive valid time-series information from CPI results and therefore TI has only been able to draw limited conclusions regarding progress or setbacks in the countries listed.

There is, nevertheless, a growing demand for trend data. The causes and consequences of corruption, as well as the success of anti-corruption efforts, can be better addressed and investigated when time-series information is available.[2] The following analysis of the CPI and its component data provides initial findings relating to country trends over the period 1995–2004.

Data sources

Five sources used in the CPI contain sufficient data to be included in an assessment of trends as they have been used on a continuous basis for at least seven years and the methodology used to produce them has not changed significantly.[3] These are:

- the Economist Intelligence Unit (EIU), 1996–2004
- the Institute for Management Development, Lausanne (IMD), 1995–2004
- the World Economic Forum (WEF), 1996–2004
- the Political and Economic Risk Consultancy (PERC) in Hong Kong, 1995–2004
- Freedom House Nations in Transit (FH). Data is available for 1998, 1999/2000, 2001–04.

Constructing time series

As with the CPI, all data must be placed in common units. Once this is achieved, we must observe how the time-series information of individual sources interact with each other. One source may be slow in responding to real changes; another might be more topical. This can be determined by disregarding differences across countries and analysing only time-series information. Simple (fixed effect) panel regressions are used to observe whether delaying a time series improves its correlation with other sources.

Taking EIU as the dependent variable, we observe that the time-series information inherent in EIU data is well explained by IMD data, but less so by WEF data, for example. The explanatory power of the variables increases when using one period lagged values. This implies that EIU provides assessments of perceived levels of corruption with a one-year time lag. This may be because the local business people surveyed by the IMD and WEF gather topical information more quickly and are thus better placed to assess the current state of affairs. The strength of EIU data, on the other hand, may relate to its in-depth, but more time-consuming, country analysis.

When assessed against the other indices, the FH figures did not provide significant results, and so were left out of subsequent analyses. This may have been because of the different method used by FH to define and quantify corruption: FH tries to assess the governments' anti-corruption efforts, the success of which is difficult to evaluate.

Constructing panel data

Based on the above findings, the EIU data was entered in lagged form. A corruption trend was determined for a country when the four data sources provide at least 15 observations. In order to avoid confusion with the original CPI data, all data for 2004 are set at zero. Table 10.1 shows the data for each year, ranked on a scale of 0 (very corrupt) to 10 (very clean). Bulgaria, for example, obtains –1.4 in 1995, implying an improvement to 0 in 2004. As revealed by the scores for 1996–2003, this was not an even development, but involved an initial deterioration to –2.4 before improvements were perceived.

Interpreting the data

Given the inherent imprecision of subjective indicators, how certain can we be that a country improved or deteriorated? An improvement between 1995 and 2004 of 0.5 might be significant if observed similarly by all sources, while an improvement by 1 may be insignificant if only few and contradictory observations are available. To control for this, a test for the significance of a simple linear trend was conducted.[4] The usefulness of this test can be seen from Figure 10.1 for Argentina. The slope of this line is –0.16, indicating that Argentina experienced an annual drop in the CPI by 0.16. Statistical analysis allows us to determine the precision of the estimated slope. The standard error for this coefficient is 0.03, about a fifth of the slope. This factor (5 in the case of Argentina) is known as the *t*-statistic and provides statistical confidence that the slope is indeed positive (or negative).

Table 10.1 reports the annual change as determined by the test outlined above, the corresponding standard error and *t*-statistic. In cases where there was a significant trend,

Table 10.1: Trends in perceived levels of corruption

Trends 1995–2004	Observations	1995	1996	1997	1998	1999	2000	2001	2002	2003	2004	Annual change	Standard error	t-statistics
Argentina	28	0.7	0.6	0.6	0.4	0.4	0.4	-0.1	-0.6	-0.4	0.0	-0.16	0.03	-4.6
Australia	28	-0.7	-0.8	-1.0	-0.6	-0.7	-0.6	-0.5	-1.1	-0.1	0.0	0.05	0.02	**2.4**
Austria	27	-0.4	-0.5	-0.6	-0.5	-0.3	-0.8	-0.7	-0.4	0.2	0.0	0.08	0.05	1.8
Belgium	28	-0.1	-0.1	-1.4	-1.3	-1.5	-0.4	0.0	-0.1	0.0	0.0	0.08	0.06	1.4
Brazil	28	0.2	-0.2	0.2	0.2	0.0	-0.1	-0.1	0.3	-0.3	0.0	-0.02	0.03	-0.7
Bulgaria	15	-1.4	-2.4	-2.4	-1.0	-1.0	-1.0	-0.6	0.0	-0.4	0.0	0.15	0.05	**3.3**
Canada	28	0.6	0.6	0.4	0.5	0.5	0.3	0.4	0.3	-0.1	0.0	-0.07	0.03	-2.3
Chile	28	-0.3	-0.4	-0.5	-0.5	0.2	0.1	-0.2	-0.2	-0.5	0.0	0.01	0.03	0.3
China	27	-0.5	-0.8	0.2	1.2	-0.1	0.3	0.4	0.5	0.1	0.0	-0.02	0.03	-0.5
Colombia	27	-0.2	0.0	-1.3	-0.9	-0.4	-0.2	-0.3	0.0	0.1	0.0	0.11	0.04	**2.9**
Costa Rica	15	–	-0.7	-0.9	-0.8	-0.7	-0.5	-0.5	-0.7	-0.4	0.0	0.05	0.02	**2.4**
Czech Republic	28	0.3	0.6	1.1	0.2	0.1	0.0	-0.3	0.0	0.2	0.0	-0.10	0.03	-3.2
Denmark	28	-0.1	0.0	-0.2	-0.1	-0.1	-0.2	-0.2	-0.2	0.0	0.0	0.01	0.01	0.8
Ecuador	15	1.5	0.5	0.5	0.5	0.5	0.2	0.2	0.2	0.2	0.0	-0.08	0.03	-2.7
Estonia	16	–	-2.2	-1.0	-0.9	-0.8	-0.8	-0.8	-0.9	-0.7	0.0	0.15	0.03	**4.3**
Finland	28	-0.4	-0.3	-0.1	-0.1	-0.1	0.0	-0.1	0.0	0.0	0.0	0.03	0.01	**3.1**
France	28	-0.3	-0.3	-0.3	-0.2	-0.2	-0.4	-0.8	-0.8	0.1	0.0	0.01	0.03	0.2
Germany	28	-0.7	-0.6	-0.7	-0.2	-0.1	-0.8	-0.7	-0.6	0.2	0.0	0.06	0.04	1.5
Greece	28	0.3	0.1	0.7	0.8	1.0	-0.1	0.3	-0.1	0.1	0.0	-0.04	0.05	-0.7
Hong Kong	28	-1.4	-1.4	0.3	0.1	0.2	0.7	-0.3	-0.6	0.6	0.0	0.12	0.04	**3.2**
Hungary	28	-0.9	-0.9	-0.4	-0.4	0.2	0.2	0.0	-0.3	0.0	0.0	0.03	0.04	0.8
Iceland	19	-0.8	-0.8	-2.9	-1.4	-1.5	-0.7	0.0	-0.3	-0.1	0.0	0.22	0.10	**2.3**
India	28	0.5	1.1	0.0	0.9	0.3	-0.1	0.3	0.2	0.0	0.0	0.00	0.02	-0.2
Indonesia	28	1.0	1.5	0.1	0.1	-0.2	-0.1	0.6	-0.4	-0.2	0.0	-0.07	0.03	-2.7
Ireland	28	0.7	0.7	0.4	0.2	-0.4	-0.4	-1.3	-0.3	-0.6	0.0	-0.17	0.04	-3.9
Israel	28	1.5	1.8	1.2	0.0	0.6	1.2	1.4	0.5	0.9	0.0	-0.10	0.06	-1.6
Italy	28	-0.9	-0.8	-0.7	-0.5	-0.5	-0.2	0.2	-0.1	-0.3	0.0	0.09	0.03	**3.5**
Japan	28	-0.3	-0.3	-1.5	-1.9	-1.4	-0.3	-0.8	-1.0	-1.3	0.0	0.02	0.03	0.5
Jordan	19	–	0.1	-1.4	-1.1	-0.7	-0.8	-1.0	-1.1	-0.1	0.0	0.03	0.07	0.5
Luxembourg	16	–	0.8	0.7	0.5	1.0	1.2	1.0	0.6	0.0	0.0	-0.02	0.06	-0.3

Trends 1995–2004	Observations	1995	1996	1997	1998	1999	2000	2001	2002	2003	2004	Annual change	Standard error	t-statistics
Malaysia	28	1.2	2.4	2.2	1.9	0.3	1.8	1.5	2.2	1.5	0.0	–0.07	0.04	*–1.9*
Mexico	28	–0.2	–0.2	0.3	0.1	0.3	0.3	0.3	0.4	0.5	0.0	0.06	0.02	**3.3**
Netherlands	28	0.3	0.6	0.6	0.4	0.7	0.7	0.7	0.6	0.4	0.0	–0.02	0.02	–1.0
New Zealand	27	–0.2	–0.4	–0.3	–0.1	–0.3	–0.1	–0.2	–0.1	–0.1	0.0	0.02	0.01	1.5
Norway	28	–0.4	–0.2	–0.4	–0.1	–0.1	–1.1	–0.8	0.0	–0.9	0.0	–0.02	0.05	–0.3
Peru	18	–0.9	0.7	0.7	0.6	0.4	–0.3	0.6	0.1	0.0	0.0	–0.05	0.06	–0.9
Philippines	28	1.1	1.0	1.7	1.3	3.2	1.2	0.7	0.7	1.0	0.0	–0.06	0.03	*–2.2*
Poland	27	1.3	1.5	1.4	1.1	1.3	1.7	1.1	0.9	0.5	0.0	–0.12	0.03	*–3.4*
Portugal	28	–0.2	0.1	0.9	0.8	0.6	0.6	0.1	0.6	–0.1	0.0	–0.01	0.06	–0.2
Romania	15	0.3	0.6	–0.7	–0.7	–0.8	–0.7	0.6	0.3	–0.1	0.0	0.03	0.06	0.6
Russia	28	–0.4	–0.3	–0.2	0.4	0.0	0.1	0.2	0.6	0.0	0.0	0.06	0.03	**2.1**
Singapore	27	–0.1	–0.1	–0.2	–0.3	–0.1	–0.2	–0.3	–0.1	0.1	0.0	0.00	0.01	–0.4
Slovakia	21	0.7	0.7	0.5	–0.1	–1.2	–0.8	–0.3	–0.8	–0.2	0.0	–0.03	0.05	–0.6
Slovenia	18	–	0.4	0.2	0.4	0.3	–0.5	–0.8	–0.4	–0.3	0.0	–0.14	0.07	*–2.0*
South Africa	28	–0.7	–0.2	–0.6	–0.4	–0.9	–0.8	–0.8	–0.8	–0.7	0.0	–0.04	0.03	–1.2
South Korea	28	1.0	0.3	–1.9	–1.5	–1.8	–1.5	–1.1	0.1	0.9	0.0	0.01	0.04	0.3
Spain	28	–2.4	–2.2	0.3	0.4	0.4	0.7	0.1	0.3	0.8	0.0	0.25	0.06	**3.9**
Sweden	28	0.1	–0.1	0.1	0.0	–0.5	0.0	0.1	0.1	0.1	0.0	0.01	0.02	0.6
Switzerland	28	–0.1	–0.3	–0.2	0.0	–0.3	–0.2	–0.7	–0.2	0.0	0.0	0.02	0.03	0.6
Taiwan	28	–1.5	–2.5	–1.1	0.0	–0.7	–0.8	–0.3	–1.7	–1.0	0.0	0.07	0.03	**2.4**
Thailand	27	0.1	–0.2	–0.5	–1.3	–0.3	–0.2	–0.3	–1.3	–0.9	0.0	0.02	0.03	0.7
Turkey	28	0.7	0.4	0.4	0.4	0.6	0.7	0.2	–0.2	0.1	0.0	–0.07	0.03	*–2.5*
Ukraine	17	0.7	0.8	0.8	0.0	0.1	0.2	0.0	0.4	0.2	0.0	–0.02	0.03	–0.6
United Kingdom	28	0.4	0.4	0.3	0.2	0.1	0.3	–0.2	–0.1	0.2	0.0	–0.05	0.02	*–2.9*
USA	27	–0.5	–0.5	–0.4	–0.5	–0.8	–0.3	0.2	0.4	0.3	0.0	0.00	0.02	–0.2
Venezuela	28	0.6	0.1	0.4	0.2	0.5	0.4	0.1	0.3	0.2	0.0	–0.03	0.02	–1.5
Vietnam	17	–0.9	0.6	1.3	0.9	1.3	1.1	0.1	1.2	1.0	0.0	0.03	0.04	0.7
Zimbabwe	16	–	1.6	0.2	–0.2	0.2	–0.3	–0.8	–0.4	–0.8	0.0	–0.17	0.06	*–3.0*

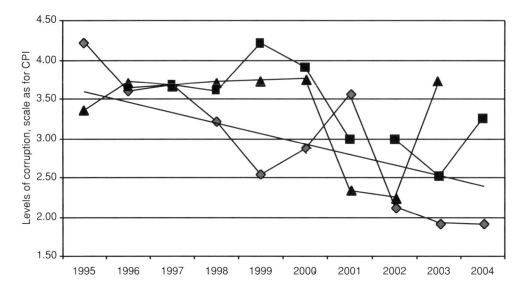

Figure 10.1: Levels of corruption, Argentina, individual data as reported by EIU, IMD and WEF

the *t*-statistics reported are emphasised in bold in the case of decreasing corruption, or italics in the case of increasing corruption.

The values for the annual change range between 0.25 and –0.17, which suggests that lowering perceived levels of corruption – achieving improvements in the CPI – is a long-term undertaking. A decade of substantial effort might improve the score by 1 point on a scale from 0 to 10. Only in rare instances will improvements be more pronounced.

Overall, our findings indicate that significant improvements between 1995 and 2004 occurred (in descending order of significance) in Estonia, Spain, Italy, Bulgaria, Mexico, Hong Kong, Colombia, Costa Rica, Taiwan, Australia, Iceland and Russia. A deterioration, on the other hand, was significant in Argentina, Ireland, Poland, Czech Republic, Zimbabwe, United Kingdom, Ecuador, Indonesia, Turkey, Canada and the Philippines.

This data mark a first approach to determining composite time-series information for a sample of 58 countries. Due to the short time horizon, the level of significance is still limited. As data on levels of corruption become available for future periods, the precision of the underlying measurement is likely to increase. The data presented here may prove useful in determining the causes and consequences of corruption, where research has until now been limited to cross-section analysis.

Notes

1. Johann Graf Lambsdorff is chair in economic theory at the University of Passau and a research consultant to Transparency International, for whom he has coordinated and carried out the CPI since 1995.

2. Björnskov and Paldam determine time series by processing only the ordinal changes in the data over time, that is, whether a country improves its rank relative to others. With this approach, one-shot changes of a purely methodological nature play a minor role as compared to actual trend information. They conclude that generalised trust is about the only explanatory variable with significant impact. See C. Björnskov and M. Paldam, 'Corruption Trends' in J. Graf Lambsdorff, M. Schramm and M. Taube (eds) *The New Institutional Economics of Corruption – Norms, Trust, and Reciprocity* (London: Routledge, 2004), pp 59–75.
3. Minor variations in the phrasing of questions have taken place over time, however. For instance, in 2002–04, IMD asked respondents to assess whether 'bribing and corruption prevail or do not prevail in the economy'. Previously, respondents had been asked whether 'bribing and corruption prevail or do not prevail in the public sphere'. This change seemed to have little impact on the data, however, allowing inferences to be made over time.
4. Separately for each country, k, I seek to determine the coefficient a_k, which depicts the influence of a simple time trend (Trend$_{1995}$ = 1, Trend$_{1996}$ = 2 …) on the dependent variables, which are our source's values for country k. The coefficient a_k thus resembles an estimate for the annual change in the CPI. All four subsequent regressions were run simultaneously.

$$IMD_{ik} = a_k \cdot Trend_i + b_{k,\,IMD} \cdot d_{IMD} + e_i$$
$$WEF_{ik} = a_k \cdot Trend_i + b_{k,WEF} \cdot d_{WEF} + e_i$$
$$PERC_{ik} = a_k \cdot Trend_i + b_{k,\,PERC} \cdot d_{PERC} + e_i$$
$$EIU_{i+1,k} = a_k \cdot Trend_i + b_{k,\,EIU} \cdot d_{EIU} + e_i.$$

We allow for our sources to differ systematically and capture this difference with the help of a dummy variable for each source, for example d_{IMD}. Thus, if IMD is more favourable in its assessment of country k as compared to WEF, this is captured by the dummy and its associated coefficient, $b_{k,IMD}$. A random error term is added, e_i. The intention of this system of regressions was to find a joint trend in each of the sources for a given country k. OLS was employed for estimating the coefficients.

11   Corruption Perceptions Index 2005

Johann Graf Lambsdorff[1]

The Corruption Perceptions Index, now in its eleventh year, aims to provide data on extensive perceptions of corruption within countries. These perceptions enhance our understanding of real levels of corruption from one country to another. The CPI is a composite index, making use of surveys of business people and assessments by country analysts.

Overall, 16 sources were included in the 2005 CPI, originating from 10 independent institutions and using data compiled between 2003 and 2005. The sources used were: (1) Columbia University; (2) the Economist Intelligence Unit; (3) Freedom House; (4) Information International from Beirut (Lebanon); (5) the International Institute for Management Development (in Lausanne); (6) the Merchant International Group Limited (in London); (7) the Political and Economic Risk Consultancy (in Hong Kong); (8) the United Nations Economic Commission for Africa; (9) the World Economic Forum; (10) the World Markets Research Centre (in London). The number of countries in the CPI 2005 increased to 159 from 146 in 2004.

For an analysis of the medium-term corruption trends that can be discerned from the CPI data series, see Chapter 10 in this volume. A more detailed description of the methodology is available at www.transparency.org/surveys/index.html#cpi or at www.icgg.org.

Table 11.1: Corruption Perceptions Index 2005

Country Rank	Country	2005 CPI score[a]	Surveys used[b]	Standard deviation[c]	High–low range[d]	Confidence range[e]
1	Iceland	9.7	8	0.2	9.3 – 9.8	9.5 – 9.7
2	Finland	9.6	9	0.2	9.3 – 9.8	9.5 – 9.7
	New Zealand	9.6	9	0.2	9.3 – 9.7	9.5 – 9.7
4	Denmark	9.5	10	0.3	8.7 – 9.8	9.3 – 9.6
5	Singapore	9.4	12	0.2	9.0 – 9.7	9.3 – 9.5
6	Sweden	9.2	10	0.3	8.7 – 9.6	9.0 – 9.3
7	Switzerland	9.1	9	0.3	8.5 – 9.4	8.9 – 9.2
8	Norway	8.9	9	0.6	7.9 – 9.5	8.5 – 9.1
9	Australia	8.8	13	0.8	6.7 – 9.5	8.4 – 9.1

Country Rank	Country	2005 CPI score[a]	Surveys used[b]	Standard deviation[c]	High–low range[d]	Confidence range[e]
10	Austria	8.7	9	0.5	8.1 – 9.3	8.4 – 9.0
11	Netherlands	8.6	9	0.5	7.8 – 9.4	8.3 – 8.9
	United Kingdom	8.6	11	0.5	7.7 – 9.3	8.3 – 8.8
13	Luxembourg	8.5	8	0.7	7.7 – 9.6	8.1 – 8.9
14	Canada	8.4	11	0.9	6.5 – 9.4	7.9 – 8.8
15	Hong Kong	8.3	12	1.1	5.5 – 9.4	7.7 – 8.7
16	Germany	8.2	10	0.6	7.5 – 9.2	7.9 – 8.5
17	USA	7.6	12	1.0	5.3 – 8.5	7.0 – 8.0
18	France	7.5	11	0.8	5.5 – 9.0	7.0 – 7.8
19	Belgium	7.4	9	0.9	5.6 – 9.0	6.9 – 7.9
	Ireland	7.4	10	1.0	5.5 – 8.7	6.9 – 7.9
21	Chile	7.3	10	0.9	5.5 – 8.7	6.8 – 7.7
	Japan	7.3	14	1.2	5.5 – 9.0	6.7 – 7.8
23	Spain	7.0	10	0.7	5.6 – 8.1	6.6 – 7.4
24	Barbados	6.9	3	1.2	5.7 – 8.1	5.7 – 7.3
25	Malta	6.6	5	1.6	5.1 – 9.0	5.4 – 7.7
26	Portugal	6.5	9	1.2	5.0 – 7.8	5.9 – 7.1
27	Estonia	6.4	11	1.1	5.1 – 9.0	6.0 – 7.0
28	Israel	6.3	10	1.2	4.2 – 8.5	5.7 – 6.9
	Oman	6.3	5	1.5	4.2 – 8.0	5.2 – 7.3
30	United Arab Emirates	6.2	6	1.4	4.5 – 8.2	5.3 – 7.1
31	Slovenia	6.1	11	1.2	4.8 – 8.7	5.7 – 6.8
32	Botswana	5.9	8	1.4	4.4 – 8.1	5.1 – 6.7
	Qatar	5.9	5	0.6	5.5 – 6.9	5.6 – 6.4
	Taiwan	5.9	14	1.0	3.7 – 7.7	5.4 – 6.3
	Uruguay	5.9	6	0.6	5.5 – 6.9	5.6 – 6.4
36	Bahrain	5.8	6	0.7	4.7 – 6.9	5.3 – 6.3
37	Cyprus	5.7	5	0.5	4.9 – 6.2	5.3 – 6.0
	Jordan	5.7	10	1.0	3.4 – 6.9	5.1 – 6.1
39	Malaysia	5.1	14	1.2	3.4 – 8.0	4.6 – 5.6
40	Hungary	5.0	11	0.5	4.1 – 5.7	4.7 – 5.2
	Italy	5.0	9	0.8	4.1 – 6.2	4.6 – 5.4
	South Korea	5.0	12	0.7	3.8 – 5.8	4.6 – 5.3
43	Tunisia	4.9	7	1.1	3.7 – 6.9	4.4 – 5.6
44	Lithuania	4.8	8	0.6	4.0 – 5.5	4.5 – 5.1
45	Kuwait	4.7	6	1.0	3.4 – 5.7	4.0 – 5.2
46	South Africa	4.5	11	0.6	3.4 – 5.6	4.2 – 4.8
47	Czech Republic	4.3	10	1.4	2.7 – 7.7	3.7 – 5.1
	Greece	4.3	9	0.8	3.7 – 5.7	3.9 – 4.7
	Namibia	4.3	8	1.0	3.4 – 6.2	3.8 – 4.9

Country Rank	Country	2005 CPI score[a]	Surveys used[b]	Standard deviation[c]	High–low range[d]	Confidence range[e]
	Slovakia	4.3	10	1.0	3.2 – 5.7	3.8 – 4.8
51	Costa Rica	4.2	7	0.9	3.4 – 5.5	3.7 – 4.7
	El Salvador	4.2	6	1.1	2.6 – 5.5	3.5 – 4.8
	Latvia	4.2	7	0.7	3.6 – 5.5	3.8 – 4.6
	Mauritius	4.2	6	1.2	2.5 – 5.7	3.4 – 5.0
55	Bulgaria	4.0	8	1.1	2.7 – 5.6	3.4 – 4.6
	Colombia	4.0	9	0.8	2.7 – 5.6	3.6 – 4.4
	Fiji	4.0	3	1.0	3.4 – 5.1	3.4 – 4.6
	Seychelles	4.0	3	0.4	3.5 – 4.2	3.5 – 4.2
59	Cuba	3.8	4	1.6	1.7 – 5.5	2.3 – 4.7
	Thailand	3.8	13	0.6	2.6 – 4.7	3.5 – 4.1
	Trinidad and Tobago	3.8	6	1.0	2.7 – 5.5	3.3 – 4.5
62	Belize	3.7	3	0.4	3.4 – 4.1	3.4 – 4.1
	Brazil	3.7	10	0.5	2.7 – 4.4	3.5 – 3.9
64	Jamaica	3.6	6	0.3	3.4 – 4.1	3.4 – 3.8
65	Ghana	3.5	8	0.8	2.6 – 5.1	3.2 – 4.0
	Mexico	3.5	10	0.5	2.7 – 4.5	3.3 – 3.7
	Panama	3.5	7	0.8	2.6 – 5.1	3.1 – 4.1
	Peru	3.5	7	0.6	2.6 – 4.1	3.1 – 3.8
	Turkey	3.5	11	1.0	2.2 – 5.3	3.1 – 4.0
70	Burkina Faso	3.4	3	0.7	2.7 – 4.2	2.7 – 3.9
	Croatia	3.4	7	0.4	3.0 – 4.2	3.2 – 3.7
	Egypt	3.4	9	0.8	2.3 – 5.1	3.0 – 3.9
	Lesotho	3.4	3	0.8	2.6 – 4.1	2.6 – 3.9
	Poland	3.4	11	1.0	2.5 – 5.7	3.0 – 3.9
	Saudi Arabia	3.4	5	1.0	2.0 – 4.5	2.7 – 4.1
	Syria	3.4	5	1.1	2.2 – 5.1	2.8 – 4.2
77	Laos	3.3	3	2.0	2.1 – 5.5	2.1 – 4.4
78	China	3.2	14	0.6	2.2 – 4.1	2.9 – 3.5
	Morocco	3.2	8	0.7	2.2 – 4.1	2.8 – 3.6
	Senegal	3.2	6	0.6	2.5 – 4.2	2.8 – 3.6
	Sri Lanka	3.2	7	0.7	2.2 – 4.1	2.7 – 3.6
	Suriname	3.2	3	1.0	2.2 – 4.1	2.2 – 3.6
83	Lebanon	3.1	4	0.4	2.7 – 3.5	2.7 – 3.3
	Rwanda	3.1	3	1.7	2.1 – 5.1	2.1 – 4.1
85	Dominican Republic	3.0	6	0.8	2.0 – 4.2	2.5 – 3.6
	Mongolia	3.0	4	0.8	2.2 – 4.2	2.4 – 3.6
	Romania	3.0	11	0.9	2.0 – 5.1	2.6 – 3.5
88	Armenia	2.9	4	0.5	2.4 – 3.4	2.5 – 3.2

Country Rank	Country	2005 CPI score[a]	Surveys used[b]	Standard deviation[c]	High–low range[d]	Confidence range[e]
	Benin	2.9	5	1.3	1.7 – 5.1	2.1 – 4.0
	Bosnia and Herzegovina	2.9	6	0.4	2.4 – 3.4	2.7 – 3.1
	Gabon	2.9	4	1.0	2.1 – 4.1	2.1 – 3.6
	India	2.9	14	0.5	2.1 – 3.5	2.7 – 3.1
	Iran	2.9	5	0.8	1.7 – 3.5	2.3 – 3.3
	Mali	2.9	8	1.2	1.5 – 5.1	2.3 – 3.6
	Moldova	2.9	5	1.1	1.9 – 4.6	2.3 – 3.7
	Tanzania	2.9	8	0.5	2.1 – 3.5	2.6 – 3.1
97	Algeria	2.8	7	0.7	2.0 – 4.2	2.5 – 3.3
	Argentina	2.8	10	0.6	1.8 – 3.5	2.5 – 3.1
	Madagascar	2.8	5	1.2	1.7 – 4.2	1.9 – 3.7
	Malawi	2.8	7	0.9	2.0 – 4.6	2.3 – 3.4
	Mozambique	2.8	8	0.6	2.1 – 3.5	2.4 – 3.1
	Serbia and Montenegro	2.8	7	0.7	2.2 – 4.1	2.5 – 3.3
103	Gambia	2.7	7	0.7	1.7 – 3.9	2.3 – 3.1
	Macedonia	2.7	7	0.7	2.2 – 4.1	2.4 – 3.2
	Swaziland	2.7	3	0.7	2.0 – 3.4	2.0 – 3.1
	Yemen	2.7	5	0.5	2.2 – 3.6	2.4 – 3.2
107	Belarus	2.6	5	1.4	1.7 – 5.1	1.9 – 3.8
	Eritrea	2.6	3	1.3	1.7 – 4.2	1.7 – 3.5
	Honduras	2.6	7	0.6	1.6 – 3.5	2.2 – 3.0
	Kazakhstan	2.6	6	0.8	1.8 – 4.1	2.2 – 3.2
	Nicaragua	2.6	7	0.4	2.1 – 3.0	2.4 – 2.8
	Palestine	2.6	3	0.5	2.1 – 3.1	2.1 – 2.8
	Ukraine	2.6	8	0.3	2.2 – 3.0	2.4 – 2.8
	Vietnam	2.6	10	0.6	1.7 – 3.5	2.3 – 2.9
	Zambia	2.6	7	0.5	2.1 – 3.4	2.3 – 2.9
	Zimbabwe	2.6	7	0.8	1.4 – 3.6	2.1 – 3.0
117	Afghanistan	2.5	3	1.1	1.6 – 3.7	1.6 – 3.2
	Bolivia	2.5	6	0.5	2.0 – 3.5	2.3 – 2.9
	Ecuador	2.5	6	0.6	1.9 – 3.5	2.2 – 2.9
	Guatemala	2.5	7	0.6	1.7 – 3.5	2.1 – 2.8
	Guyana	2.5	3	0.4	2.0 – 2.7	2.0 – 2.7
	Libya	2.5	4	0.7	1.8 – 3.4	2.0 – 3.0
	Nepal	2.5	4	0.7	1.7 – 3.4	1.9 – 3.0
	Philippines	2.5	13	0.6	1.5 – 3.5	2.3 – 2.8
	Uganda	2.5	8	0.5	2.0 – 3.5	2.2 – 2.8
126	Albania	2.4	3	0.4	2.1 – 2.8	2.1 – 2.7
	Niger	2.4	4	0.3	2.1 – 2.7	2.2 – 2.6

Country Rank	Country	2005 CPI score[a]	Surveys used[b]	Standard deviation[c]	High–low range[d]	Confidence range[e]
	Russia	2.4	12	0.3	1.9 – 3.0	2.3 – 2.6
	Sierra Leone	2.4	3	0.5	2.1 – 3.0	2.1 – 2.7
130	Burundi	2.3	3	0.3	2.1 – 2.7	2.1 – 2.5
	Cambodia	2.3	4	0.5	1.7 – 2.7	1.9 – 2.5
	Congo, Republic	2.3	4	0.4	2.0 – 3.0	2.1 – 2.6
	Georgia	2.3	6	0.5	1.7 – 2.7	2.0 – 2.6
	Kyrgyzstan	2.3	5	0.4	1.9 – 2.7	2.1 – 2.5
	Papua New Guinea	2.3	4	0.5	1.7 – 2.7	1.9 – 2.6
	Venezuela	2.3	10	0.2	2.0 – 2.5	2.2 – 2.4
137	Azerbaijan	2.2	6	0.5	1.7 – 3.0	1.9 – 2.5
	Cameroon	2.2	6	0.4	1.8 – 2.7	2.0 – 2.5
	Ethiopia	2.2	8	0.4	1.7 – 2.8	2.0 – 2.5
	Indonesia	2.2	13	0.4	1.7 – 3.3	2.1 – 2.5
	Iraq	2.2	4	1.0	1.4 – 3.6	1.5 – 2.9
	Liberia	2.2	3	0.1	2.1 – 2.4	2.1 – 2.3
	Uzbekistan	2.2	5	0.2	2.0 – 2.5	2.1 – 2.4
144	Congo, Democratic Republic	2.1	4	0.4	1.6 – 2.5	1.8 – 2.3
	Kenya	2.1	8	0.5	1.4 – 3.0	1.8 – 2.4
	Pakistan	2.1	7	0.7	1.3 – 3.4	1.7 – 2.6
	Paraguay	2.1	7	0.4	1.6 – 2.7	1.9 – 2.3
	Somalia	2.1	3	0.4	1.6 – 2.4	1.6 – 2.2
	Sudan	2.1	5	0.2	1.7 – 2.3	1.9 – 2.2
	Tajikistan	2.1	5	0.4	1.7 – 2.7	1.9 – 2.4
151	Angola	2.0	5	0.2	1.6 – 2.2	1.8 – 2.1
152	Cote d'Ivoire	1.9	4	0.3	1.6 – 2.2	1.7 – 2.1
	Equatorial Guinea	1.9	3	0.3	1.6 – 2.2	1.6 – 2.1
	Nigeria	1.9	9	0.3	1.4 – 2.2	1.7 – 2.0
155	Haiti	1.8	4	0.5	1.4 – 2.5	1.5 – 2.1
	Myanmar	1.8	4	0.2	1.6 – 2.2	1.7 – 2.0
	Turkmenistan	1.8	4	0.2	1.6 – 2.2	1.7 – 2.0
158	Bangladesh	1.7	7	0.5	1.0 – 2.4	1.4 – 2.0
	Chad	1.7	6	0.6	1.0 – 2.7	1.3 – 2.1

a. '2005 CPI score' relates to perceptions of the degree of corruption as seen by business people, academics and risk analysts, and ranges between 10 (highly clean) and 0 (highly corrupt).

b. 'Surveys used' refers to the number of surveys that assessed a country's performance. A total of 16 surveys were used from 10 independent institutions, and at least three surveys were required for a country to be included in the CPI.

c. 'Standard deviation' indicates differences in the values given by the sources: the greater the standard deviation, the greater the differences in perceptions of a country among the sources.

d. 'High–low range' provides the highest and lowest values given by the different sources.

e. 'Confidence range' provides a range of possible values of the CPI score. This reflects how a country's score may vary, depending on measurement precision. Nominally, with 5 per cent probability when few sources are available, an unbiased estimate of the mean coverage probability is lower than the nominal value of 90 per cent. It is 65.3 per cent for 3 sources; 78.4 per cent for 5 sources; 80.2 per cent for 6 sources and 81.8 per cent for 7 sources.

Note

1. Johann Graf Lambsdorff is chair in economic theory at the University of Passau (Germany) and a research consultant to Transparency International, for whom he has coordinated and carried out the CPI since 1995.

12   Governance matters IV: new data, new challenges

Daniel Kaufmann, Aart Kraay and Massimo Mastruzzi[1]

In this new study, we present a set of governance indicators covering 209 countries over the period 1996–2004. For 2004, these indicators are based on 352 different underlying variables measuring perceptions of a wide range of governance issues.[2] The variables are drawn from 32 separate data sources constructed by 30 different organisations worldwide. The indicators that capture the six key dimensions of institutional quality or governance are as follows: voice and accountability, political stability and lack of violence, government effectiveness, regulatory quality, rule of law and control of corruption.

The precision of the aggregate governance indicators in this updated analysis has increased since we have substantially increased the number of sources and individual variables used in the aggregate indices. We do stress, however, that comparisons across countries and across time should be treated with caution since the margins of error are not negligible. These margins of error are not unique to the perceptions-based measures of governance we use, but are an important feature of any measure of governance, objective or subjective.[3]

Is there an economic development dividend for better governance, or are governance improvements mostly a by-product of higher incomes?

There is by now a strong consensus among both academics and policy-makers that good governance provides the fundamental basis for economic development. Academic research has focused on the effects of institutional quality on growth in the long run, noting that there is a strong causal impact of institutional quality on per capita incomes worldwide. Figure 12.1 shows a representative set of estimates of this 'development dividend' of good governance. These estimates suggest that a realistic one-standard-deviation improvement in governance would raise incomes in the long run by about two- to threefold.[4] Of course, there is variation around these relationships, since governance is not the only thing that matters for development – but it certainly is a very important factor deserving policy-makers' attention.

Given the strong positive effect of governance on development, and its importance for effective aid delivery, it is a matter of considerable concern that governance performance in sub-Saharan Africa is on average quite weak. Altogether, 38 out of 46 countries in the region lie in the bottom-left quadrant of the graph, meaning that they are both

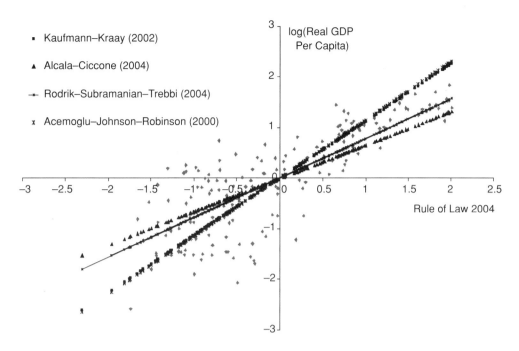

poorer than the world average and also exhibit worse governance than the world average. Some observers have argued that we should discount the poor governance performance of the region based on the fact that these countries have very low income levels – arguing that good governance costs money to provide. Yet recent research provides very little evidence in support of the proposition that poor governance in Africa is attributable to poverty. Rather, most of the causality is in the opposite direction, from better governance to better development outcomes.

Is governance in some countries improving and how do we know that a significant change has actually taken place?

Reformers in many governments as well as civil society and investors increasingly view governance as key for development and the investment climate, which in turn has increased the demand for monitoring the quality of governance in a country over time. Further, aid donors have also come to the view that aid flows have a stronger impact on development in countries with good institutional quality.

In light of this, it is important to measure trends over time, as well as levels of governance. Our new indicators now span an eight-year period from 1996 to 2004, which is sufficiently long to begin looking for meaningful trends in governance. Over the eight-year period, we find that in about 10 per cent of countries we can be highly confident (at the 90 per cent significance level) that governance has changed substantially, while at a lower 75 per cent significance level, roughly 20 per cent of all observed changes stand out as significant.[5] Importantly, we show that there is a great deal of agreement among our many data sources about the direction of change in governance in these countries. Overall this reminds us that, while in general institutional quality changes only gradually, there are also countries where one can point to sharp improvements or deteriorations over an eight-year period. This finding is of particular interest, given the common perception that while deterioration in a particular country can take place rather quickly, improvements are always very slow and incremental.

For instance, since 1996 there has been significant improvement in 'voice and accountability' in a number of countries, such as in Bosnia, Croatia, Serbia, Ghana, Indonesia, Sierra Leone, Slovak Republic and Peru, while a significant deterioration has taken place in countries such as the Ivory Coast, Zimbabwe, Kyrgyz Republic, Nepal, Haiti and Israel. With these aggregate indicators it is also possible to ascertain that some countries have experienced significant changes in briefer time spans, such as the case of the major improvement in the 'voice' variable for Senegal, Turkey and Nigeria during 1998–2004, or its deterioration in Pakistan, Belarus, Russia and Venezuela.

In general, it is of concern that there is little evidence of systematic improvements in regional averages for governance in most regions, including Africa. However, new governance indicators for trends in three dimensions of governance for the period 1996–2004 in Africa show that roughly as many countries show declines in governance as show improvements. Focusing only on those changes that are sufficiently large as to suggest that there are significant trends in institutional quality, the story is much the same: as many countries show significant improvements as declines.

Looking ahead

We argue that governance *can* be measured, using a variety of types of data, both the subjective information on which we rely as well as more objective indicators. But it is essential that indicators on governance and investment climate take margins of error into account and are complemented with in-depth in-country governance diagnostics, based on micro-surveys of households, firms, and public officials within the country. The lessons being drawn from these combined aggregate and micro datasets point to the importance of moving concretely to the next stage of governance reforms.

Given the lack of worldwide progress on governance, coupled with its importance for development, a case can be made for redoubling our analysis of this connection, as well as for questioning the effectiveness of some traditional approaches to improving governance, such as creating additional anti-corruption commissions and laws. In particular, the importance of political factors (including 'state capture' and political commitment from the top) has been underplayed, as have many 'second generation' institutional reforms supporting political, economic and financial transparency. Examples include natural resource revenue transparency mechanisms, disclosure of assets by politicians, voting records of parliamentarians, political campaign contributions, and fiscal accounts.

Notes

1. Daniel Kaufmann is the director for global governance and regional learning at the World Bank Institute, United States. Contact: dkaufmann@worldbank.org. Aart Kraay is a lead economist in the development research group at the World Bank. Contact: akraay@worldbank.org. Massimo Mastruzzi is a research analyst at the World Bank. Contact: mmastruzzi@worldbank.org. The views expressed here are the authors' and do not necessarily reflect the official position of the World Bank, its executive directors, or the countries they represent.
2. For the full paper, see www.worldbank.org/wbi/governance/pubs/govmatters4.html. The data and a graphical interface are available at www.worldbank.org/wbi/governance/govdata/
3. For more in-depth discussions of the issues of margins of error and the usefulness of perceptions-based measures, see our paper in the *Global Corruption Report 2004*, pp. 302–6.
4. The estimates come from Alcala and Ciccone (2004), Acemoglu, Johnson and Robinson (2001), Kaufmann and Kraay (2002), and Rodrik, Subramanian and Trebbi (2004). References available in the full paper at: www.worldbank.org/wbi/governance/pubs/govmatters4.html
5. Nine statistically significant changes per indicator were found using a 'rule of thumb' labelling of those countries for which the change in estimated governance over the 1996–2004 period is sufficiently large that the 90 per cent confidence intervals for governance in the two periods do not overlap. These were compared with a dynamic formal statistical model, which turned up more or less the same set of significant changes in governance, although it is important to note that the magnitude of these changes is substantially smaller in the formal dynamic model.

13   Corruption in the United States of America

Edward Glaeser and Raven Saks[1]

Corruption is not just something that happens to poor countries. Between 1990 and 2002, federal prosecutors in the United States convicted more than 10,000 government officials of acts of corruption including fraud, campaign-finance violations, and obstruction of justice. While corruption in the United States is bad news for the country, it is a mixed blessing for researchers, whose analysis of corruption has been hampered by lack of data. Most studies of corruption have relied on international opinion surveys that ask private individuals about the level of corruption in a nation. While these opinion surveys contain valuable information, they do not provide a full picture of corruption in a country.

As a complement to the international evidence, recent research on corruption in the United States examines the determinants of corruption using information on the number of public officials convicted for corruption in each of the 50 US states.[2] Because the individuals were all prosecuted by the same federal agency, the data can be compared across states, in contrast to the available international survey data.[3] Measuring corruption as the number of federal corruption convictions per capita, this research explores the state characteristics that predict corruption and the extent that corruption deters economic growth at the state level. Although these conviction data have been used in other contexts, prior research has not examined the effects of the level of income or ethnic heterogeneity on corruption, nor has it discussed the effect of corruption on economic growth.[4] Moreover, in contrast to earlier work, this research explores alternative identification strategies by examining changes in corruption over time and taking account of income and education using historical variables.

Table 13.1 lists the most and least corrupt states ranked by the average number of convictions per capita from 1976 to 2002. The ranking lines up reasonably well with general notions about the areas in the United States that are more corrupt, and is positively correlated with a 1998 survey of congressional reporters' perception of public corruption.[5]

The report finds that states with higher incomes and a larger share of college-educated population are less corrupt. In a simple OLS regression, the 1970 levels of education and income in each state are negatively correlated with the average corruption rate from 1976 to 2002 (see Table 13.2).[6] The same negative correlations exist when estimating the effect of the initial level of education and income on changes in corruption in each state over the past 25 years. Thus, this relationship cannot be attributed to omitted variables that might lead to a spurious correlation among the levels of income, education and corruption across states.

Table 13.1: US states with most and least convictions per capita, 1976–2002

Most convictions		Least convictions	
State	Average annual convictions per 100,000 people	State	Average annual convictions per 100,000 people
Alaska	0.643	Colorado	0.151
Mississippi	0.612	Wisconsin	0.150
Louisiana	0.513	Nebraska	0.133
South Dakota	0.472	Utah	0.130
Tennessee	0.464	Iowa	0.127
Illinois	0.458	New Hampshire	0.125
New York	0.439	Minnesota	0.121
Oklahoma	0.415	Vermont	0.115
Montana	0.414	Washington	0.104
North Dakota	0.398	Oregon	0.074

Table 13.2: Effect of income and education on average corruption rate, 1976–2002

	OLS		IV	
	(1)	(2)	(3)	(4)
Ln (Income)	−.203		−.470**	
	(.144)		(.179)	
Share with 4+ years of college		−2.91**		−5.03**
		(1.18)		(2.27)
Adj. R^2	.27	.34	.11	.16
No. Observations	50	50	48	45

Note: All regressions also control for the following state characteristics in 1970: the logarithm of state population, the share of government employment, the share of urban population, dummy variables for each census region, and a constant. The instruments used in column 3 are the logarithm of median household income in 1940 and quadratic functions of longitude and latitude. The instrument used in column 4 is the fraction of church members who are Congregationalist from the 1890 census.

The magnitude of the coefficients reported in Table 13.2 suggest that a one standard deviation increase in income would lead to about one-sixth of a standard deviation decrease in corruption. The effect of education is larger, as a one standard deviation increase in the fraction of the population with a college degree would lead to a decrease in the corruption rate of one-half of a standard deviation.

An alternative interpretation of these results is that high income and education levels may be the result, rather than the cause, of lower corruption. To address this concern, the third and fourth columns of Table 13.2 use historical data to predict the levels of income and schooling in 1970. Income is predicted using a state's geographic location and income in 1940. The level of education in each state is predicted using the fraction of Congregationalist church members in 1890.[7] These factors are all strong predictors of income and education today, and yet are unlikely to have been influenced by the level of corruption at the end of the twentieth century. Using this method, the negative effect of income and education on corruption becomes even stronger.

The report also investigates several other theories concerning the determinants of corruption. Income inequality and racial heterogeneity are found to be associated with higher corruption rates.[8] In contrast, there is only weak evidence that states with larger local governments are more corrupt. Finally, the report examines the effect of corruption in 1976–1980 on economic growth during the subsequent 20 years. States with higher corruption rates have experienced lower income growth from 1980 to 2000, but there is no evidence that corruption has led to lower employment growth or lower housing values.

In general, the patterns documented in the data for US states reveal the same basic relationships that have been found using international evidence. This similarity is particularly interesting given that, here, corruption is measured using federal conviction data rather than the type of opinion survey that is the norm in the cross-country literature. This suggests that both methods can provide useful information concerning the amount of corruption in a particular location. A second important implication of this research is that improving the education system in a state or country can help reduce corruption in government.

Notes

1. Edward Glaeser is a professor of economics at Harvard University and Raven Saks is an economist at the Federal Reserve Board of Governors. Contact information: eglaeser@harvard.edu and raven.e.saks@frb.gov. The views presented are solely those of the authors and do not necessarily represent those of the Federal Reserve Board or its staff.
2. Edward Glaeser and Raven E. Saks, 'Corruption in America', National Bureau of Economic Research Working Paper No. 10821, October 2004.
3. One disadvantage of using convictions to measure corruption is that the intensity of investigation or prosecution might be lower in places that are more corrupt. This concern is mitigated by the fact that these convictions are all prosecuted by the same federal agency. Nonetheless, this data may still provide an inaccurate view of the degree of corruption, if the Department of Justice (DOJ) treats richer or more corrupt states differently, or if the types of corruption not covered by the DOJ are more prevalent in richer states.
4. Daniel Berkowitz and Karen Clay, 'Initial Conditions, Institutional Dynamics and Economic Performance: Evidence from American States', William Davidson Institute Working Paper No. 615, 2003. Raymond Fisman and Robert Gatti, 'Decentralization and Corruption: Evidence from U.S. Federal Transfer Programs', *Public Choice* 113(1), 2002. Rajeev K. Goel and Michael A. Nelson, 'Corruption and Government Size: A Disaggregated Analysis', *Public Choice* 97(1–2), 1998.
5. Richard T. Boylan and Cheryl Long, 'A Survey of State House Reporters' Perception of Public Corruption', *State Politics and Policy Quarterly*, 2003.

6. Each regression includes the following 1970 state characteristics as additional controls: the logarithm of state population, the share of urban population, the fraction of employment in the government sector, and dummy variables for the four census regions.
7. Congregationalism was almost never a dominant religion during this time period, but it is generally associated with elites and their commitment to education. As a result, education developed more quickly in states with more Congregationalists and those states remain more educated today.
8. The hypothesis, associated with Paolo Mauro, 'Corruption and Growth', *Quarterly Journal of Economics*, MIT Press, vol. 110(3): 681–712, 1995, and Alberto Alesina, Reza Baqir and William Easterly, 'Redistributive Public Employment', *Journal of Urban Economics* 48: 219–41, 2002, is that ethnic heterogeneity increases corruption. As voters become more diverse along ethnic or income lines, then voting will inevitably focus on redistribution rather than on the honesty of government officials.

14   Transparency and its impact on financial fragility

Saadia Zahidi[1]

In recent decades, many countries have experienced some form of banking crisis, either small borderline crises or systemic ones, typically involving widespread bank insolvencies, liquidity squeezes and depositor withdrawals. The crises have been expensive, not only through their effects on government budgets and taxes, but also due to forgone economic output. The economic literature investigating the causes of banking crises has focused mainly on macroeconomic factors, such as growth rates and inflation, financial factors, such as liquidity and credit growth, and only more recently on the role of institutions. This work is an attempt to probe further into the role of institutions by examining the empirical relationship between financial fragility and the *transparency* of financial institutions.

While crises may erupt in a relatively short period of time, they are usually the result of long-term fundamental problems in a country's financial institutions. Weak, inefficient institutions lead to fragile financial systems, where a small event or trigger may lead to a large effect (that is, a full-blown crisis). The mechanism of a banking crisis becomes obvious if one recalls the fundamental characteristics of finance: information asymmetries, intertemporal trade and demandable debt. Providers of funds (lenders) have difficulties monitoring intermediaries, who in turn face the same problem with users of funds (borrowers). Those receiving funds know better how they will utilise them than providers, and this is further complicated by the exchange of money today for money in the future.[2]

As a result, banking systems with poor transparency are particularly vulnerable. Literature on the subject has shown that they can become increasingly fragile through two ways: first, investments (loans) are made on the basis of incorrect or misrepresented information, and second, once bad loans are discovered, there is a strong incentive to roll them over rather than to declare them as non-performing. Since banking crises can erupt where there are bad investments and mismatched balance sheets, we would predict that countries with poor transparency should be prone to a higher number of banking crises.

Using a multivariate logit model, the hypothesis that high levels of transparency (that is, high scores on the 'institutional' variables) significantly decrease the probability of a crisis when other factors are controlled for, was tested. The dependent variable, the banking crisis dummy, is equal to zero if there is no banking crisis, and it is equal to one if there is a crisis.[3] The set of control variables covers macroeconomic developments that affect bank performance (the rate of growth of real GDP, the external terms of trade, the rate of inflation and the real short-term interest rate); characteristics of the banking system (vulnerability to sudden capital outflows, liquidity, exposure to the private sector and credit growth); and other relevant factors (financial liberalisation and GDP per capita).[4] Unique qualitative perceptions data[5] for 41 countries across a period of 11 years is used as a proxy for the transparency of institutions (see Table 14.1).

Table 14.1: Perceptions data on the transparency of institutions

Variable name	Question detail
Corruption	Improper practices (such as bribing, corruption, and irregular payments): (1 = prevail in the public sphere; 7 = do not prevail in the public sphere)
Favouritism	When deciding upon policies and contracts, government officials (1 = usually favour well connected firms and individuals, 7 = are neutral among firms and individuals)
Independence of the judiciary	The judiciary in your country is independent from influences of members of government, citizens, or firms (1 = no, heavily influenced, 7 = yes, entirely independent)
Insider trading	Insider trading is not common in the domestic stock market (1 = strongly disagree; 7 = strongly agree)
Regulation of the financial system	Regulation and supervision of financial institutions in your country is among the world's most stringent (1 = strongly disagree; 7 = strongly agree)

Transparency variables are indeed significant in explaining the probability and severity of banking crises, perhaps more so than several traditional explanatory variables. The clearly negative and significant relationship between transparency variables and banking crises remains robust to several specification changes. Some cautious but interesting insights can be obtained from the analysis undertaken in this research. Transparency variables consistently display far better significance levels than several of the control variables.[6] Second, we find that a one-unit increase in the scores for corruption, favouritism, judicial independence, insider trading and regulation decreases the *odds* in favour of a country having a banking crisis by 74 per cent, 86 per cent, 89 per cent, 69 per cent and 76 per cent respectively; whereas one-unit increases in inflation, credit ratio and the real interest rate increase the odds in favour of crises by 4–11 per cent, 2–4 per cent and 3–5 per cent, and one-unit increases in credit growth and GDP growth decrease the odds by 6–9 per cent and 12–26 per cent respectively (see Table 14.2). Clearly, transparency is important in preventing financial crises and the role of the judiciary appears to be particularly important. This is not surprising given the inherent need for contract enforcement in all areas of finance.

These results have substantial policy implications, providing support for strong national financial sector regulation, as well as global, standardised frameworks, such as those developed by the Bank of International Settlements.[7] Transparency in general is indispensable to the financial sector, providing access, timeliness, relevance and quality, and developing institutional infrastructure, standards, auditing and accounting practices that promote transparency, implementing incentives for disclosure and installing countervailing regulations to minimise the perverse incentives generated by safety-net arrangements, is absolutely imperative.[8] The challenge lies in creating the type of public–private partnership and cooperation that are necessary for implementing effective regulation.

Table 14.2: Transparency variables explaining probability of banking crises

Variable name	Percentage effect on the odds in favour of a crisis due to a one-unit increase in the variable
Corruption	−74
Favouritism	−86
Independence of the judiciary	−89
Insider trading	−69
Regulation of the financial system	−76
Inflation	4 to 11
Credit ratio	2 to 4
Real interest rate	3 to 5
Credit growth	−6 to −9
GDP growth	−12 to −26

Notes

1. Saadia Zahidi is an economist at the World Economic Forum. This research was carried out at the Graduate Institute of International Studies in Geneva.
2. Charles Wyplosz, 'Globalized Financial Markets and Financial Crises', April 1998.
3. Gerard Caprio and Daniela Klingebiel, 'Database on Banking Crises', World Bank, October 2003. See: http://www1.worldbank.org/finance/html/sfd_home.html
4. These are taken from a previous study with a similar focus. Asli Demirguc-Kunt and Enrica Detragiache, 'The Determinants of Banking Crises in Developing and Developed Countries', IMF Staff Papers 45(1), March 1998.
5. World Economic Forum, *Global Competitiveness Reports 1992–2002.*
6. Having corrected for multicollinearity.
7. 'Core Principles for Effective Banking Supervision', developed by the Basel Committee on Banking Supervision at the Bank of International Settlements.
8. Daniel Kaufmann and Tara Vishwanath, 'Toward Transparency: New Approaches and their Application to Financial Markets', *World Bank Observer* 16(1), Spring 2001.

15   Budget transparency survey

Pamela Gomez[1]

As part of the global movement towards more open government, citizens around the world have become increasingly concerned with obtaining access to accurate, comprehensive, and timely information on the financial activities of their governments. This is not surprising. Comprehensive financial information, which should be disclosed in a country's budget documents, allows the public to evaluate a government's policy intentions, its policy priorities, and their implementation. Public access to such documents is essential to ensure both that government is financially accountable and that civil society can participate effectively in budget debates.

The International Budget Project (IBP) was established at the Washington, DC-based Center on Budget and Policy Priorities in 1997 to assist non-governmental organisations and researchers in developing and transitional countries in their efforts to analyse budget policies, to open budget processes and to strengthen budget-related institutions.

In 2004, the IBP published the findings of a pilot study to evaluate public access to budget information in 36 countries. The IBP, along with several partner organisations in developing countries, had designed a questionnaire, the Open Budget Questionnaire, to evaluate the public availability of budget documents at the central government level, the presentation of budget information in a manner suitable for policy analysis, and the extent to which public and legislative involvement in the budget debate is encouraged. The IBP expanded the project following the pilot in 2004, and will publish results from 60 countries in September 2006.

During the pilot phase of the project, civil society researchers from 36 developing and transitional countries completed the *Open Budget Questionnaire*. The questionnaire results were intended to offer an independent, non-governmental view of the state of budget transparency in the countries studied. All of the researchers who completed the questionnaire were from academic or other non-governmental organisations. One researcher (or one group of researchers within an organisation) from each of the countries represented was responsible for submitting a single questionnaire with the results for that country.

The questionnaire contained 122 questions. All of the questions were constructed with the intention that they should capture easily observable and replicable phenomena.[2] The questionnaire drew on the efforts of multilateral organisations for many of the criteria it used in evaluating best and good practice. Specifically, it used criteria from the Organisation for Economic Co-operation and Development's (OECD) *Best Practices for Budget Transparency*, the International Monetary Fund's (IMF) *Code of Good Practices on Fiscal Transparency*, and the International Organization of Supreme Auditing Institutions' (INTOSAI) *Lima Declaration of Guidelines on Auditing Precepts*.

Findings from the questionnaire

Table 15.1 shows the questionnaire results. The researchers in the 36 countries studies found that in all but one of the countries studied, governments made their main policy document, the executive's budget proposal, available to the public. But lack of public access to other types of essential budget documents raised concerns. Nine of the 36

Table 15.1: Summary results by major category

Country	Executive budget documents (%)	Country	Monitoring and evaluation reports (%)	Country	Public and legislative involvement (%)
Czech Republic	86	Slovenia	99	Slovenia	86
Slovenia	86	Poland	97	South Africa	77
Botswana	84	South Africa	82	Czech Republic	65
South Africa	83	Czech Republic	76	Poland	63
Poland	79	Russia	74	Brazil	57
Peru	77	Mexico	70	Uganda	54
Kenya	72	Kenya	64	Indonesia	52
Namibia	68	Peru	64	Romania	51
Jordan	68	Bulgaria	57	Peru	49
Ghana	64	Romania	55	Argentina	49
Azerbaijan	64	Georgia	53	Burkina Faso	48
Russia	63	Croatia	51	Mexico	48
Mexico	62	Brazil	49	Kenya	46
Brazil	61	Uganda	48	Costa Rica	46
Argentina	61	Jordan	46	Russia	45
Uganda	59	Indonesia	45	Bangladesh	40
India	59	El Salvador	44	Colombia	38
Bangladesh	58	Burkina Faso	43	India	37
El Salvador	58	Argentina	42	El Salvador	37
Colombia	57	Botswana	42	Croatia	36
Costa Rica	56	Bangladesh	40	Botswana	36
Nepal	56	Kazakhstan	36	Bulgaria	34
Burkina Faso	56	Colombia	36	Malawi	33
Malawi	52	Nicaragua	34	Namibia	33
Georgia	52	Ghana	34	Ghana	33
Romania	51	Nepal	32	Jordan	31
Kazakhstan	48	Costa Rica	31	Kazakhstan	28
Indonesia	47	Zambia	31	Azerbaijan	27
Bulgaria	45	India	30	Honduras	25
Honduras	43	Ecuador	25	Georgia	24
Zambia	35	Namibia	14	Nicaragua	20
Ecuador	31	Bolivia	12	Zambia	19
Croatia	28	Azerbaijan	10	Mongolia	19
Bolivia	21	Honduras	7	Bolivia	18
Nicaragua	19	Malawi	6	Ecuador	14
Mongolia	0	Mongolia	0	Nepal	7
Average	56	Average	44	Average	40

Note: The shading groups countries according to their average score. Scores of 67 per cent or above generally indicate 'positive' practices, and scores of 50–66 per cent reflect 'mostly positive' practices. In contrast, scores of 33–49 per cent indicate 'mostly negative' practices, and scores of less than 33 per cent reflect 'negative' practices.

countries did not release routine reports during the year allowing for the monitoring of expenditure, revenue collection and borrowing. At the same time, 12 of the 36 countries did not make audit reports available to the public. (See Table 15.2.)

Table 15.2: Budget documents made available to the public

(out of 36 countries completing the questionnaire)

	Number of countries	Percent of total
Pre-budget statement	19	53
Executive budget proposal	35	97
Citizens budget	6	17
In-year monitoring reports	27	75
Mid-year review	17	47
Year-end evaluation reports	29	81
Audit reports	24	67

Significantly, the researchers found that many governments could substantially improve budget transparency in their countries by taking the simple step of releasing to the public documents they are already producing for internal use. The researchers found that in all of the countries that did not release routine monitoring reports except one – Namibia – these reports were in fact prepared, but only for internal use. Similarly, in the 12 countries that did not make audit reports available to the public, all of the countries except one – Nicaragua – were preparing the audits, but simply not releasing them to the public.

In addition to examining the public availability of the documents as noted above, the survey also evaluated the comprehensiveness of the content of the documents. Each country's performance for the executive's budget proposal, and for its monitoring and evaluation reports, are shown in the first two columns in Table 15.1. The third column shows the extent to which the country's executive makes available information and the legislature provides opportunities to facilitate public discourse and understanding of the budget.

The results from the pilot project included the following:[3]

- The countries surveyed fare best in the first of the three main areas examined: the executive's budget proposal. Documents related to the executive's budget are routinely released to the public and typically contain significant amounts of information on at least the budget year and the year before it.
- Far fewer countries report positive practices in the second area examined: issuing public reports that monitor the budget while it is being implemented or evaluate the budget once the fiscal year has been completed. Governments typically fall short of international best practices in this area. Without these documents, the public and civil society cannot easily assess budgetary outcomes, including how well public funds are being spent.
- The weakest scores, in most of the countries surveyed, concern the final area examined: efforts by the executive to facilitate public discourse and understanding

of the budget. Most executives fail to provide information to the public and to legislatures that can help make the budget (and the policies it embodies) more understandable. Without such information, a broad and informed debate on a nation's fiscal priorities is impossible. In addition, official avenues for legislative and public input, such as legislative hearings or public consultation periods, tend to be lacking.

The IBP made these results from the pilot study available in October 2004 to promote discussion of the study's methodology. Following the release, the IBP collected feedback on the study from academics, non-governmental organisations, public expenditure management experts, and international financial institutions and other organisations. The IBP used the feedback to refine the questionnaire and the study's methodology, and expects to have results from 60 countries available in September 2006.

Notes

1. Pamela Gomez is an international policy analyst at the International Budget Project at the Center on Budget and Policy Priorities in Washington, DC.
2. Most of the questions on the questionnaire required the researcher to choose among five responses. Responses 'a' and 'b' reflected best or good practice regarding the subject matter of the question, 'c' and 'd' reflected poor practices, and 'e' reflected *not applicable*. For the purposes of aggregating the responses in the three major categories, an 'a' response was awarded a score of 100 per cent, 'b' was worth 67 per cent, 'c' was worth 33 per cent, and 'd' was marked as 0 per cent. Responses of 'e' *not applicable* were not considered in the scoring.
3. For full details of the study, please see the International Budget Project's website at http://www.internationalbudget.org/openbudgets/index.htm

16 Beyond the rhetoric: measuring revenue transparency in the oil and gas industry

Elizabeth Lort-Phillips and Vanessa Herringshaw[1]

There has been growing recognition that transparent disclosure of revenues from extractive industries is vital for responsible use of oil and gas and the avoidance of the 'resource curse'. This insight has been strongly endorsed by those committing to schemes such as the Extractive Industries Transparency Initiative (EITI).[2] But beyond the rhetoric, what concrete action has been taken to improve transparency in the oil and gas sectors?

Save the Children UK (SC UK) has been very proactive in tackling this question. In 2005, it created a framework for measuring revenue transparency and developed a set of indices to set transparency standards for key actors, to evaluate their current performance and to track progress over time. The standards can be readily incorporated into regulations, policies and guidelines relating to revenue transparency in the extractive industries, such as for reporting requirements, investor guidelines or company policies.

SC UK published two reports in 2005 measuring revenue transparency in the oil and gas sectors. The first report ranked 25 *companies* in terms of their performance in the disclosure of revenues paid to host governments by the oil and gas industries, based on their company-wide policies, their management systems and their transparency performance in six host countries – Nigeria, Angola, Azerbaijan, Indonesia, Timor Leste and Venezuela. The second report ranks 10 *home countries* (that is, countries in which companies are registered or raising finance) – the United Kingdom, the United States, Canada, France, the Netherlands, Italy, Norway, Australia, South Africa and Russia – according to their measures to regulate and support company reporting of revenue payments to host governments.

As the research relates to transparency and accountability, the methodology used to carry out both of these reports consisted largely of surveying data available in the public domain. This included websites, annual reports, statements of policy, press releases, accounting standards and financial regulations. Company performance was assessed in three categories: revenue payments transparency (disclosure of benefit streams from companies to host governments); supportive disclosure (disclosure of other information necessary to judge the accuracy of the revenue information and predict future revenues); and anti-corruption and whistleblowing measures. Home government performance was assessed in four categories: revenue payments transparency; supportive disclosure; access to information (from public, parastatal and private bodies); and the broad governance environment. The overall methodology was developed through consultation with a reference group involving government, civil society, investors and industry experts.

The report on companies found that the majority of companies were not disclosing revenue payments to host governments. More than half the companies scored zero on this category. Existing disclosure was mostly made known by geographic segment (such as a region, or 'rest of the world' category), which is of little use to citizens wishing to find out information on company payments to their governments. However, systematic disclosure across countries was shown to be possible, as Talisman disclosed royalties, taxes and bonuses paid in all countries of operation.

Some companies are disclosing some information in a few countries but this is usually limited and variable. For example, Shell had the highest country score for its progressive disclosure practices in Nigeria (82 per cent), yet its overall performance (29 per cent) was weakened by its lack of disclosure practices in Venezuela. Performance also varied within single countries between different companies. In Azerbaijan, only BP disclosed any payments to the government; eight other companies operating there have yet to do so. There was great variation between companies disclosing in Nigeria and Indonesia. This clearly shows that companies can do more in particular countries and that there is a need for them to take a globally systematic approach to improving their transparency. (See Figure 16.1.)

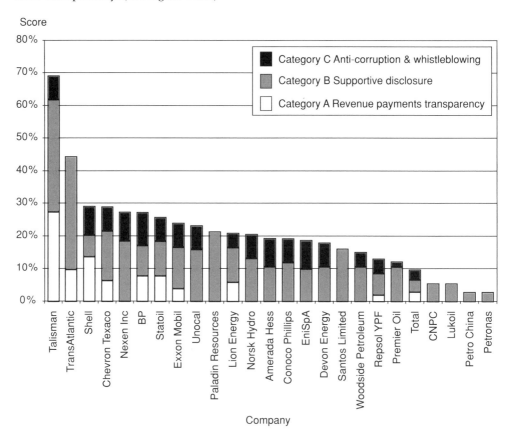

Figure 16.1: Overall company performance

Companies based in home countries with mandatory disclosure requirements lead in performance results on transparency. Canadian government disclosure requirements are stronger than the nine other governments assessed, and three of the top five companies were Canadian (Talisman, Nexen and TransAtlantic). Perhaps surprisingly, there was uneven transparency performance by the voluntary EITI signatories. Of the seven companies listed as EITI participants, only four publicly disclosed any payments to the governments. Total, Exxon and Repsol did not disclose in any of the countries researched. This poor performance illustrates the limitations of the voluntary process.

The assessment of home government action in supporting transparency in the oil and gas industries revealed disappointing performance, despite their stated commitments to transparency. Almost no home country had any requirement that companies disclose their revenues on a host country-by-country basis in their regulations on corporate reporting. (See Figure 16.2.)

As indicated above, overall leadership is shown by Canada, a non-EITI country, which is the only country with any requirement for disclosure of royalty payments at a host country level through its securities legislation. Leadership on access to information also came from a non-EITI country, South Africa, which had the most progressive law allowing access to private sector information 'where access is necessary for the protection or exercise of another right'. Furthermore, the research indicated that there was a distinct lack of 'joined-up' policies. Many countries reported a lack of coordination between different government departments about disclosure commitments in the extractive sector.

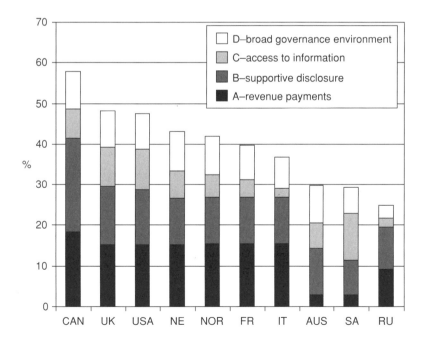

Figure 16.2: Overall home government performance

The findings of these reports produced some key policy recommendations. Home governments must require companies to publish what they pay to governments wherever they operate, commit to global standards for disclosure in the extractive industry and actively engage the EITI in the implementation of those standards. Companies too must move beyond the rhetoric and publish what they pay to governments wherever they operate on a country-by-country basis in a systematic way. Companies must lobby home governments to mainstream disclosure requirements into accounting and listing standards, actively participate in the EITI and work collaboratively with other actors to build disclosure agreements. This is important and advantageous, as such regulation would afford investment protection and ensure a more level playing field in the oil and gas markets.

For the full text of the reports, including key recommendations and standards for inclusion in policies and guidelines, see www.savethechildren.org.uk/measuring transparency.

Notes

1. Elizabeth Lort-Phillips is a consultant with Save the Children UK. Vanessa Herringshaw is head of economic policy with Save the Children UK.
2. The EITI 'supports improved governance in resource-rich countries through the full publication and verification of company payments and government revenues from oil, gas and mining. Many countries are rich in oil, gas, and minerals and studies have shown that when governance is good, these can generate large revenues to foster economic growth and reduce poverty. However when governance is weak, they may instead cause poverty, corruption, and conflict – the so called "resource curse". The EITI aims to defeat this "curse" by improving transparency and accountability.' www.eitransparency.org

17 Benchmarking corporate reputation: an incentive for good anti-corruption practice

Transparencia Mexicana

The reputation of private companies is highly sensitive to news or suspicion of corrupt behaviour. The financial collapses of powerful corporations such as Enron and Parmalat are examples of the dire consequences companies face when their reputation is damaged by actions that are corrupt or that unfairly damage the interests of competitors or shareholders. Conversely, corporations that demonstrate positive good business practices and values in their relationships with their community and stakeholders can boast of a commitment to a less corrupt society. With this in mind, Transparencia Mexicana, the Mexican chapter of Transparency International, in collaboration with market research company Consulta-Mitofsky, developed a tool, the Mexican Corporate Reputation Index (MECRI), to highlight companies' good practices. The aim is to provide corporations with a positive incentive to enhance their reputation as well as information about which areas to improve, at the same time as generating public awareness about the reputations of major corporations operating in the country.

The MECRI is based on the opinions of a total of 32 managers and executives from the following professions: stockbrokers, publicists, economics analysts, financial risk analysts, external auditors, certifiers, civil servants, corporate lawyers and entrepreneurs.[1] Participants were required to be very well acquainted with the sectors and corporations under investigation, but were precluded from assessing corporations they had any kind of relationship with.

Respondents were asked which factors determine whether a company has a good or a bad reputation. Eight factors were selected on the basis of these responses: concern for the shareholders, investors, and partners; compliance with current laws and standards; service to customers and suppliers; environmental responsibility; respect for workers' rights; involvement with the community; nature and quality of relationships with competitors; and commitment to the development of Mexico. A closed question was asked about each of the areas of concern. For example: 'How well do you think the following companies treat their clients and providers? Very well (1)/ Well (2)/ Average (3)/ Badly (4)/ Very badly (5)'. The MECRI has a scale of values between one and zero: the higher the value, the better the standing of a firm's reputation.

The MECRI evaluated 108 corporations, which were selected on the basis of total revenues declared by the corporation. The companies are amongst the 500 largest Mexican corporations, as listed in *Expansión* magazine, and operate in one of the following 12 industries: food and non-alcoholic beverages; higher education; automotive; pharmaceutical; alcohol and tobacco; self-service and department stores; public works and construction; financial services; information technology and telecommunications; mass media; tourism and transportation; and energy resources. (See Table 17.1.)

Table 17.1: Best-standing corporations according to the MECRI 2004

Ranking	Corporation	MECRI 2004
1	Grupo Industrial Bimbo	0.90
2	Instituto Tecnológico y de Estudios Superiores de Monterrey	0.88
3	PEMEX	0.86
4	Nestlé	0.85
5	Universidad Iberoamericana	0.84
6	Grupo Modelo	0.83
6	Instituto Tecnológico Autónomo de México	0.83
6	Universidad de las Américas, Puebla	0.83
9	Vitro	0.81
9	Coca-Cola FEMSA	0.81
9	Cervecería Cuauhtémoc Moctezuma	0.81

Transparencia Mexicana decided to provide a positive incentive to corporations to improve by publicly acknowledging the good standing of the 10 firms with the strongest reputation, rather than publishing the names of the worst performers or measuring perceived corruption levels. Companies with the best reputation in each of the 12 sectors under examination and those with the highest index for each of the eight variables measured were also publicly acknowledged. Information about all of the 108 corporations is open to the governing bodies and high-level executives of each corporation concerned in order to help them identify areas for improvement. The information is not available to the general public, since the idea behind the exercise is to provide positive incentives for companies to improve by striving to be included on the list of top-performing companies.

For more information see: www.transparenciamexicana.org.mx

Note

1. The MECRI 2004 survey interviews were conducted between 15 November and 7 December 2003.

18 Officials' asset declaration laws: do they prevent corruption?

Ranjana Mukherjee and Omer Gokcekus[1]

Requiring public officials to declare their wealth and assets is widely considered an effective measure to prevent corruption. It has been included as an article of agreement in the United Nations, the African Union, and the Inter-American conventions against corruption. But how effectively can officials' asset declaration laws reduce corruption? Are there any features in the laws' design and implementation that act as stronger antidotes to corruption than others?

To address these questions, we examined various countries' asset declaration laws to find common aspects within such laws. Using a method similar to that of Transparency International's National Integrity Systems Survey, we then constructed a list of seven different aspects of such laws: (1) the date of implementation and whether there is a constitutional mandate; (2) the coverage, or who must file a declaration (for example, only the highest level officials, or both high- and low-level officials); (3) the filing frequency; (4) the specificity of the declaration's content (for example, must the declaration include the value of the assets, assets held outside the country?); (5) the details of the declaration's processing (for example, is there a separate body which receives and verifies the declaration's contents; does the law describe the verification process?); (6) the punishment for breach; and (7) whether or not there is public access to declarations. Next, we collected the laws from 16 different countries and systematically analysed the laws according to the seven common aspects listed above.

This project was initiated both to evaluate current laws designed to reduce corruption, and as a tool for governments designing or improving their own laws. In order to facilitate this process, the World Bank has created a website which contains a database of the laws used in this study and tools for comparing the different aspects of these countries' laws.[2] To highlight the most significant aspects of these laws and their effectiveness in reducing corruption, we performed a series of statistical tests to measure the association between the possession of these countries' laws and their perceived level of corruption. These results are presented below. In all cases, Transparency International's 2004 Corruption Perceptions Index (CPI) was used as the measure of corruption inside each country. To perform the statistical tests, we divided the countries into quartiles based on their CPI scores. Accordingly, countries with the highest scores are in the *least corrupt* quartile and countries with the lowest scores are in the *most corrupt* quartile.

Findings

1. *Is there an association between the inclusion of asset declaration laws within the constitution and reduced corruption?* No. In six of the examined countries, officials' asset declarations followed from constitutional directives. But these countries had lower average CPI scores, implying higher perceived corruption, than countries that did not have asset declaration within their constitutions (2.69 versus 3.39). Additionally, four of those six countries' laws did not require full transparency concerning officials' wealth, as they did not include directions on how the public could access officials' asset statements. Thus, although a constitutional provision is intended to signal the high value placed by a nation on its officials' integrity, our analysis finds that this intention does not necessarily translate into reduced corruption.

2. *Is there an association between the level of corruption and the amount of time that the law has been in effect?* Yes. Countries with a longer tradition of officials' asset declaration laws had significantly lower corruption than countries with newer laws. Among the countries examined, the quartile with the oldest laws (where the average age of the law was 17 years) had average CPI scores of 5.2, which was nearly three times higher than the average CPI (1.8) of the quartile of countries with newest laws (where the age was 1.7 years). (See Figure 18.1.)

3. *Is there an association between the level of corruption and which level of officials must declare their assets?* No. In 7 of the 16 countries examined, asset disclosure was required of all public officials. The average CPI scores for this group of countries was not significantly

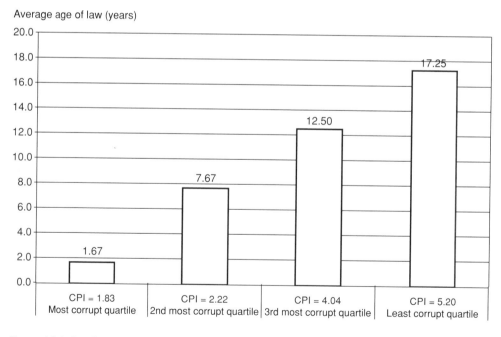

Figure 18.1: It takes time for officials' wealth declaration law to demonstrate results

lower than countries that had adopted a more top-down approach. In the latter group of countries, the list of officials that are required to submit asset statements started at the very top of the executive pyramid, and extended downwards to the senior or middle level. This could imply that corruption reduction at top executive levels has a powerful demonstrative effect on other officials and that transparent behaviour at the top can deter administrative corruption. Additionally or alternatively, it could imply that petty administrative corruption affects CPI ratings less than grand corruption. Thus our findings suggest that instead of simply requiring all officials to submit declarations, a pragmatic recognition of internal enforcement capacity and the selection of who should declare wealth could be more useful.

4. *Is there an association between the level of corruption and the threat of prosecution for those who do not follow the laws?* Yes. Perceived corruption was lower in countries whose declaration laws also permitted the government or anti-corruption body to prosecute the offending official. In the least corrupt quartile, all countries' asset declaration laws also provided for prosecution for offenders. In the second lowest quartile, three-quarters of the countries' laws had prosecution provisions. Only half the countries in the bottom two quartiles had prosecution provisions in their asset declaration laws.

5. *Is there an association between lower corruption levels and verification mechanisms within the various laws?* Yes. In this respect, two practices were observed. In some countries, every official's submission was verified by the recipient body; in others, the declaration was stored untouched, to be retrieved only if corruption allegations were received against the official. Countries that verified officials' statements have significantly lower corruption than countries that do not verify declaration content. The average CPI of the verifiers (3.72) was higher than that of the do-nothings (2.48).

6. *Is there an association between lower corruption and public access to asset disclosure laws?* Yes. Some countries' laws required that asset disclosures be placed in the public domain, either through website posting, or by informing where and when these documents were available for public inspection. In others, only a designated organisation of government could view the officials' declarations. Countries that gave public access to officials' asset declaration had significantly lower corruption (average CPI = 3.61) than the other group that restricted public access (average CPI = 2.46).

Our analysis further demonstrated that the combination of content verification and public access to the declarations demonstrated an even greater association of reduced corruption. Where full verification and public access to declarations is allowed, the average CPI score (4.13) is double that of countries that neither verify statements' contents nor allow public access to them (2.07). Countries that either verify or allow public access have perceived corruption levels in between these two extremes (with average CPI scores of 3.4 and 2.5 respectively). (See Figure 18.2.)

Conclusion

These preliminary results were supported by regression analyses with the variables described above, along with other country characteristics. Since the conclusion of these preliminary analyses, we have expanded our dataset to include 42 countries. Our

Average CPI in this group

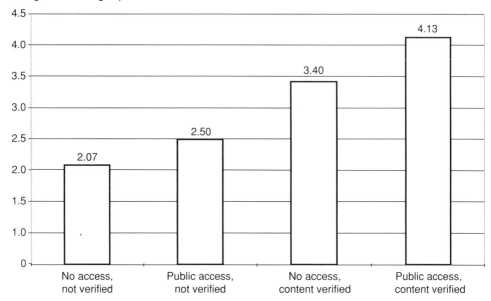

Figure 18.2: Effectiveness of content verification and public access in officials' asset declaration laws

initial analysis of this expanded dataset corroborates our findings from the original dataset. In addition, we are currently examining the different aspects of conflict of interest laws and their ability to reduce corruption. The expanded database for asset declaration laws and a new database for conflict of interest laws will be available at the above-mentioned World Bank website.

Notes

1. Ranjana Mukherjee is senior public sector specialist in the South Asia Region of Poverty Reduction and Economic Management Network at the World Bank (contact: rmukherjee@ worldbank.org). Omer Gokcekus is an associate professor at the John C. Whitehead School of Diplomacy and International Relations, Seton Hall University, United States (contact: gokcekom@shu.edu).
2. See http://www1.worldbank.org/publicsector/civilservice/assets.htm

19 Tax evasion, fines and corruption in Mozambique

Ralf Lanwehr[1]

A survey on the investment climate in the Mozambican province of Inhambane was conducted in March 2004.[2] Its aim was to describe and explain cooperation problems between the public and private sectors, and it unveiled a systemic network of major tax evasion, compensatory fining and fine-related bribery.

Although Inhambane has great economic potential, investors are currently hesitant regarding further investment and are dissatisfied with the status quo, because of serious disruptions in cooperation between the private and public sector. These disruptions hamper the climate for new investment and thereby threaten the province's economic development.

To describe, explain and quantify problem areas of investor–government relations, a survey on the provincial investment climate was conducted. In order to establish an initial understanding of the situation and to construct a survey, 25 key investors and their public counterparts were interviewed utilising the critical incident technique.[3] The sample of the main survey was drawn on the basis of a nationwide business census of the National Institute of Statistics Mozambique.[4] The sample size was set to 100 firms in the formal sector.[5]

Public officials suspect massive tax evasion

The preliminary interviews revealed that the primary source for disruptions in cooperation between the public and private sector are systemic. Public officials claim that the vast majority of provincial firms illegally evade tax payments by not declaring their full revenues. The applied government strategy to counter perceived tax evasion is heightened vigilance in the auditing of more easily identifiable and/or minor transgressions. When such transgressions are exposed, the maximum force of the law is imposed on the individual firm, with the aim of balancing out suspected tax evasion. The result is often disproportionately harsh fines for nearly all provincial firms.

The business community feels misjudged

What might be called 'heightened vigilance' from public officials is not well received by the provincial business community. The latter claims that many fines are exorbitant, arbitrary and counterproductive to economic development. Also, investors strongly defend themselves against being prejudged for tax fraud. They state that many provincial firms are not underreporting their gross revenues, but that they are nonetheless heavily targeted by government.

Many business operators strongly emphasise that they are willing to contribute their tax share in accordance with Mozambican law, but feel that the current practice of exaggerated, non-selective fining actually rewards 'cheaters' among the business community. From a rational point of view, they argue, it would be wiser to underreport gross revenues because, regardless of the correctness and honesty of their accounting, their firm will be heavily fined in any case.

It is interesting to note that the preliminary interviews showed surprising accuracy and unanimity in the perception of the situation between the public and the private sector. The decisive difference is quantitative rather than qualitative, with respect to the proportion of the overall value of fines issued in relation to the amount of tax debts evaded.

Sixty-four per cent of taxes evaded on average in the tourism sector

One of the main 'disruptions' in Inhambane, as seen by both business and government, is in the area of taxation. Unfortunately, it is quite difficult to confirm, let alone quantify, the amount of tax evasion by firms there. In the tourism sector, though, reliable figures on the maximum capacity of accommodation do exist from the provincial delegation of the National Institute of Statistics. At the same time, it is well known that the occupation rate during the last two weeks of December is nearly 100 per cent. Based on this information, estimation of the amount of tax evasion can be attempted by comparing the 'reported reality' of room nights spent with the 'real reality' of available hotel beds during the last two weeks of December.

The 'reported reality' was an occupation rate of 18 per cent for December.[6] If we assume that the low number of tourists in the first half of December is made up for by almost full occupancy in the second half of the month, and if we factor in the suboptimal use of space, we might expect an occupation rate of approximately 50 per cent for December. The difference between the reported and the probable reality is therefore 32 per cent unreported occupation.

Only figures for room nights have been included in this calculation. Additional potential income from restaurants or diving schools, as well as systematic underreporting of accommodation costs is not addressed. Thus the estimate for tax evasion based on underreporting of occupation should be considered to be at the lower boundary of real tax evasion. In summary, the overall amount of underreported gross revenue of the province's firms is 64 per cent,[7] thereby lending credence to the claim by public officials of massive tax evasion.

Besides negatively influencing the quality of interprovincial cooperation and seriously hampering provincial tax income, the current practice of fining to balance out tax evasion facilitates corruption on a massive scale. This is demonstrated by the fact that a public official encouraged to issue heavy fines might be tempted to cancel these fines, or turn a blind eye to exposed transgressions, in exchange for a bribe.

Corruption is the biggest obstacle to business development

The results of the survey show that firms spend a total of about 10 per cent of their gross revenue on corruption, and 64 per cent reported being subjected to corrupt actions by public officials (82 per cent in the tourism centre of Vilanculo). Corruption is perceived as the biggest obstacle for business development, followed by government bureaucracy and insufficient infrastructure.

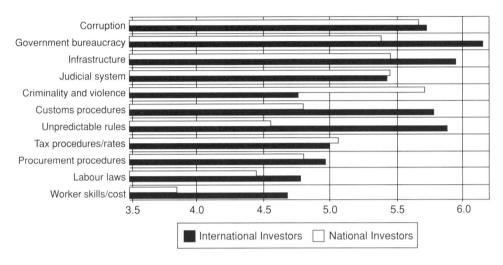

Figure 19.1: Perceived obstacles to business development for national and international investors on a scale ranging from 1 ('No obstacle') to 7 ('Extreme obstacle')

Differences between national and international investors

On a closer look, a principal component analysis[8] revealed a latent pattern in the data. Four factors underlying obstacles to business development were identified as:

1. corruption, bureaucracy and an unreliable judicial system
2. business environment (containing worker skills, labour laws, unpredictable rules and inadequate infrastructure)
3. government procedures (procurement procedures, tax collection procedures and customs procedures)
4. criminality and violence.

There are remarkable differences between national and international investors. 'Business environment' is a far greater obstacle for international than for national investors.[9] One interpretation of this finding might be that foreign investors often originate from developed countries and thus have more difficulty adapting to developing country conditions. Criminality and violence, however, are greater obstacles for national investors.[10]

Outlook

It is difficult to assess and quantify the origins and causal relationships in the vicious circle of tax evasion, fining and bribery in Inhambane. The system is, however, clearly self-supporting. As long as firms keep underreporting their revenues and the government continues its harsh fining strategy, no changes in current practice can be expected, resulting in a loss of the majority of the province's tax income and severely reduced future investments.

Notes

1. Ralf Lanwehr is a research associate at the Berlin University of Technology (contact: lanwehr@epix.de). He would like to thank Mike MacDonald and Ulrike Beuing for their advice and support in the course of the project as well as Marie Wolkers and Robin Hodess from TI for their valuable suggestions.
2. The survey was financed by the German Technical Cooperation Agency (GTZ).
3. J. C. Flanagan, 'The Critical Incident Technique', *Psychological Bulletin* 51(28), 1954.
4. Instituto Nacional de Estatística, *Censo de Empresas* (Survey of Businesses) (Maputo, 2003).
5. To analyse the fact that future business development in the province will depend heavily on investment in the tourism sector, 50 firms from that area were randomly drawn, alongside 50 firms from the commercial and industrial sectors. Two versions of the questionnaire were used, with the order of the questions altered.
6. The 15 tourism companies offer a combined total of 1,252 beds.
7. 100 per cent – reported reality of 18 per cent/expected reality of 50 per cent = 64 per cent underreported gross revenue.
8. Principal component analysis (PCA) is a standard procedure of data reduction. Its aim is to reduce the dimensionality of a given set of data and to clarify the correct classification of the items to their underlying factors.
9. $F = 11.1$; $df = 1/48$; $p = 0.002$.
10. $F = 7.7$; $df = 1/49$; $p = 0.008$.

20   The V4 index: corruption propensity in four Visegrád capitals

Michal Štička[1]

The V4 Index is a Transparency International Czech Republic research project that was completed in the first half of 2004. The goals of the project were to design a survey methodology that would establish the existence and evaluate the functionality of anti-corruption institutions ('corruption propensity') in the public administration at local/regional levels. That is, in the public administrations of the four Visegrád (V4) capitals: Bratislava, Budapest, Prague and Warsaw. A major outcome of the project was to rank the capitals' administrations according to the quality of their anti-corruption institutions. By doing this, the index raised public awareness with respect to the problem of corruption in the public administrations of V4 capitals.

The research project focused on anti-corruption tools and mechanisms in five areas: public procurement tenders, internal audit and control mechanisms, codes of ethical behaviour, conflicts of interest, and public administration information policies/public accessibility of information.

The survey was conducted in two stages. The first stage involved gathering objective, hard data on the existing anti-corruption tools and mechanisms in the public administration of each of the V4 capitals. The data were gathered through interviews with the representatives of the municipal councils of each capital and through content analysis of relevant documents. For the interviews, the head of the office and head of the legal department (or head of the internal audit department) were asked yes/no questions concerning the existence of anti-corruption mechanisms. For the content analysis, the relevant laws, ordinances and instructions (internal norms effective in the offices) were examined, if interviewees were unable to provide the requested data. The objective data were aggregated to form the V4 Objective Index.

In the second, subjective stage of the survey, perceptions of the efficiency of anti-corruption tools and mechanisms in each of the five above-mentioned areas of the public administration were studied, from the perspective of selected and well informed members of the public. Interviews were conducted among employees and elected members of the municipal councils of the V4 capitals, journalists, businessmen and NGO representatives. In each of the cities, a minimum of 100 respondents were interviewed. The subjective data were aggregated to form the V4 Subjective Index.

The scale of the Objective V4 Index ranges from 0 to 1, where '0' indicates the absence of anti-corruption tools and measures in the public administration and '1' indicates that all the elements measured exist. The results of the objective part of the V4 Index show that most anti-corruption tools in the examined fields are present in Budapest, with a score of 0.87. (See Table 20.1.)

Table 20.1: Objective V4 Index

	Bratislava	Prague	Warsaw	Budapest
Overall index	**0.55**	**0.60**	**0.64**	**0.87**
Public procurement tenders	0.36	0.61	0.90	0.96
Internal audit and control mechanisms	0.93	0.73	0.62	0.76
Codes of ethical conduct	0.22	0.80	0.00	0.93
Conflicts of interest	0.64	0.37	0.86	0.79
Open information policies	0.61	0.50	0.83	0.90

(Range from 0 to 1)

Note: Zero in the intersection of 'Warsaw' and 'Codes of ethical conduct' is due to the fact that none of the examined anti-corruption tools in the field of codes of conduct were in place in Warsaw.

The results of the second stage of the research project, based on the subjective perceptions of the respondents, showed that the operation and functionality of anti-corruption tools used in the public administration of individual capitals were less positive than in the objective part of the survey. This difference, however, met expectations: similar research results comparing reality with perception have shown that public opinion is more critical than the objective situation.

On a scale of 0 to 1 (where 0 indicates 'very bad'; 0.33 indicates 'somewhat bad'; 0.66 indicates 'somewhat good'; and 1 indicates 'very good'), Budapest retained its position from the objective part of the survey, and finished in first position, with a score of 0.49 (See Table 20.2). In Budapest, respondents rated public procurement tenders and information accessibility, such as the open information policies of municipal authorities, highest. These results correlated fully with the data generated by the objective part of the survey, which indicated that Budapest had most anti-corruption tools in these areas.

Table 20.2: Subjective V4 Index

	Prague	Bratislava	Warsaw	Budapest
Overall index	**0.40**	**0.44**	**0.44**	**0.49**
Public procurement tenders	0.40	0.46	0.47	0.55
Internal audit and control mechanisms	0.38	0.40	0.39	0.46
Codes of ethical conduct	0.47	0.51	0.51	0.50
Conflicts of interest	0.29	0.32	0.40	0.42
Open information policies	0.46	0.51	0.43	0.52

(Range from 0 to 1)

Despite scoring lowest in terms of objective anti-corruption tools and mechanisms, Bratislava came second according to respondents' opinions, with a score of 0.44. It is striking that Bratislava achieved above average results in terms of its codes of ethical conduct. In fact, most of the individuals interviewed consider the environment in Bratislava's public administration to be ethical, despite the fact that the city's executive authority had not implemented any code of ethical conduct. The greatest need for improvement in Bratislava, in the view of respondents, was in the area of preventing conflicts of interest.

In Warsaw, which came third of the V4 capitals (also at 0.44, but just behind Bratislava), respondents rated the area of codes of ethical conduct highest, although, in objective terms, there are no such codes in the Warsaw public administration. Compared to the other cities, Warsaw respondents perceived public procurement tenders quite positively. Internal audits and the operation of control mechanisms, however, were considered to be rather dysfunctional.

Prague was placed fourth out of the cities studied, with a score of 0.40. If the partial indices between the different capitals were compared, Prague did not exceed the average in any of the areas under consideration. The respondents who had dealings with the public administration did not believe that anti-corruption tools were implemented with much efficiency. The best results in Prague were achieved in the area of codes of ethical conduct, where more than half of the respondents considered the environment in the Czech capital's public administration to be ethical. As in the case of Bratislava, Prague residents were most critical of the way in which conflict of interest provisions were implemented.

Note

1. Michal Štička is project manager, Transparency International Czech Republic.

21 Efficiency of federal transfers to municipalities in Brazil

Marcos Jose Mendes[1]

This study aims to analyse irregularities uncovered by the Office of the Inspector General (Controladoria Geral da União, CGU) in the administration of the Fund for Development and Maintenance of Elementary Teaching and for Professional Improvement of Teachers (FUNDEF). In order to inspect FUNDEF and other federal transfers, the CGU has maintained, since 2003, a systematic programme for conducting random audits in municipalities across the country. For the purposes of this work, only federal transfers are analysed, since CGU does not audit the use of state and municipal funds.

Federal funds are an important part of municipal budgets representing 62 per cent of municipal revenue. Municipal accounts are regularly audited by state audit courts, but these are reputed to provide only weak supervision – by municipal citizen councils, which also have a poor reputation since they are often controlled by the local authorities they are supposed to audit; and by federal agencies that supervise the use of federal funds transferred to municipalities, which tend to conduct more efficient audits. One of those federal agencies is the CGU, which randomly chooses municipalities to audit. These audits cover all of the federal programmes financed by the federal government in the chosen municipality.

By looking in depth at one instrument of public education funding, the FUNDEF, we aim to identify weaknesses in the management of municipal funds. The analysis covers 67 municipalities of the states of Bahia (22), Maranhão (14), Pará (15) and Piauí (16) that received federal subsidies to finance their local educational system. These municipalities are among the poorest in the country and were randomly chosen by CGU, the agency which sent the auditors to the cities. The auditors analysed financial records, but also visited schools, interviewing teachers, public workers and students, and compared prices paid by the government for goods and services with those in effect in local markets. The auditors' reports were used to classify the most common irregularities found in the municipalities. Table 21.1 shows the most common irregularities and the percentage of municipalities in which those irregularities were observed.

The many irregularities identified appear to seriously harm the quality and efficiency of the programme. Furthermore, irregularities are spread across almost all of the municipalities in the sample. Only 1 per cent of this sample does not present any irregularity. This diagnosis is confirmed when we analyse the amount of money involved in the irregularities, as shown in Table 21.2. The total amount of FUNDEF allocations audited was 161.4 million reais (US $54 million). The various irregularities listed in the table were responsible for total losses equivalent to 13 per cent of the budget. Fraud in public procurement was the most costly type of irregularity.

Table 21.1: Main irregularities in terms of the number of municipalities where they were observed

Irregularities	Municipalities (%) where irregularity observed
The community council created to supervise funds does not work properly or is in practice controlled by the mayor (the authority that should be inspected by the council)	73
Embezzlement (or evidence of embezzlement) of resources by means of fraud (false fiscal documents, goods bought but not received by schools, purchases at prices above the market, etc.)	63
Use of funds in expenditures not characterised as fundamental to education	60
Low quality and organisation of the financial resources management (poor accounting; emission of cheques with no funds; cash withdrawals from bank accounts, which makes it difficult for auditors to check how the money was used, etc.)	52
Evidence of fraud in public procurement (mainly through the creation of 'ghost' competitor companies to create the illusion of a competitive bidding process; or through the division of a single contract into a number of smaller contracts that are below the threshold to hold a competitive contracting process)	43

Table 21.2: Percentage of the total amount of funds received by the municipality from FUNDEF that was embezzled, according to type of irregularity

Irregularity	Mean %	Max. %
Evidence of fraud in procurement	13	55
Embezzlement (or evidence of embezzlement) of resources by means of fraud (false fiscal documents; goods bought but not received by schools; purchases at above-market prices, etc.)	12	45
Embezzlement of funds earmarked to pay teachers (money received by persons other than teachers; fraud and illegal practices in the hiring of teachers, etc.)	11	42
Illegal payment of teachers and other workers ('ghost teachers'; illegal bonuses, etc.)	3	6
Use of funds on expenditures not characterised as fundamental to education	3	12

The high level of irregularities in the management of FUNDEF funds indicates that community councils lack the power and resources necessary to ensure that local authorities manage FUNDEF funds honestly and effectively. It is necessary to create another body of supervision or to create sanctions for those members of community councils who fail to carry out their duty. In order to remedy the lack of staff capable of managing procurement, distribution and bookkeeping tasks in poorer municipalities, state governments should be required to provide municipal governments with an electronic procurement system for services and goods.

Note

1. Marcos Jose Mendes is a consultant at the Brazilian senate.

22   Integrity Index for Public Institutions: evaluating Colombia's health sector

Transparencia por Colombia[1]

Since 2002, Transparencia por Colombia, the Colombian chapter of Transparency International, has produced an annual Integrity Index for Public Institutions, comparing levels of corruption risks in the country's public institutions. The aim of the index is to provide a tool for civil society to monitor transparency, integrity and efficiency of public institutions. Since institutions are individually evaluated, it is possible to use the index to assess vulnerabilities to corruption of a particular sector. Here we provide an overview of the index and examples of how it can be used to assess corruption risks in the health sector.

The index ranks public institutions according to 20 indicators, all of which are objective measures.[2] The indicators fall into three groups:

- *Transparency*. This measures visibility of the organisation to the general public, assessed using the following indicators: information found on the institution's web page; mechanisms for filing complaints; transparency of contracting processes; compliance with the national contracting information system (SICE); accountability mechanisms; transparency, accessibility and clarity of bureaucratic processes; anti-corruption efforts and access to information.
- *Control and punishment*. This measures the level of sanctions or decisions taken by control bodies against officials of public bodies by looking at sanctions for fiscal irregularities; disciplinary sanctions; and value of decisions signalling fiscal irregularities as a proportion of the organisation's budget. The underlying premise is that a higher number of dishonest practices is associated with institutional scenarios where preventative mechanisms are deficient or non-existent.
- *Efficiency and institutionality*. This measures efficient compliance with the objectives and missions of the body. The indicators look closely at simplicity of organisational processes, and clarity and knowledge of rules and controls, as these factors limit the margin for discretion by personnel and therefore risk of corruption. The indicators include: number of complaints presented and investigations opened by public auditor and public prosecutor as a proportion of the number of officials employed; procedures for hiring staff; incentives for employees; performance of the internal control function; and evaluation of management.

Each of the three components is made up of a simple average of the indicators in the category, and the index is an average of the three, weighted against the number of indicators that make up each component.

The 2004 index evaluates 80 per cent of public entities at central government level (182 central government bodies are assessed). For the first time state government bodies are also evaluated.[3]

Risks of corruption in the health sector

Some 12 per cent of the public institutions assessed in the National Index correspond to the health sector. The risk of corruption is considered high in 59 per cent of these. Of particular concern are the results of health delivery bodies such as the Social State Enterprises (ESE), which were recently created in an attempt to overcome the inefficiencies and poor quality services offered by the centralised Social Security Institute (ISS). While the results for the health sector are slightly better than recorded by the 2003 index, they are poor in two of the three categories: transparency (45 on a scale of 1 to 100, where 100 indicates a low risk of corruption) and efficiency and institutionality (55 out of 100). (See Figure 22.1.)

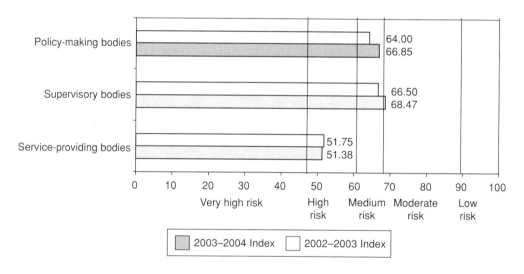

Figure 22.1: National public health institutions

At the state level a number of problems were also identified: the average score of health agencies responsible for directing, coordinating and monitoring the health and social security services in each jurisdiction is 49.2 out of 100, which is lower than the average score per sector. More than 35 per cent of these health agencies are considered to face a high or very high risk of corruption, while only 12.5 per cent show a moderate risk.

A comparison of data on risks of corruption in state health authorities and infant mortality rates[4] suggests a correlation between corruption and health outcomes,[5] as

Figure 22.2 suggests. The data is by no means conclusive: we cannot omit the possibility of reverse causality (that is, that poor health leads to higher levels of corruption), or that a third variable, such as low income per head, might be driving both infant mortality and corruption.

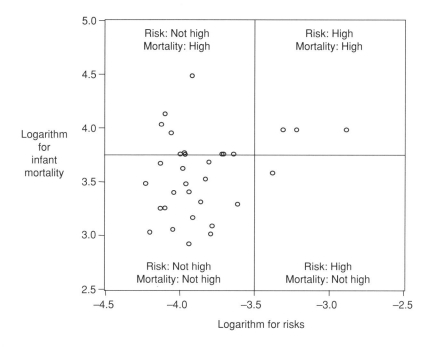

Figure 22.2: Comparison of data on corruption risks and infant mortality rates at state level

Conclusions

The simple exercise above shows how the index can be used to explore costs of corruption in specific sectors and to identify vulnerabilities to corruption that should be taken into account when formulating public policies. The results on health authorities alerted Transparencia por Colombia to the need to develop new indicators to measure the performance of the authorities responsible for coordinating, regulating and operating health systems.

After three editions of the index, it is possible to draw preliminary conclusions about its impact. The 2004 index reflects an improvement in the response by public officials to requests for information. Public institutions are interested in the index as a benchmarking tool that can help identify institutional weaknesses: more than 600 public employees representing more than 40 per cent of the national institutions evaluated have used the index to identify and rectify weaknesses. The demand for detailed and accurate information on corruption risks has grown at state level, too: half of the 32 states have organised forums to debate the results.

Notes

1. The principal researcher at Transparencia por Colombia is Martha Badel. Contact: indiceintegridad@transparenciacolombia.org.co
2. For details of the first edition, released in 2002, see *Global Corruption Report 2004*. The first index used 16 indicators, most of which were objective, with the others reflecting the opinions of a sample of public officials from each institution. The opinion survey data was published separately in 2004.
3. Colombia has three levels of government: central, state (known as 'departments' in Colombia) and municipal.
4. National Department of Statistics, 'Departmental Estimates of Infant Mortality 1985–1993: Mid-term Perspectives 1995–2005', in *Estudios Censales No. 5* (Bogota: DANE, 1998). The estimates are per 1,000 live births.
5. Infant mortality is one of the best measures of influence of social factors on health, according to Michael Grossman in 'The Human Capital Model of the Demand for Health', National Bureau of Economic Research Working Papers No. 7078, 1999.

23 Corruption in the public health service in Bangladesh

Iftekhar Zaman and Alim Abdul[1]

Health is a priority sector in the allocation of public funds in Bangladesh. In line with the 'Health for All' policy, first adopted in 2000, the government allocated 9 per cent of its development budget for the 2004–05 fiscal year to health, which was the fifth largest category of its public expenditure. The government formed a Health Watch Committee in 1998 under the ministry of health, which was aimed at making doctors and other health officials more accountable for public funds and to their patients. The new government disbanded the programme when it came to power in 2001, however. The Corruption Database created by Transparency International Bangladesh (TIB) on the basis of corruption reports in the print media, highlights a need for renewed anti-corruption efforts in the sector: the database has consistently identified health as the fourth most corrupt sector in Bangladesh since 2000.[2] TIB's 2002 and 2005 Household Corruption Surveys also found that health is considered to be the fourth most corrupt sector in the country.[3] Corruption in the health sector results in ordinary people, and especially the disadvantaged, being deprived of the benefits of basic health facilities and services.

According to the Household Corruption Survey of 2002,[4] which is based on interviews with 3,030 households, 61 per cent sought services from government hospitals, of which 47 per cent failed to gain admittance into hospitals through the prescribed procedure and instead were forced to seek 'alternative' ways of obtaining health services. In 56 per cent of these cases, a bribe was paid for health care, while in the remaining cases patients obtained the health service thanks to the assistance of influential relatives or of doctors involved in private practice. The 2005 Household Corruption Survey revealed that 60 per cent of households interviewed received services as out-patients of government hospitals, of which 29 per cent had to pay bribes to doctors worth 60 takas (US $1) on average. Some 21 per cent of households interviewed had a member who was admitted to hospital, of whom 20 per cent had paid a bribe to a public hospital doctor for medical advice. In these cases, the bribes were worth on average 478 takas (US $8). The survey also revealed that 94 per cent of patients had paid for medicines that should have been provided for free.[5]

The 2005 Household Corruption Survey also revealed that 3 per cent of households interviewed had a family member who had undergone surgery, of whom 37 per cent were asked for bribes worth on average 1,420 takas (US $24). Of the 4.5 per cent of households interviewed with a family member who needed an X-ray, 56 per cent had to pay 516 takas (US $9) on average as a bribe. Furthermore, of the 9 per cent of interviewed households that had required pathology tests, 60 per cent had paid a bribe worth on average 410 takas (US $7). In an earlier study, the bribe amount paid for delivery of newborn babies was generally reported to be between 1,000 and 5,000 takas (US $15–76).[6] (See Figures 23.1 and 23.2.)

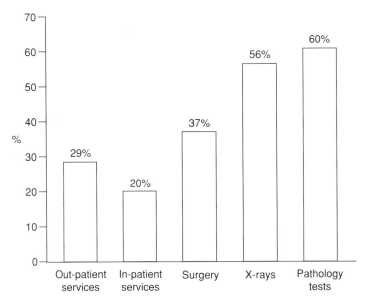

Figure 23.1: Percentage of patients forced to pay a bribe to obtain selected health services

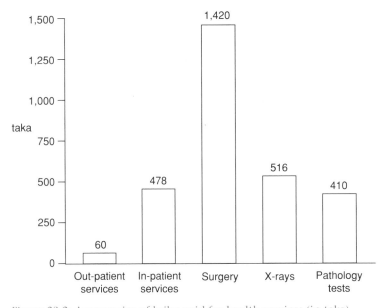

Figure 23.2: Average size of bribe paid for health services (in taka)

The 2002 TIB Report Card Survey revealed that half of the patients polled felt that doctors did not pay due attention to patients, while only 34 per cent of patients were satisfied with the service they received from doctors. Only 1 per cent of patients were satisfied with the degree of cleanliness of government hospitals.[7]

Among respondents who had paid bribes in hospitals or experienced poor service due to mismanagement, unavailability of staff, negligence or an unhelpful attitude towards patients, 56 per cent blamed doctors, 36 per cent blamed hospital staff and 5 per cent blamed nurses. Some 61 per cent of respondents who received hospital services complained that corruption in hospitals was carried out directly by service providers, while 17 per cent said corruption was practised indirectly through a third party. Some 3 per cent of respondents had offered money directly to service providers.[8]

All patients complained that they had to wait for long periods in hospitals. One reason for this was that doctors failed to arrive on time. According to a study by TIB of health services in the Nalitabari Upazilla Health Complex, the main reason for irregular attendance by hospital doctors is that they are busy with their private sector work.[9]

In TIB's 2002 survey, 67 per cent of respondents cited a lack of accountability as the major cause of corruption in hospitals that are fully or partially government owned. Discretionary power without accountability was identified as the second major cause (50 per cent), followed by lack of transparency (45 per cent), prevalence of monopoly power (28 per cent), influence of powerful people (13 per cent), and red tape (7 per cent). Corruption was considered to have the worst effects for the poor.[10]

The 2002 survey also revealed that households with members who received a service in a government hospital and became victims of corruption spent about 1,847 takas (US $28) annually on corruption. The sum was greater in urban areas (an average of 2,256 takas, over US $36) than in rural areas (an average of 1,711 takas, US $26). Extrapolating from the survey data, the amount of bribes annually paid by patients for services in public hospitals is estimated at 12,500 million takas a year (US $190 million).

Notes

1. Iftekhar Zaman is the executive director and Alim Abdul is a researcher at Transparency International Bangladesh.
2. Corruption Database, (Transparency International Bangladesh (TIB), 2000, 2001, 2002, 2003), see: www.ti-bangladesh.org
3. *Corruption in Bangladesh: A Household Survey* (TIB, 2002), *Corruption in Bangladesh: A Household Survey* (TIB, 2005).
4. In 2004, the sectors covered in the survey were: education, health, land administration, power, taxation, police, judiciary, local government, banking and pensions. The respondents were selected randomly from across Bangladesh. Additional conclusions about this data are drawn from TIB's Corruption Database; a household survey conducted in 2002, a Report Card Survey on Health conducted in 2002 by TIB's Committees of Concerned Citizens; and focus group discussions with patients who sought or received services in Nalitabari Health Complex.
5. *Corruption in Bangladesh: A Household Survey*, 2005.
6. *The Quality of Health Services in Nalitabari Upazilla Health Complex* (TIB, 2003).
7. *Report Card Survey on Health* (TIB, 2002).
8. *Corruption in Bangladesh: A Household Survey*, 2002.
9. *The Quality of Health Services in Nalitabari Upazilla Health Complex*, 2003.
10. Ibid.

24   Governance in Bulgaria's pharmaceutical selection and procurement systems

Patrick Meagher[1]

The selection and procurement of pharmaceuticals in health care systems presents a host of governance challenges. Technically sound decisions about the cost-effectiveness of drugs, and objective evaluations of bids, must be made in a political environment fraught with contending pressures from domestic and foreign companies, patients' and physicians' lobbies, and policy-makers with strong views. In this field, both politics and profits create strong pressures towards rent-seeking and corrupt behaviour.

This research has two components, the first concerning the central processes of drug selection for the health system, and the second focusing on procurement of pharmaceuticals by hospitals throughout Bulgaria. The *drug selection* component focuses primarily on the two major selection processes: the Positive Drug List (PDL) and the National Health Insurance Fund (NHIF) Reimbursement List. The *procurement* component deals with medicines that are chosen from the PDL for hospital formularies and purchased from suppliers.

Findings

The government pays for the bulk of health care through direct Ministry of Health spending and, increasingly, the National Health Insurance Fund (NHIF). The government was estimated to have covered about three-quarters of (formal) medicinal drug expenditures in 2002, about US $375 million. Gaining access to this market for their products requires drug producers to pass through a series of regulatory hurdles – from market authorisation to price regulation and selection for the central drug lists – before they can bid for sales to government, hospitals or pharmacies. The system of drug selection, reimbursement and procurement has undergone major change since 2000, with a raft of reforms implemented for the first time in 2004.

Our research indicates a struggle by international and local drug producers to exert influence at several levels of the system, from policy-makers at the Ministry of Health and NHIF to parliamentarians, associations and parties, hospitals and physicians.

Regarding the selection processes, we found ample – if indirect – evidence of procedural irregularity, including corruption. This evidence comes from interviews, official filings and hearings, and a comprehensive review of media reports (some 5,000 items) for the period from mid-2003 to the end of 2004. Several scandals involving shell companies and conflicts of interest were reported, in addition to more mundane allegations of bribery.

Furthermore, we asked pharmacy experts to evaluate the Positive List and NHIF Reimbursement List against international benchmarks. A comparison of drug choices against World Health Organization Essential Drugs criteria showed a number of cases of under-inclusion, where older drugs with proven benefits were excluded in favour of newer, more expensive ones. Several cases were also found of over-inclusion, where a high number of alternative name brands were selected, some of them redundant, others of questionable efficacy. Price comparisons with neighbouring countries also suggest that Bulgaria may not be getting the best value for its drug expenditure. These outcomes show weak implementation of essential drugs policy, consistent with (but not proof of) perceptions that corruption plays a role.

Regarding drug procurements by hospitals, we carried out a survey of supplier firms and persons knowledgeable about drug tenders in 148 hospitals, and looked at hospital records. Some evidence was found of incorrect procedure in such areas as bid-ranking, discretionary exemptions of bidders from documentation requirements (which were in any case excessive), and the frequent granting of price adjustments in post-procurement contract amendments. Ethical lapses were also reported, including the use of drug donations by supplier firms to influence subsequent procurements (see Table 24.1, showing perceptions of knowledgeable hospital personnel).

Table 24.1: Influence of drug donations on procurement

Amount of influence (%)	None	A little	Some	A lot	Enormous
Doctors	21.2	36.8	29.2	9.5	3.3
Nurses	26.8	30.3	28.9	10.7	3.3
Pharmacists	59.4	26.1	11.6	0.0	2.9

Institutional integrity

Here, we investigated the following attributes: transparency, accountability, prevention, enforcement and education (that is, on ethics and integrity standards). In the research on selection processes, we gave rankings to these processes with respect to each factor. The information came from responses given in structured interviews, our examination of official documents and records, and direct testing by means of some 15 information requests that our researchers filed under the Bulgarian Access to Public Information Act (APIA). Using international (not regional) best practice benchmarks, we assessed each factor and gave a ranking – most of these rankings for Bulgaria were poor.

The integrity findings broadly matched up with our information on corruption and procedural regularity in the different selection processes. In particular, selection criteria were found to be broad and sometimes quite vague, and there were needless constraints on the openness of selection processes and information access. There appeared to be little rigour or accountability in selection, since multiple name-brands could be listed and it was acknowledged that independent clinical trials and pharmaco-economic studies were rarely done in Bulgaria. Also, there was little effective oversight of selection and very limited public input. Rules and implementation mechanisms concerning appointments, ethics standards and conflicts of interest appear insufficiently robust to constrain abuses. The extent of integrity (and conversely, vulnerability) varied across selection processes. Bulgaria has taken several important steps to strengthen selection processes, such as defining the Positive List procedure and imposing some level of transparency. Unfortunately, the pressures on the selection system as a whole are considerable, and reforms in particular areas cannot constrain potential abuses in others.

In the procurement component, we found significant variation across hospitals on most factors – but there were no detectable patterns of co-variance (for example, high transparency correlating with high accountability). While respondents tended to give the 'correct' (high integrity) response, we did find patterns such as a paucity of ethics training, along with generally low expectations about whistleblowing or punishment in cases of corruption (see Table 24.2, showing what respondents expected that actual sanctions would be for taking an informal payment).

Table 24.2: Likely punishment for taking an informal payment (% of respondents)

Possible punishments in decreasing order of punishment	Evaluation committee	Pharmacist	Hospital director
Arrest	2.8	0.0	2.4
Dismissal	24.8	27.3	40.0
Suspension	4.3	9.1	7.1
Demotion	2.8	3.6	7.1
Fined	7.5	7.3	5.9
Warning	18.5	32.7	7.1
Dropped from next year's committee	23.2	9.1	24.7
No punishment	5.1	5.5	1.2

Conclusion

This study, using combined methods to examine governance at two levels in Bulgaria's pharmaceutical system, offers a potential model for corruption assessment. In particular, the study shows that a focus on institutional integrity is helpful but requires complementary analysis of social and political-economic factors. The recommendations that flow from these findings point to a range of needed steps in such areas as transparency and oversight, process streamlining, moving parts of the process to independent commissions (or outsourcing), making international standards mandatory in selection processes, and improving corporate governance of hospitals.

Note

1. Patrick Meagher is associate director of the IRIS Center, University of Maryland, United States. The research was sponsored by the US Agency for International Development. The author's views expressed in this publication do not necessarily reflect the views of USAID or

the US government. This summary draws on the author's collaboration with, and on analysis done by, Omar Azfar and Diana Rutherford of IRIS. This work also includes expert background analysis by Jillian Clare Cohen and Judith Fisher of the University of Toronto; and research and survey implementation by Denitsa Sacheva, Roza Evtimova and Mina Popova of the International Healthcare and Health Insurance Institute, Sofia, and its survey affiliate, FACT Marketing.

25 Survey research sheds light on Latin Americans' experience with corruption

Eric Kite and Margaret Sarles[1]

The United States Agency for International Development (USAID) is increasingly using citizen surveys to improve its democracy and governance programmes and measure their impact. In Latin America, USAID completed 11 surveys in 2004, comprising Bolivia, Colombia, Costa Rica, the Dominican Republic, Ecuador, El Salvador, Guatemala, Honduras, Mexico, Nicaragua and Panama.[2] The surveys probe perceptions of corruption behaviour, and corruption victimisation, all of which can be disaggregated by personal attributes (gender, region, age, ethnicity, income, and so on) and cross-tabulated with political behaviour.

The survey results enable analysis of the depth and effects of corruption, determining the corruption problems most important to particular kinds of citizens, identifying potential constituencies for reform, and suggesting promising approaches for anti-corruption reform. In some countries, these surveys have by now been conducted two or three times, allowing study of corruption and democracy trends. Comparison over time also provides a tool to assist in better matching USAID programmes to the evolving nature of the problem.

The surveys provide compelling quantitative evidence of the corroding effect of corruption on citizens' support for democracy and democratic institutions. Among all of the factors examined, *corruption, along with citizen security concerns, has the most detrimental impact on citizens' confidence in democracy and democratic institutions.* There is a strong negative correlation between the number of times one is victimised by corruption and one's level of support for democratic institutions (see Figure 25.1). Only crime has a similar impact.

In Nicaragua, for example, 'system support' for democracy falls almost by half for a citizen who has frequently (four times or more) been pressed to pay a bribe. In these cases, citizens are willing to consider abandoning democracy as a political system in favour of more authoritarian options. The implication of these findings for governments and those supporting democratic reform is that serious and carefully targeted anti-corruption reforms should play a critical role in the strategy for democratic consolidation.

A second general finding relates to the overall level of bribery in each country, here assessed by corruption 'victimisation'. In general, in Central America and Colombia the figure was around 15 per cent (see Figure 25.2). In contrast, the citizens of Bolivia, Mexico and Ecuador reported experiencing bribery far more frequently.

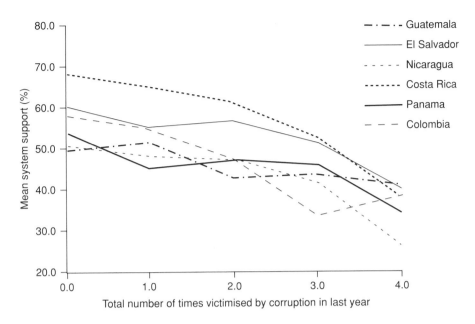

Figure 25.1: Impact of corruption victimisation on system support

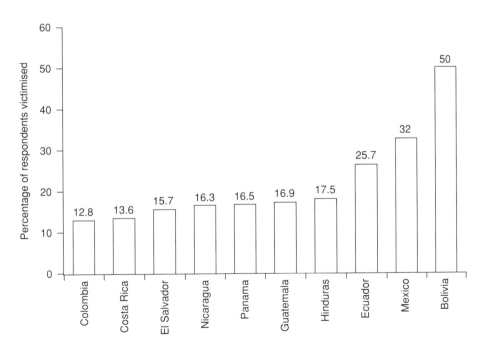

Figure 25.2: Total index of corruption victimisation

The surveys also asked citizens what specific governmental institutions demanded bribes from them. The results varied widely across countries and institutions, and provide rich data for anyone trying to target anti-corruption programmes effectively. Table 25.1 looks at nine countries, summarising citizen responses on whether they faced demands for bribes in different institutional settings: to avoid a false accusation by police; other demands by police, public employees, municipal employees, courts, health services, schools or employers.

Table 25.1: Percentage of respondents who were victimised by bribery, by source of request

	Accused by police	Police demanded bribe	Public employee bribe	Municipal bribe	Bribe at work	Courts	Health service bribe	School bribe
Mexico	9.4	18.0	12.9	20.7	10.3	13.5	9.5	12.7
Guatemala	4.2	6.9	3.3	8.2	6.5	5.0	6.7	8.7
El Salvador	4.7	5.5	4.3	5.3	5.4	4.0	6.6	7.3
Honduras	3.7	5.3	2.7	10.2	9.9	6.6	7.2	11.3
Nicaragua	3.5	3.7	3.4	12.9	12.6	15.5	10.7	9.5
Costa Rica	3.1	3.5	3.2	5.6	4.2	2.7	3.8	8.6
Panama	4.5	6.9	6.0	9.3	6.2	6.5	5.7	6.7
Colombia	4.8	3.8	2.7	5.3	5.6	5.1	7.7	5.5
Ecuador	4.6	9.7	14.8	15.0	11.3	20.5	12.8	23.8

In Ecuador, for example, citizens reported twice the level of demands for bribes from the education sector than in any other country. In Mexico, the police were a greater source of bribery demands than in other countries. Perhaps not too surprising, municipal governments, as the level of government most directly and most frequently in contact with citizens, appeared to be a major locus of demands for bribes.

Some results vary from the results of Transparency International's Corruption Perceptions Index, probably reflecting the purposes and methodology of each of these tools. Indices such as TI's CPI capture perceptions and attitudes related to grand or systematic corruption among high-level public officials, but do not capture the vast majority of citizens' experience in their daily lives. In contrast, the USAID surveys capture some attitudes and perceptions at the national level, but are more squarely focused on the views and experiences of all citizens. Both types of measures have their place, and can be used by policy-makers and researchers to complement each other in examining the phenomenon of corruption in a given country.

Experience with these surveys has been very positive. Citizens have been open to answering very detailed questions about the sources of corruption they experience in their daily lives. USAID plans to provide this survey data to the widest possible community of reformers, policy-makers and researchers for further analysis, by posting it on the Internet in both Spanish and English. Making this publicly funded survey data openly available allows anyone to scrutinise the survey methods and results and, more importantly, to use the data to improve public policy, better target reform efforts and accurately measure progress.

Notes

1. Eric Kite is a democracy officer for USAID in Kabul, Afghanistan and Margaret Sarles is based at the Office of Democracy and Governance, USAID. Contact details: mekite@usaid.gov and msarles@usaid.gov
2. The 2004 surveys were undertaken by Latin American survey firms and research institutions under the technical supervision of Dr Mitchell Seligson of Vanderbilt University. See his paper 'The University of Pittsburgh Latin American Public Opinion Project's Corruption Victimisation Scale' in the *Global Corruption Report 2004*. Seligson's definition of 'corruption victimisation' refers to citizens' actual experience with public sector corruption.

26 Corruption in Palestinian society

TI Palestine/the Coalition for Accountability and Integrity (AMAN)

In late 2004, TI Palestine/the Coalition for Accountability and Integrity (AMAN) commissioned the Palestinian Centre for Political Studies and Surveys to conduct an opinion poll focusing on levels and forms of corruption in the Palestinian Territories of the West Bank and the Gaza Strip. Questions assessed the extent of *wasta*, the practice of people making inappropriate interventions on behalf of individuals, who do not possess the requisite qualifications or demonstrated work ethics, often resulting in appointments being made on the basis of family connections or party affiliation. *Wasta*, usually translated as 'nepotism', is viewed as a significant source of corruption in the Middle East. The survey was conducted in December 2004, among a random sample of 1,319 adults in 120 residential areas. The statistical margin of error was 3 per cent.

Wasta considered most blatant form of corruption

According to the survey, *wasta* was perceived to be the most common form of corruption in Palestinian society today. Consensus on this point crossed gender, age, education and socio-economic lines. *Wasta* was followed by bribery and personal use of public resources as common forms of corruption. There was a general impression that bribery was more common in the Gaza Strip than in the West Bank.[1] (See Table 26.1.) Nepotism was viewed to be higher in the West Bank than in Gaza.

Nearly a quarter of those surveyed indicated that they, one of their family members, or friends had been asked to intervene by exerting influence over a public official in the Palestinian Authority in order to secure provision of a required public service. From among those surveyed, approximately two-thirds of those working in the public sector indicated that they were asked to intervene, compared with about 46 per cent of those employed in the private sector. Among supporters of Fatah, the ruling party, the figure was 46 per cent, compared with 35 per cent of Hamas supporters who were asked to intervene.

The purpose of nearly one-third of all interventions was to acquire a job. A similar amount of interventions dealt with the police or the security establishment. The rate of interventions related to job-seeking was higher in the districts of Deir Al-Balah, Nablus and the refugee camps, and lower in Tulkarem and Jerusalem. The rate of intervention was higher in the Gaza Strip than in the West Bank for job-seeking (37 per cent compared with 28 per cent) and in relation to the police or one of the security establishments (37 per cent compared with 19 per cent). In the education sector, however, the rate of intervention was much higher in the West Bank (18 per cent) than in Gaza (5 per cent).

Table 26.1: Locating corruption

'If you, a family member or a friend intervened with a public official or a person responsible in the Palestinian Authority to have a public service delivered, in what organisation/sector or field did this intervention take place? (Choose the most suitable answer).'

	Total %	West Bank %	Gaza Strip %
1. Regulatory offices for business and workplaces	3.7	5.5	1.6
2. Law courts	2.0	1.8	2.3
3. Customs	1.0	1.2	0.8
4. Education (government and private schools, universities, colleges)	12.6	18.2	5.4
5. Public utilities	1.0	0.6	1.6
6. Medical services	4.8	3.6	6.2
7. Passports, IDs and immigration	5.8	7.3	3.9
8. Police or security forces	26.9	18.8	37.2
9. Political party, elected representatives	1.0	1.8	0.0
10. Private sector	1.0	1.2	0.8
11. Social services	6.1	9.1	2.3
12. Tax revenue	0.3	0.6	0.0
13. Employment-seeking	32.0	27.9	37.2
14. No opinion/do not know	1.7	2.4	0.8

Of those who intervened, 52 per cent of men requested a personal favour from a government employee (a public official), compared with only 19 per cent of women. Women more frequently relied on family members to request a personal favour from a public official rather than asking directly: 55 per cent of women surveyed asked family members to seek the personal favour, compared with 28 per cent of men.

A majority of people surveyed – 63 per cent of men and 46 per cent of women – believes *wasta* will become less prevalent in the next few years. Of those who believe that corruption will increase, more live in the West Bank (47 per cent) than in the Gaza Strip (33 per cent).

Locating corruption – employment and the police are most corrupt

Most people surveyed (82 per cent) believe that corruption is most prevalent in the public sector. Only 6 per cent believe corruption is most prevalent in the private sector, while 5 per cent singled out civil society as the most corrupt sector. Gender differences were significant, however, with 75 per cent of women compared with 87 per cent of men indicating that they believe there is corruption in public sector institutions.

When asked from which public institution or sector they would most like intervention to be removed, the top choices of those surveyed were job-seeking and the police/

security sectors, followed by education – the same areas identified as most riddled by *wasta*. More men would like to see *wasta* eliminated from the police and security services than from any other field, while more women would like to see it eliminated from the employment field.

The response to the survey data from public officials was initially negative, on the grounds that the results were not convincing. A number of ministries responded more positively. The Ministry of Health and Higher Education has formed special committees to propose ways of combating *wasta* and has encouraged AMAN to carry out similar surveys on an annual basis.

Note

1. Previous surveys conducted for AMAN revealed that bribery is believed to be concentrated in the higher levels of the Palestinian National Authority. See the findings of the national chapter's report on the Coalition for Accountability and Integrity (AMAN), 'Opinion Poll on Corruption in the Palestinian Society'; http://www.transparency.org/surveys/#palestine

Index

Compiled by Sue Carlton

Bulgaria, health sector corruption 65–6, 67, 68, 289–90, 346–9
Burke, Ray 174
Burkina Faso 136–9
  anti-corruption measures 136–7
  judiciary 120, 137–8
Bush, George W. 162

Calderón, Rafael Angel 26, 27, 147, 156
Cambodia, health sector corruption xvi, 22–4, 55, 108
Cameroon 119, 139–42
  and EITI 141
  procurement 140–1
Canada 11, 12, 288
  oil and gas industry 319, 321
Cape Verde 53–4
Central and Eastern Europe (CEE), health sector corruption 39–43, 63–74
Chávez, Hugo 28
Chile 12
  health sector corruption 52, 81
China 142–6
  anti-corruption measures 143–4
  banking system 144–5
  corruption of party officials 144
  counterfeit medicines 84, 99
  health sector corruption 12
civil society xx, 132, 136, 138, 170, 207, 267, 272, 339, 355
  and budget transparency 315, 317
  and HIV/AIDs treatment 105, 106–7, 108, 115
  interaction with governments 119, 121, 127, 190, 194, 247–8
  and judiciaries 153, 215, 219, 281
  Mexican CSOs 44–5
  and oil revenue transparency 141, 319
  and pharmaceutical sector 77, 80
  and police corruption 202
  and political financing 147, 150, 221, 239, 240, 275
  and public contracting 159, 169, 186
  see also non-governmental organizations (NGOs)
codes of conduct
  health sector xix
    hospitals 9, 11, 59–60
  judiciaries 143
  pharmaceutical sector 83, 93
  public contracting 132, 160, 192, 193
  public officials 120, 245, 249, 251
Colombia 350
  health sector corruption 3, 14–15, 289, 339–42
Commonwealth of Independent States (CIS), informal payments for health care 63–71
Compaoré, Blaise 137
complaints 143, 201, 218, 278, 339
  about access to information 170
  about oil industry 282
  about political finance 274, 275
  against judiciaries 219, 272–3
  against police 174, 202
  health sector 11, 28, 55, 64, 93, 101, 102

conflicts of interest 119, 130–1, 204, 239, 260, 269, 272–3
  health sector 13, 28, 59, 81, 83, 89–90, 94–6, 97
  pharmaceutical sector 81, 83, 87–9, 90, 94–6, 97
  regulation 120, 131, 151, 178, 233, 236, 237–8, 248–9, 250–1, 276, 328
corruption
  definition of xvii
  obstacle to business development 119, 331
  perceptions of 25, 29, 36, 38, 40–3, 65, 108, 290, 292–7, 313
Corruption Perceptions Index 108, 119, 155, 210, 287, 292–303, 325, 352
Costa Rica 146–8, 350
  access to information 147–8
  corruption scandals 119, 146–7
  health sector corruption 4, 26–9, 53, 82
Cote d'Ivoire, and counterfeit ARVs 106
counterfeit medicines xvi, 13, 25, 76, 77, 83–4, 92, 96–100, 104, 105–6
Croatia 120, 149–52, 306
  hospital waiting lists 55
  Imostroj affair 151–2
  political financing 150–1
Cuba 12
Czech Republic 289
  anti-corruption institutions 333–5
  informal payments for health care 65–6, 68, 69

Dashiki, Alberto 153
Deuba, Sher Bahadur 207–8
development assistance 23, 107, 108–9
doctors
  hospital referrals 9, 19, 20, 50, 56, 57, 68
  and pharmaceutical sector 82–3, 86–7, 92–3, 94–6
  role in fighting corruption 94–6
  wages 65–6, 69
Dominican Republic 350
DRC, and counterfeit ARVs 106

e-government 192, 193
Ecuador 119, 120, 152–4, 350
  democratic crisis in 153–4
Egypt 4
El Salvador 350
embezzlement 137–8, 143, 153, 193, 204, 205, 214, 263–4, 337
  Baikonur case 185–6
  in health sector 8, 13, 21, 49–50, 52–4, 59, 104, 112–13
ethics 143, 333–5, 347–8
  and health sector 9, 24, 84, 89, 90, 93, 94–5
  and judiciaries 282
  legislative 272–3
  and plea bargaining 162
  and public sector 132, 160, 201, 212, 218, 229, 248–9
Ethiopia 4, 106, 107
Europe, perceptions of corruption 40–1
European Union
  cross-border judicial system 157–8
  regulation of pharmaceutical sector 110

New Partnership for African Development
    (NEPAD) 111
New Zealand 119, 210–13
    misuse of public funds 210–11
    promoting integrity in public sector 211–12
    promoting transparency abroad 212–13
Nicaragua 213–16, 350
    anti-corruption efforts 214–15
Nigeria
    and counterfeit medicines 84, 96–9
    health sector corruption 31, 34, 35
    and HIV/AIDS treatment 106–7, 110
    National Agency for Food and Drug
        Administration and Control (NAFDAC) 84,
        97–9
    and oil and gas industry 319, 320
Noboa, Gustavo 153
non-governmental organizations (NGOs) 12, 24,
    44–5, 92, 93, 100, 101, 113–15, 161–2, 194,
    205, 271, 281
    see also civil society
Noriega, Manuel Antonio 218
Norway, and oil and gas industry 319

OECD 124
    Anti-Bribery Convention 121, 156, 268–9
    Anti-Corruption Network for Transition
        Economies 162
    Financial Action Task Force (FATF) 258
oil and gas industry, revenue transparency 141,
    319–22
organised crime 18, 97, 251–2, 269
Ortega, Daniel 214, 215

Pacheco, Abel 147
Pakistan 4, 306
Palacio, Alfredo 154
Palestine 290, 354–6
Panama 216–20, 350
    'Pact for Justice' 219
    promoting transparency 217–18
Papua New Guinea 220–3
    by-elections audit 221–2
    health sector corruption 31
    police corruption 119, 202, 208–9, 222
Pavlov, Alexander 186
Peru 223–6, 306
    fight against corruption 224–5
    health sector corruption 32, 54, 56
    and signature falsification 225–6
pharmaceutical sector xvi, 8, 10, 27, 46, 76–102
    advertising 80, 87, 99
    distribution 79, 82, 96
    drug selection 79, 80–1, 346–9
    enticements to doctors 51, 86–7, 92–3
    key decision points 79–82
    and medical research 87–90, 95
    procurement 51, 79, 81–2, 92, 100–1, 289, 346–9
    registration 79, 80, 98
    and regulation 78, 79, 84, 91–3, 95, 110
    service delivery 79, 82–3
    susceptibility to corruption 77–9

and WHO criteria 27, 80, 81, 83
    see also counterfeit medicines
Philippines, health sector corruption xvi, 37–9
Poland 227–30
    civil service recruitment 228–9
    health sector corruption 64, 65, 69
    MPs and corruption scandals 229–30
    reform of judiciary 228
police
    corruption in 119, 129, 138, 174–5, 190, 202,
        208–9, 233, 290, 352, 355–6
    reform of 163–4, 174–5, 222, 266
political finance 150–1, 159, 177–8, 182–3, 239–40,
    260, 274–5
poverty xvi, 75, 77, 121, 196, 305
press 52, 83, 99, 123–4, 125, 137, 193, 197, 204,
    207
privatisation 12, 128, 131, 182, 198
privileges 10, 50, 101, 131, 133, 134, 198
procurement 23, 124–5, 132, 158–60, 185–6, 188,
    189, 201, 275–6, 331, 333–5
    health sector 7, 9, 10, 11, 23, 26–8, 30, 49, 50,
        51–2, 59
    and HIV/AIDS treatment 104, 106–7, 111, 112,
        199
    and pharmaceutical sector 51, 79, 81–2, 92,
        100–1, 289, 346–9
    and transparency 24, 52, 59, 79, 82, 100, 120,
        140–1
Public Expenditure Tracking Surveys (PETS) 29–36
Publish What You Pay campaign 288

Rodríguez, Miguel Angel 146
Roh Moo-Hyun 248
Romania 120, 230–4
    and EU accession 232–3
    health sector corruption 65, 67, 69, 106
    infrastructure 233–4
Russia 306
    health sector corruption 64
    and oil and gas industry 319
Rwanda
    health sector corruption 30, 32, 34
    and HIV/AIDS treatment programmes 108

Saaskashvili, Mikheil 161, 162–3
al-Sabah, Sheikh Jabir al-Ahmad al-Jabir 192
Sanader, Ivo 151
Sánchez de Lozada, Gonzalo 131
Schering-Plough 78
Senegal, health sector corruption 32, 34
Serbia 235–8, 306
    access to information 235–6
    salaries of public officials 236–7
Sharon, Ariel 177, 178–9
Shevardnadze, Eduard 161
Sierra Leone 306
Silva, Luis Inácio Lula da 133
Slovakia 239–42, 306
    health sector corruption 64, 65–6, 69
    political finance 239–40
    senior officials and corruption 240–1